T0259591

Pediatric Gastroenterology

Editors

STEVEN J. CZINN
SAMRA S. BLANCHARD

PEDIATRIC CLINICS
OF NORTH AMERICA

www.pediatric.theclinics.com

Consulting Editor
BONITA F. STANTON

June 2017 • Volume 64 • Number 3

ELSEVIER

1600 John F. Kennedy Boulevard • Suite 1800 • Philadelphia, Pennsylvania, 19103-2899

http://www.theclinics.com

THE PEDIATRIC CLINICS OF NORTH AMERICA Volume 64, Number 3
June 2017 ISSN 0031-3955, ISBN-13: 978-0-323-53023-1

Editor: Kerry Holland
Developmental Editor: Casey Potter

The Pediatric Clinics of North America (ISSN 0031-3955) is published bimonthly by Elsevier Inc., 360 Park Avenue South, New York, NY 10010-1710. Months of issue are February, April, June, August, October, and December. Periodicals postage paid at New York, NY and additional mailing offices. Subscription prices are $208.00 per year (US individuals), $589.00 per year (US institutions), $281.00 per year (Canadian individuals), $784.00 per year (Canadian institutions), $338.00 per year (international individuals), $784.00 per year (international institutions), $100.00 per year (US students and residents), and $165.00 per year (international and Canadian residents and students). To receive students/resident rare, orders must be accompanied by name of affiliated institution, date of term, and the signature of program/residency coordinator on institution letterhead. Orders will be billed at individual rate until proof of status is received. Foreign air speed delivery is included in all *Clinics* subscription prices. All prices are subject to change without notice. **POSTMASTER:** Send address changes to *The Pediatric Clinics of North America*, Elsevier Health Sciences Division, Subscription Customer Service, 3251 Riverport Lane, Maryland Heights, MO 63043. **Customer Service: 1-800-654-2452 (US and Canada). From outside of the US and Canada: 1-314-447-8871. Fax: 1-314-447-8029. For print support, E-mail: JournalsCustomerService-usa@elsevier.com. For online support, E-mail: JournalsOnlineSupport-usa@elsevier.com.**

Reprints. For copies of 100 or more, of articles in this publication, please contact the Commercial Reprints Department, Elsevier Inc., 360 Park Avenue South, New York, NY 10010-1710. Tel.: 212-633-3874; Fax: 212-633-3820; E-mail: reprints@elsevier.com.

The Pediatric Clinics of North America is also published in Spanish by McGraw-Hill Inter-americana Editores S.A., Mexico City, Mexico; in Portuguese by Riechmann and Affonso Editores, Rua Comandante Coelho 1085, CEP 21250, Rio de Janeiro, Brazil; and in Greek by Althayia SA, Athens, Greece.

The Pediatric Clinics of North America is covered in *MEDLINE/PubMed (Index Medicus), Excerpta Medica, Current Contents, Current Contents/Clinical Medicine, Science Citation Index, ASCA, ISI/BIOMED,* and *BIOSIS.*

PROGRAM OBJECTIVE

The goal of the *Pediatric Clinics of North America* is to keep practicing physicians and residents up to date with current clinical practice in pediatrics by providing timely articles reviewing the state-of-the-art in patient care.

TARGET AUDIENCE

All practicing pediatricians, physicians and healthcare professionals who provide patient care to pediatric patients.

LEARNING OBJECTIVES

Upon completion of this activity, participants will be able to:

1. Review topics in gastroesophageal reflux, pediatric inflammatory bowel disease, and other gastroenterological disorders in children.
2. Discuss updates in treating pancreatic and liver conditions in children.
3. Recognize developments in the management of pediatric abdominal pain and disorders.

ACCREDITATION

The Elsevier Office of Continuing Medical Education (EOCME) is accredited by the Accreditation Council for Continuing Medical Education (ACCME) to provide continuing medical education for physicians.

The EOCME designates this enduring material for a maximum of 15 *AMA PRA Category 1 Credit*(s)™. Physicians should claim only the credit commensurate with the extent of their participation in the activity.

All other healthcare professionals requesting continuing education credit for this enduring material will be issued a certificate of participation.

DISCLOSURE OF CONFLICTS OF INTEREST

The EOCME assesses conflict of interest with its instructors, faculty, planners, and other individuals who are in a position to control the content of CME activities. All relevant conflicts of interest that are identified are thoroughly vetted by EOCME for fair balance, scientific objectivity, and patient care recommendations. EOCME is committed to providing its learners with CME activities that promote improvements or quality in healthcare and not a specific proprietary business or a commercial interest.

The planning committee, staff, authors and editors listed below have identified no financial relationships or relationships to products or devices they or their spouse/life partner have with commercial interest related to the content of this CME activity:

Naim Alkhouri, MD; Samra S. Blanchard, MD; Máire A. Conrad, MD, MS; Steven J. Czinn, MD, FAAP, FACG, AGAF; Punyanganie S.A. de Silva, MBBS, MPH, MRCP(UK); Lisa M. Fahey, MD; Douglas S. Fishman, MD; Laurie N. Fishman, MD, FAGA; Anjali Fortna; Maheen Hassan, MD; Kerry Holland; Mohammad Nasser Kabbany, MD; Marsha Kay, MD; Indu Kumari; Jacob A. Kurowski, MD; Erin Lane, MD; Chris A. Liacouras, MD; Hayat Mousa, MD, AGAF; Valerio Nobili, MD; Samuel Nurko, MD, MPH; Anita K. Pai, MD; Nidhi Rawal, MD; Joel R. Rosh, MD; Praveen Kumar Conjeevaram Selvakumar, MD; Bonita F. Stanton, MD; Aliye Uc, MD; Runa D. Watkins, MD; Katie Widmeier; Amy Williams; Nada Yagizi, MD; Shamila Zawahir, MD; Donna K. Zeiter, MD.

The planning committee, staff, authors and editors listed below have identified financial relationships or relationships to products or devices they or their spouse/life partner have with commercial interest related to the content of this CME activity:

Victor L. Fox, MD is a consultant/advisor for Medtronic.

Wikrom Karnsakul, MD has research support from Gilead.

Karen F. Murray, MD has stock ownership in Merck & Co., Inc., and has research support from Gilead and the National Institute of Diabetes and Digestive and Kidney Diseases, part of the US Department of Health and Human Services.

Kathleen B. Schwarz, MD is a consultant/advisor for UptoDate, Inc and The American Board of Pediatrics, and has research support from Gilead; Bristol-Myers Squibb Company; and Genentech, A Member of the Roche Group.

UNAPPROVED/OFF-LABEL USE DISCLOSURE

The EOCME requires CME faculty to disclose to the participants:

1. When products or procedures being discussed are off-label, unlabelled, experimental, and/or investigational (not US Food and Drug Administration [FDA] approved); and

2. Any limitations on the information presented, such as data that are preliminary or that represent ongoing research, interim analyses, and/or unsupported opinions. Faculty may discuss information about pharmaceutical agents that is outside of FDA-approved labelling. This information is intended solely for CME and is not intended to promote off-label use of these medications. If you have any questions, contact the medical affairs department of the manufacturer for the most recent prescribing information.

TO ENROLL

To enroll in the *Pediatric Clinics of North America* Continuing Medical Education program, call customer service at 1-800-654-2452 or sign up online at http://www.theclinics.com/home/cme. The CME program is available to subscribers for an additional annual fee of USD 290.

METHOD OF PARTICIPATION

In order to claim credit, participants must complete the following:
1. Complete enrolment as indicated above.
2. Read the activity.
3. Complete the CME Test and Evaluation. Participants must achieve a score of 70% on the test. All CME Tests and Evaluations must be completed online.

CME INQUIRIES/SPECIAL NEEDS

For all CME inquiries or special needs, please contact elsevierCME@elsevier.com.

Contributors

CONSULTING EDITOR

BONITA F. STANTON, MD
Founding Dean and Professor of Pediatrics, Seton Hall-Hackensack Meridian School of Medicine, President, Academic Enterprise, Hackensack Meridian Health, Professor of Pediatrics, South Orange, New Jersey

EDITORS

STEVEN J. CZINN, MD, FAAP, FACG, AGAF
The Drs. Rouben and Violet Jiji Endowed Professor and Chair, Department of Pediatrics, Division of Pediatric Gastroenterology and Nutrition, University of Maryland School of Medicine, Baltimore, Maryland

SAMRA S. BLANCHARD, MD, FACG
Division Chief, Pediatric Gastroenterology and Nutrition, University Maryland Medical Center, Associate Professor of Pediatrics, University of Maryland School of Medicine, Baltimore, Maryland

AUTHORS

NAIM ALKHOURI, MD
Department of Pediatric Gastroenterology and Hepatology, Digestive Disease Institute, Cleveland Clinic Cleveland, Cleveland, Ohio

MÁIRE A. CONRAD, MD, MS
Attending Physician, Division of Gastroenterology, Hepatology and Nutrition, The Children's Hospital of Philadelphia, Instructor, Perelman School of Medicine, University of Pennsylvania, Philadelphia, Pennsylvania

PUNYANGANIE S.A. DE SILVA, MBBS, MPH, MRCP(UK)
Division of Gastroenterology, Hepatology and Endoscopy, Brigham and Women's Hospital, Harvard Medical School, Boston, Massachusetts

LISA M. FAHEY, MD
Senior Fellow Physician, Division of Gastroenterology, Hepatology, and Nutrition, The Children's Hospital of Philadelphia; Department of Pediatrics, Perelman School of Medicine, University of Pennsylvania, Philadelphia, Pennsylvania

DOUGLAS S. FISHMAN, MD
Associate Professor of Pediatrics, Section of Pediatric Gastroenterology, Hepatology and Nutrition, Texas Children's Hospital, Baylor College of Medicine, Houston, Texas

LAURIE N. FISHMAN, MD, FAGA
Division of Pediatric Gastroenterology, Boston Children's Hospital, Harvard Medical School, Boston, Massachusetts

VICTOR L. FOX, MD
Division of Gastroenterology, Hepatology, and Nutrition, Boston Children's Hospital, Associate Professor of Pediatrics, Harvard Medical School, Boston, Massachusetts

MAHEEN HASSAN, MD
Pediatric Gastroenterology Fellow, University of California, San Diego, Rady Children's Hospital, San Diego, California

MOHAMMAD NASSER KABBANY, MD
Department of Pediatric Gastroenterology and Hepatology, Cleveland Clinic, Cleveland, Ohio

WIKROM KARNSAKUL, MD
Associate Professor, Pediatric Liver Center, Department of Pediatrics, Johns Hopkins University School of Medicine, Baltimore, Maryland

MARSHA KAY, MD
Chair, Director Pediatric Endoscopy, Department of Gastroenterology, Hepatology, and Nutrition, Cleveland Clinic, Cleveland, Ohio

JACOB A. KUROWSKI, MD
Clinical Assistant Professor of Pediatrics, Department of Gastroenterology, Hepatology, and Nutrition, Cleveland Clinic, Cleveland, Ohio

ERIN LANE, MD
Fellow, Division of Pediatric Gastroenterology and Hepatology, Seattle Children's Hospital, Seattle, Washington

CHRIS A. LIACOURAS, MD
Attending Physician, Co-director of the Center for Pediatric Eosinophilic Disorders, Division of Gastroenterology, Hepatology, and Nutrition, The Children's Hospital of Philadelphia, Professor, Department of Pediatrics, Perelman School of Medicine, University of Pennsylvania, Philadelphia, Pennsylvania

HAYAT MOUSA, MD, AGAF
Professor in Pediatrics, University of California, San Diego, Director of Neurogastroenterology and Motility Center, Medical Director of Pediatric Gastroenterology, Hepatology, and Nutrition, Rady Children's Hospital, San Diego, California

KAREN F. MURRAY, MD
Division Chief of Pediatric Gastroenterology and Hepatology, Professor, Seattle Children's Hospital, Seattle, Washington

VALERIO NOBILI, MD
Liver Unit, IRCCS Bambino Gesù Children's Hospital, IRCCS, Rome, Italy

SAMUEL NURKO, MD, MPH
Professor of Pediatrics, Harvard Medical School, Center for Motility and Functional Gastrointestinal Disorders, Boston Children's Hospital, Boston, Massachusetts

ANITA K. PAI, MD
Fellow, Division of Gastroenterology, Hepatology, and Nutrition, Boston Children's Hospital, Instructor of Pediatrics, Harvard Medical School, Boston, Massachusetts

NIDHI RAWAL, MD
Pediatric Gastroenterologist, Division of Gastroenterology, Hepatology and Nutrition, Department of Pediatrics, University of Maryland Medical Center, Baltimore, Maryland

JOEL R. ROSH, MD
Director, Pediatric Gastroenterology; Vice Chairman, Clinical Development and Research Affairs, Goryeb Children's Hospital/Atlantic Health System, Professor of Pediatrics, Icahn School of Medicine at Mount Sinai, Morristown, New Jersey

KATHLEEN B. SCHWARZ, MD
Professor, Pediatric Liver Center, Department of Pediatrics, Johns Hopkins University School of Medicine, Baltimore, Maryland

PRAVEEN KUMAR CONJEEVARAM SELVAKUMAR, MD
Department of Pediatric Gastroenterology and Hepatology, Cleveland Clinic, Cleveland, Ohio

ALIYE UC, MD
Professor of Pediatrics and Radiation Oncology, Stead Family Department of Pediatrics, Stead Family Children's Hospital, University of Iowa Carver College of Medicine, Iowa City, Iowa

RUNA D. WATKINS, MD
Assistant Professor, Fellowship Director, Pediatric Gastroenterology & Nutrition, University of Maryland, Baltimore, Maryland

NADA YAZIGI, MD
Pediatric Transplant Hepatology, Department of Transplantation, MedStar Georgetown University Hospital, MedStar Georgetown Transplant Institute, Washington, DC

SHAMILA ZAWAHIR, MD
Assistant Professor, Pediatric Gastroenterology & Nutrition, University of Maryland, Baltimore, Maryland

DONNA K. ZEITER, MD
Assistant Professor, Department of Pediatrics, Division of Pediatric Gastroenterology, Hepatology and Nutrition, University of Maryland School of Medicine, Baltimore, Maryland

Contents

Eosinophilic esophagitis (EoE) is an atopic disease that is characterized by an isolated infiltration of eosinophils into the epithelium of the esophagus and is triggered by specific allergens. Patients should undergo an upper endoscopy with biopsy after 6 to 8 weeks of treatment with a proton pump inhibitor in order to make the diagnosis of EoE. Eosinophilic gastroenteritis is a pathologic eosinophilic infiltration of any portion of the gastrointestinal tract, and eosinophilic proctocolitis is an eosinophilic infiltration in the colon alone.

Gastroesophageal reflux (GER) is a normal physiologic process. It is important to distinguish GER from GER disease (GERD) since GER does not require treatment. Although a diagnosis of GERD can largely be based on history and physical alone, endoscopy and pH impedance studies can help make the diagnosis when there in atypical presentation. In children and adolescents, lifestyle changes and acid suppression are first-line treatments for GERD. In infants, acid suppression is not effective, but a trial of hydrolyzed formula can be considered, as milk protein sensitivity can be difficult to differentiate from GER symptoms.

Children inevitably swallow foreign material accidentally or intentionally. Each type of ingestion carries their own set of risks and complications, short and long term, some requiring immediate attention while others close monitoring. Alkalotic household cleaning products and lithium button batteries are increasingly common and damage the esophagus quickly. While many toys with rare-earth metals are banned, they are already present in many households and can cause necrosis of bowel that is between the magnets. This article reviews the incidence and assessment along with current literature to provide guidelines for management of pediatric patients with suspected caustic or foreign body ingestion.

Samuel Nurko

Gastrointestinal motility disorders in the pediatric population are common and can range from benign processes to more serious disorders. Performing and interpreting motility evaluations in children present unique challenges. There are primary motility disorders but abnormal motility may be secondary due to other disease processes. Diagnostic studies include radiographic scintigraphic and manometry studies. Although recent advances in the genetics, biology, and technical aspects are having an important impact and have allowed for a better understanding of the pathophysiology and therapy for gastrointestinal motility disorders in children, further research is needed to be done to have better understanding of the pathophysiology and for better therapies.

Nidhi Rawal and Nada Yazigi

The past decade has seen major advances in the field of transplantation; it is the treatment of choice for many with intestinal failure. One-year mortality from pediatric intestinal transplantation has significantly declined, from 30% to 10% to 15% nationally, mainly due to a multidisciplinary approach in transplant centers. Pediatric age carries special considerations along the spectrum of care that continue to cause challenges but also offers growth opportunities. Pediatric intestinal transplantation indications and timing are changing as a result of new developments in diagnostic and treatment tools. This article reviews updates on pediatric intestinal transplantation and highlights future directions.

Erin Lane and Karen F. Murray

Neonatal jaundice is common and usually not concerning when it is secondary to unconjugated hyperbilirubinemia, below the neurotoxic level, and resolves early. Primary care providers should be vigilant, however, about evaluating infants in whom jaundice presents early, is prolonged beyond 2 weeks of life, or presents at high levels. Even in well-appearing infants, fractionated (direct and indirect) bilirubin levels should be obtained in these clinical scenarios to evaluate for potential cholestasis. This review presents an approach to the evaluation of a jaundiced infant and discusses diagnosis and management of several causes of neonatal cholestasis.

Wikrom Karnsakul and Kathleen B. Schwarz

Chronic viral hepatitis is a global health threat and financial burden. Hepatitis B and C viruses (HBV and HCV) are the most common causes of chronic viral hepatitis in the United States. Most cases are asymptomatic before adulthood. Research has resulted in effective therapy for HCV and the promise of effective therapies for HBV. For HCV, therapy is pegylated interferon and ribavirin. Clinical trials with effective direct-acting antiviral agents are underway in pediatrics. For HBV, approved agents are alpha-interferon, lamivudine, adefovir, tenofovir, and entecavir. However, treatment seldom results in functional cure and more effective therapies are urgently needed.

Nonalcoholic fatty liver disease (NAFLD) is considered the hepatic manifestation of metabolic syndrome and has become the most common form of chronic liver disease in children and adolescents. The histologic spectrum of NAFLD is broad ranging, from the relatively benign form of simple steatosis to the aggressive form of nonalcoholic steatohepatitis, eventually leading to fibrosis and cirrhosis. NAFLD has also been recognized as an independent risk factor for extrahepatic complications, such as cardiovascular disease, type 2 diabetes mellitus, sleep disorders, and osteoporosis. In this review, we discuss both the hepatic and extrahepatic complications of NAFLD in children.

Excellent outcomes over the last 3 decades have made liver transplantation the treatment of choice for many advanced liver disorders. This success also opened liver transplantation to new indications such as liver tumors and metabolic disorders. The emergence of such new indications for liver transplantation is bringing a new stream of patients along with disease-specific challenges. The cumulative number of liver transplant recipients is peaking, requiring novel systems of health care delivery that meet the needs of this special patient population. This article reviews updates and new development in pediatric liver transplantation.

Once considered uncommon, pancreatic diseases are increasingly recognized in the pediatric age group. Acute pancreatitis, acute recurrent pancreatitis, and chronic pancreatitis occur in children with an incidence approaching that of adults. Risk factors are broad, prompting the need for a completely different diagnostic and therapeutic approach in children. Although cystic fibrosis remains the most common cause of exocrine pancreatic insufficiency, other causes such as chronic pancreatitis may be as common as Shwachman Diamond syndrome. Long-term effects of pancreatic diseases may be staggering, as children suffer from significant disease burden, high economic cost, nutritional deficiencies, pancreatogenic diabetes, and potentially pancreatic cancer.

Transition is the long process of developing independent self-management skills whereas transfer is the actual move from pediatric to adult-centered provider. Structured anticipated transition works best with timelines of tasks to master and discussion of the stylistic differences between pediatric and adult practices. Disease-specific issues need to be addressed, such as earlier timelines for diet-based therapies, parental support for critical illnesses, and differences in therapeutic strategies.

PEDIATRIC CLINICS OF NORTH AMERICA

THE CLINICS ARE AVAILABLE ONLINE!
Access your subscription at:
www.theclinics.com

Foreword

The Remarkable Gastrointestinal Tract

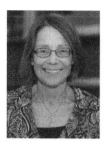

Bonita F. Stanton, MD
Consulting Editor

While arguably there is some competition for this role, I assert that among all organ systems, the pediatric gastroenterologic system offers the greatest range of pleasure-producing and distressing experiences, with enormous direct and indirect impacts on a child's physical and psychosocial well-being. The neonate's immediate and obvious comfort from suckling, leading to ever closer ties with his or her mother, starkly contrasts with the great distress felt by both mother and infant in the presence of gastroesophageal reflux disease. The joy and excitement in discovering new foods are contrarily matched by the despair and anxiety associated with food allergies. Physical and mental growth and development—so impactful on a child's ability to thrive in society—are greatly influenced by the integrity and function of the gastrointestinal (GI) system. Malabsorption, anorexia, and motility problems can greatly disrupt this critical platform for normal development. Given the importance of the GI system and the many ways in which dysfunction can be easily detected, it is not surprising that GI manifestations are often the presenting symptoms in a multiorgan disease process.

Therefore, we are fortunate that the last few decades have witnessed many advances in our understanding of pathophysiology of gastroenterologic disorders at the molecular level, leading to many new diagnostic, prevention, and treatment options. In this issue, the authors present and discuss these important breakthroughs. They also devote considerable attention to those disorders for which major breakthroughs are yet to come, but outline the smaller successes that have allowed for earlier detection and treatment that at least modify the associated discomfort and adverse effects. This is a field of practice that is rapidly changing, and the authors have done a wonderful job of capturing the important events therein. General

Pediatr Clin N Am 64 (2017) xv–xvi
http://dx.doi.org/10.1016/j.pcl.2017.03.016
0031-3955/17/© 2017 Published by Elsevier Inc.

pediatricians, pediatric gastroenterologists, and other pediatric practitioners will have much to learn from the content of this issue.

Bonita F. Stanton, MD
Seton Hall-Hackensack
Meridian School of Medicine
Academic Enterprise
Hackensack Meridian Health
400 South Orange Avenue
South Orange, NJ 07079, USA

E-mail address:
Bonita.stanton@shu.edu

Preface

Pediatric Gastroenterology

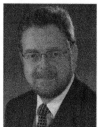

Steven J. Czinn, MD, FAAP, FACG, AGAF   Samra S. Blanchard, MD, FACG

Editors

We are excited to present this special gastroenterology issue of *Pediatric Clinics of North America*. By editing this issue, we had the opportunity to collaborate with numerous specialists in the field, each bringing their expertise to a variety of topics that are important to today's pediatric gastroenterologists.

The past decade has resulted in medical advances that many of us thought impossible. Our understanding of genomics, proteomics, and metabolomics has given the practitioner insights into the pathophysiology of gastroenterologic disorders at the molecular level. The end result is targeted therapies that are allowing us to achieve long-term remission of chronic gastrointestinal (GI) inflammatory disorders, cure hepatitis C, and make liver and small bowel transplant almost routine. In parallel to these discoveries, endoscopic and radiologic improvements have also enhanced our ability to diagnose and treat GI disorders that previously required surgical exploratory laparotomy. Despite these medical breakthroughs, a large subset of children continues to be diagnosed with both acute and chronic gastroenterologic disorders. In this issue, we highlight in great detail the newer modalities for diagnosis, treatment, and even prevention of these disorders.

In this issue, we address issues that continue to be relevant in the field of pediatric gastroenterology. We included articles on commonly treated gastroenterologic disorders, such as gastroesophageal reflux disease (Maheen Hassan, MD and Hayat Mousa, MD), inflammatory bowel disease (Máire A. Conrad, MD, MS and Joel Rosh, MD), pancreatic disorders (Aliye Uc, MD and Douglas Fishman, MD), eosinophilic GI disorders (Lisa Fahey, MD and Chris Liacouras, MD), GI bleeding (Anita Pai, MD and Victor Fox, MD), motility disorders (Samuel Nurko, MD), and transitioning patients from pediatric to adult care (Punyanganie S.A. de Silva, MBBS, MPH, MRCP and Laurie Fishman, MD, FAGA). We also bring updates on treatment of hepatitis B and C (Wikrom Karnsakul, MD and Kathleen Schwarz, MD), abdominal pain (Donna Zeiter, MD), neonatal cholestasis (Erin Lane, MD and Karen Murray, MD), pediatric liver and small bowel transplant (Nada Yazigi, MD and Nidhi Rawal, MD), and caustic ingestions

Pediatr Clin N Am 64 (2017) xvii–xviii
http://dx.doi.org/10.1016/j.pcl.2017.03.015
0031-3955/17/© 2017 Published by Elsevier Inc.

and foreign bodies (Marsha Kay, MD and Jacob Kurowski, MD). Obesity and celiac disease continue to be at the forefront of child health, and we have included thoughtfully written pieces on nonalcoholic fatty liver disease in children (Praveen Kumar Conjeevaram Selvakumar, MD, Mohammad Nasser Kabbany, MD, Valerio Nobili, MD, and Naim Alkhouri, MD) and celiac disease and nonceliac gluten sensitivity (Runa Watkins, MD and Sharmila Zawahir, MD).

It has been a pleasure to edit the contributions of a talented group of authors, and we would like to thank them for their efforts in preparing thoughtful, concise, and relevant articles. We hope that you enjoy this special gastroenterology-focused issue of *Pediatric Clinics of North America*.

Steven J. Czinn, MD, FAAP, FACG, AGAF
University of Maryland School of Medicine
Department of Pediatrics
Division of Pediatric Gastroenterology and Nutrition
22 South Greene Street, Room N5W70
Baltimore, MD 21201, USA

Samra S. Blanchard, MD, FACG
Pediatric Gastroenterology and Nutrition
University Maryland Medical Center
Department of Pediatrics
University of Maryland School of Medicine
22 South Greene Street, Room N5W70
Baltimore, MD 21201, USA

E-mail addresses:
sczinn@peds.umaryland.edu (S.J. Czinn)
sblanchard@peds.umaryland (S.S. Blanchard)

Eosinophilic Gastrointestinal Disorders

Lisa M. Fahey, MD[a,b,*], Chris A. Liacouras, MD[a,b]

KEYWORDS

- Eosinophilic esophagitis • Eosinophilic gastroenteritis • Eosinophilic proctocolitis
- Proton pump inhibitor-responsive esophageal eosinophilia • Food allergens

KEY POINTS

- Eosinophilic esophagitis (EoE) is an atopic disease that is characterized by an isolated infiltration of eosinophils into the epithelium of the esophagus.
- A diagnosis of EoE requires an esophageal biopsy while on a proton pump inhibitor for at least 6 to 8 weeks.
- Proton pump inhibitor–responsive esophageal eosinophilia should always be differentiated from EoE.
- Both medication and dietary therapy options should be considered in patients with EoE.
- Eosinophilic gastroenteritis is described as a pathologic eosinophilic infiltration of any portion of the gastrointestinal tract, and eosinophilic proctocolitis is defined as an abnormal number of eosinophils in the colon alone.

EOSINOPHILIC ESOPHAGITIS

Introduction

Eosinophilic esophagitis (EoE) is an atopic disease that is characterized by an isolated infiltration of eosinophils into the epithelium of the esophagus. EoE is triggered by specific allergens, almost always food antigens; there has been significant research in this area over the past 30 years in order to determine the nature of these specific allergens.[1]

Definition

The 2013 revised guidelines for the diagnosis and management of this disease state that EoE is defined as a clinicopathologic disorder that meets the following criteria[1]:

1. Presence of symptoms related to esophageal dysfunction

The authors have no financial conflicts of interests to disclose.
[a] Division of Gastroenterology, Hepatology, and Nutrition, The Children's Hospital of Philadelphia, 3401 Civic Center Boulevard, 7NW, Philadelphia, PA 19104, USA; [b] Department of Pediatrics, The Perelman School of Medicine, University of Pennsylvania, 3400 Civic Center Boulevard, Philadelphia, PA 19104, USA
* Corresponding author. The Children's Hospital of Philadelphia, 3401 Civic Center Boulevard, 7NW, Philadelphia, PA 19104.
E-mail address: faheyL@email.chop.edu

2. Presence of greater than or equal to 15 eosinophils per high-power field on esophageal biopsy after a trial of a proton pump inhibitor (PPI)
3. Isolation of this mucosal eosinophilic predominance to the esophagus

Of note, symptoms of EoE are often similar to those of gastroesophageal reflux; therefore, the presence of eosinophils on esophageal biopsy is needed to make the diagnosis of EoE.

Prevalence

EoE has increased in prevalence over the past 10 years. The reported prevalence of EoE in 2003 was 4.3 per 10,000 children aged 0 to 19 years. The pediatric male to female ratio is approximately 3:1.[2]

Cause

EoE is thought to occur in genetically susceptible individuals through predominantly non–immunoglobulin E (IgE)-mediated allergic responses to allergens. These allergens are thought to be predominantly food, although other studies have suggested additional environmental allergens, such as aeroallergens, as potential triggers.[3] In general, when food allergens enter the body through a disrupted epithelial barrier, it is postulated that local esophageal antigen presenting cells interact with this antigen. Subsequently, a cascade of proinflammatory cytokines, such as interleukin (IL)-5 and IL-13, as well as chemokines, such as eotaxin-1 and eotaxin-3, are triggered. This trigger results in recruitment of eosinophils to the esophagus.[4]

The first EoE genetic susceptibility locus was recently described at locus 5 q 22.[5] One of the genes at this locus is thymic stromal lymphopoietin, a T-helper 2 proinflammatory cytokine gene that has been associated with other allergic diseases in the past.

Clinical Symptoms

Symptoms of EoE are detailed in **Table 1** and **Box 1**.[6]

Table 1 Common symptoms of eosinophilic esophagitis	
Younger Children	**Older Children and Adolescents**
Vomiting	Heart burn
Chronic nausea	Epigastric pain
Regurgitation	Dysphagia
Irritability/feeding difficulties	Nighttime cough
	Food impaction

Data from Liacouras CA, Markowitz JE. Eosinophilic esophagitis: a subset of eosinophilic gastroenteritis. Curr Gastroenterol Rep 1999;1:253–8.

Box 1 Less common symptoms of eosinophilic esophagitis
Growth failure
Hematemesis
Esophageal dysmotility
Failure to thrive
Malnutrition
Data from Liacouras CA, Markowitz JE. Eosinophilic esophagitis: a subset of eosinophilic gastroenteritis. Curr Gastroenterol Rep 1999;1:253–8.

Some children drink an overabundance of fluids with meals or chew their food excessively in order to compensate for these symptoms. Additional allergic symptoms, such as asthma, eczema, and allergic rhinitis, are present in up to 50% of patients. Complications of EoE include hiatal hernia as well as esophageal strictures, perforation, and fungal infection. Because heartburn is a common symptom of EoE, it is important to consider EoE in patients who have chronic reflux symptoms.

Diagnosis

When considering this diagnosis, patients should be placed on a PPI. After at least 6 to 8 weeks on the PPI, patients should undergo an upper endoscopy with biopsy. An esophageal biopsy is always necessary in order to diagnose EoE. Specifically, at least 15 eosinophils per high-powered field must be present on biopsy, and these eosinophils must be isolated to the esophagus. Although the distal esophagus is typically most affected, biopsies should be taken from multiple levels of the esophagus, as EoE is a patchy disease.[7] In order to make a diagnosis of EoE, biopsies must also be taken from the stomach and duodenum to be sure that excessive eosinophilia is not present. Increased eosinophilia in the stomach or duodenum would instead suggest eosinophilic gastroenteritis.

Visual endoscopic findings include concentric ring formation (called trachealization), vertical linear furrows, and white patches or plaques scattered along the mucosal surface. These findings are present in up to 70% of patients with EoE but are not pathognomonic for the disease.[8] The remaining 30% of those with EoE have visually normal esophageal mucosa. These facts reinforce the need to obtain an esophageal biopsy in order to make the diagnosis of EoE (**Box 2**).

Box 2
Differential diagnosis of eosinophilic esophagitis

Eosinophilic gastrointestinal diseases

Proton pump inhibitor–responsive esophageal eosinophilia

Celiac disease

Crohn disease

Infection

Hypereosinophilic syndrome

Achalasia

Drug hypersensitivity

Vasculitis

Pemphigus

Connective tissue diseases

Graft versus host diseases

There are no current serologic, radiologic or stool tests that have been shown to be diagnostic of EoE.

Allergy Testing

In addition to an evaluation by a gastroenterologist, consultation with an allergist is often helpful because patients often have other features of atopy including asthma, eczema, allergic rhinitis and IgE-mediated food allergies. Although allergy testing is not diagnostic of EoE, skin prick testing (SPT) should be considered in order to identify IgE-mediated food allergens and, less frequently, aeroallergens.[9] These allergens may also crossover and be potential EoE allergen triggers. In addition to SPT, atopy patch testing may be considered in order to identify non–IgE-based food allergens, as the food reactions in EoE are due to these cell-mediated reactions.

Proton Pump Inhibitor–Responsive Esophageal Eosinophilia

PPI–responsive esophageal eosinophilia (REE) should always be differentiated from EoE. PPI-REE is either related to gastroesophageal reflux, an independent disorder, or a possible subset of EoE. Despite not understanding the exact cause of PPI-REE, it is important to determine if esophageal eosinophilia do not respond to a PPI, as the following treatment approach for EoE mandates this course of action. Ngo and colleagues[10] identified several patients with esophageal eosinophilia that normalized after administration of a PPI for 1 month. Short-term aggressive dosing of the PPI should be considered; the pediatric dosage of the PPI can be up to 1 mg/kg twice daily (maximum 30–40 mg twice a day) and should be administered for 6 to 12 weeks before upper endoscopy and biopsy.

Management of Eosinophilic Esophagitis

Both medical and dietary therapy should be considered in patients with EoE. Historically, systemic steroids were the first medication that mitigated symptoms as well as normalized the number of eosinophils in the esophageal mucosa in these patients. However, chronic systemic corticosteroids cannot be used long-term because of side effects, such as decreased linear growth, increased appetite, hypertension, bone changes, and mood alterations. Although this is not currently recommended as a first-line treatment in EoE, oral corticosteroids are still a useful short-term treatment approach for patients with severe dysphagia, poor weight gain, and small-caliber esophagus.

Current first-line medical treatment of EoE is swallowed, topical corticosteroids. These medications include fluticasone propionate, which is sprayed into the pharynx and swallowed rather than inhaled, and swallowed viscous budesonide.[11] Swallowed topical corticosteroids are delivered along the surface of the esophagus, which leads to symptom improvement and histologic normalization within several weeks. Recommended dosing for fluticasone is age and weight based and varies from 110 to 880 mg twice daily; dosing for swallowed budesonide is 0.5 to 1.0 mg twice a day. Patients should not eat, drink, or rinse the mouth for 20 to 30 minutes after use. The initial treatment course is 2 to 3 months, followed by a repeat upper endoscopy. If patients have achieved histologic remission, then the steroids can be weaned (followed by another upper endoscopy). The disease almost always recurs once the medication is discontinued. The side effects of topical corticosteroids are significantly decreased compared with those of systemic steroids. However, some patients develop epistaxis, dry mouth, or esophageal candidiasis.[11–14]

Dietary modification has also been found to be an effective treatment. After identifying the appropriate dietary antigens, patients experience both an improvement in symptoms and histologic resolution. Potential dietary modifications include initiation of a hypoallergenic, elemental diet, eliminating the 6 most common food allergens (milk, eggs, wheat, soy, nuts, shellfish) or selectively eliminating particular foods from the diet. Kelly, Markowitz, and Liacouras demonstrated that greater than 95% of children completely resolve their EoE if given a strict amino acid–based formula as the sole source of dietary nutrition.[15,16] Children on this diet ingest only this formula for a period of time to allow the esophagus to heal. After the esophageal mucosa normalizes, foods are systematically reintroduced. Clinical symptoms may take up to several weeks to recur after reintroduction of a particular food. This diet is often difficult to adhere to for older children because of the large volume of formula required to meet caloric needs and the inability to eat solid foods while on the diet. Most pediatric patients on this regimen cannot tolerate this formula by mouth and instead require administration via a nasogastric tube.

Alternatively, in the mid 2000s the idea of using targeted elimination diets was introduced. Kagalwalla and colleagues[17] showed that a 6-food elimination diet without allergy testing resulted in resolution of EoE symptoms and improvement, but not elimination, of the esophageal eosinophil count in approximately 75% of patients.[17] These targeted elimination diets are executed in conjunction with serial endoscopy with biopsy. After specific foods are removed from the diet for at least 6 to 8 weeks, patients then undergo a repeat endoscopy to assess the esophageal eosinophil count. If the count has normalized, then these foods must be assessed individually to determine the exact food allergen that triggers the disease. On the other hand, if there is no improvement in the eosinophil count after removal of the foods, further dietary restriction must be initiated. This process continues for several cycles until the exact EoE food allergen triggers have been identified and removed and the esophageal eosinophil count has normalized. The most common EoE trigger foods identified through this process are dairy, eggs, soy, corn, wheat, and beef.

Other Therapy

New medications that target specific cytokines and immune mediators are being studied as potential treatment options for patients with severe EoE. These medications include anti-IL-5, very late activating antigen, and monoclonal eotaxin antibody.

EOSINOPHILIC GASTROENTERITIS (GASTROENTEROCOLITIS)
Introduction and Definition

Although there are no specific diagnostic criteria for eosinophilic gastroenteritis (EoG), it is generally described as a pathologic eosinophilic infiltration of any portion of the gastrointestinal tract. It can be superficial or infiltrative in nature.[18,19]

Cause

The cause is currently unknown; however, EoG is thought to be the result of both IgE-mediated and non–IgE-mediated processes.[20] The prevalence is unknown.

Clinical Symptoms

Common symptoms include those associated with malabsorption, including growth failure, weight loss, diarrhea, and hypoalbuminemia. Other symptoms, such as intermittent abdominal pain, vomiting, dysphagia, and bloating, can be seen as well. Severe disease manifestations are uncommon and include gastrointestinal bleeding, iron-deficiency anemia, and protein-losing enteropathy. Ascites is rare in these patients.

Diagnosis

There are currently no standard EoG diagnostic criteria. Diagnosis is typically made based on a constellation of clinical symptoms and histologic findings. Patients usually have one or more of the clinical symptoms described earlier, along with an increase in eosinophil count within the gastrointestinal tract found on endoscopic biopsy. Of note, mucosal eosinophils can be present in any portion of the gastrointestinal tract; however, these eosinophils must not be limited to the esophagus alone. Most patients have an increased antral eosinophilia. Goldman and Proujansky[21] reported that 100% of 38 pediatric patients with EoG who were studied had eosinophils present in the gastric antrum, 60% in the esophagus, 79% in the proximal small intestine, and 52% in the gastric corpus.

Approximately 70% of patients with EoG have a peripheral eosinophilia. Laboratory testing should include allergy testing (which is often unrevealing) and infectious studies including stool ova and parasite tests, serum EBV PCR, giardia antigen and stool *Helicobacter pylori* testing. These patients may also undergo D-xylose absorption tests as well as lactose hydrogen breath tests to assess possible malabsorption, which may suggest small intestinal damage.[22–27] Rheumatologic testing and inflammatory bowel disease serologies may also be considered.[28,29]

Radiologic contrast imaging may show edema, luminal narrowing, or wall thickening. Areae gastricae is a lacy mucosal pattern of the gastric antrum that is sometimes present in EoG.[30]

The differential diagnosis for EoG is expansive (**Box 3**).[31] An evaluation for other possible causes of eosinophilic infiltration should be conducted before diagnosing EoG.

Treatment

There is no consensus as to ideal treatment. In some cases, dietary therapy with an elemental formula has successfully treated this disease.[32,33] Most patients respond to systemic corticosteroids; however, although many have remittance of symptoms while on a steroid regimen, most will have recurrence of symptoms once the steroids are weaned. They may require multiple steroid courses or chronic, low-dose steroid treatment.[34] Alternatively, 6 mercaptopurine, methotrexate, and budesonide may be used.[35–37] Regardless of the treatment option chosen, endoscopy with biopsy is often required to determine the extent of disease.

EOSINOPHILIC PROCTOCOLITIS
Introduction and Definition

Eosinophilic proctocolitis (EoP) is also known as allergic proctocolitis or milk-protein proctocolitis. It is characterized by the acute onset of rectal bleeding in infants. Specifically, it is defined as an abnormal number of eosinophils in the colon. However, an endoscopy is often not performed in these infants; EoP is instead diagnosed clinically based on the gradual onset of gastrointestinal bleeding that resolves with initiation of a protein hydrolysate formula.

Cause

The mature gastrointestinal tract is typically an effective barrier to prevent intact ingested food antigens from stimulating the immune system. However, in newborns, this barrier is immature and these intact antigens are able to permeate the intestinal wall and induce an immune response.[38] Cow's milk and soy are the two most common food antigens that trigger EoP. Because most of the commercially available formula is cow's milk based or soy based, children with EoP must find an alternative nutritional formula.[39] Additionally, breastfed babies account for up to 50% of EoP cases. It is thought that these infants are having an allergic immune response to food antigens that the mother ingests and are transferred into the breast milk.[40]

Box 3
Differential diagnosis of eosinophilic gastroenteritis

Allergic diseases
Food allergies
Hypereosinophilic syndrome

Gastrointestinal diseases
Appendicitis
Celiac disease
Hypertrophic pyloric stenosis
Inflammatory bowel disease

Immunologic diseases
Chronic granulomatous disease

Rheumatologic diseases
Connective tissue disease
Systemic lupus erythematosus
Scleroderma
Dermatomyositis
Polymyositis
Polyarteritis nodosa

Other
Churg-Straus syndrome
Inflammatory fibroid polyp
Malignancy

Infectious diseases
Ancylostoma caninium (hookworm)
Anisakis
Ascaris
Epstein-Barr virus
Enterobius vermicularis (pinworm)
Eustoma rotundatum
Giardia lamblia
Helicobacter pylori
Schistosomiasis
Strongyloides Stercoalis
Toxocara canis
Trichinella spiralis

Medications

Azathioprine

Carbamazepine

Clofazimine

Enalapril

Gemfibrozil

Gold

Data from Barak N, Hart J, Sitrin MD. Enalapril-induced eosinophilic gastroenteritis. J Clin Gastroenterol 2001;33:157–8.

Clinical Symptoms

EoP typically presents in well-appearing infants. Common presenting symptoms are summarized in **Box 4**. These patients do not present with vomiting or abdominal distention. Untreated EoP with chronic blood loss often leads to anemia and/or poor growth. In addition to infants, there is a second cohort of patients that first present in adolescence or early adulthood.

Diagnosis

The differential diagnosis for EoP is noted in **Box 5**. EoP is a clinical diagnosis. However, there are several laboratory tests that may aid in diagnosis. These tests include fecal leukocytes, stool bacterial culture, and stool *Clostridium difficile* testing. Children with EoP will often have fecal leukocytes and may specifically have eosinophils; however, they should not have fecal bacterial pathogens, such as *Salmonella* or *Shigella*. If they are colonized with *C difficile*, then this testing may be positive; however, this may not be the cause of their rectal bleeding.[41] On serologic examination, these patients may have a mild peripheral eosinophilia, hypoalbuminemia, or anemia.

Some of these children undergo flexible sigmoidoscopy. Although not essential for diagnosis, this information is often helpful in determining the cause of the bleeding. Documentation of erythema, friability, or ulceration in the colon supports an EoP diagnosis. However, a grossly normal-appearing colon does not definitively rule out EoP. Histologically, patients with EoP typically have patchy, focal aggregates of eosinophils within the lamina propria with normal crypt architecture.[42–45]

SPT or serum IgE allergy testing for specific foods is unreliable in these patients.

Treatment

Ideal treatment of infants with EoP is initiation of a protein hydrolysate formula.[46] Although symptoms may resolve very quickly after discontinuing the antigenic agent

---

Box 4
Common symptoms of eosinophilic proctocolitis

Gradual-onset rectal bleeding

Diarrhea

Increased mucous production

Eczema and/or reactive airway disease

Well-appearing child

Box 5
Differential diagnosis of eosinophilic proctocolitis

Infectious disease
  Enterobius vermicularis (pinworm)
  Ancylostoma caninium (hookworm)
  Salmonella
  Shigella

Inflammatory bowel disease

Drug reactions

Vasculitis

(ie, cow's milk formula or soy formula), resolution may take 4 to 6 weeks. Specifically, grossly bloody stool should resolve within 3 to 7 days and occult blood should resolve within several weeks.[47] If symptoms persist beyond 4 to 6 weeks, alternative causative antigens and/or alternative diagnoses should be considered. In breastfed infants, the mother should restrict cow's milk and soy-containing foods. These infants have an excellent prognosis, and many of them may tolerate cow's milk and/or soy after reintroduction between 1 and 3 years of age. If a reaction occurs with milk reintroduction at 12 months old, children are often rechallenged every 3 to 6 months. If they continue to have allergic reactions, they should be referred to an allergist. Individuals who present as adolescents typically have a more chronic and relapsing disease course.

REFERENCES

1. Dellon ES, Gonsalves N, Hirano I, et al. Evidenced based approach to the diagnosis and management of esophageal eosinophilia and eosinophilic esophagitis (EoE). Am J Gastroenterol 2013;108:679–92.

2. Franciosi JP, Tam V, Liacouras CA, et al. A case-control study of sociodemographic and geographic characteristics of 335 children with eosinophilic esophagitis. Clin Gastroenterol Hepatol 2009;7(4):415–9.

3. Fahey L, Robinson G, Weinberger K, et al. Correlation between aeroallergen levels and new diagnosis of eosinophilic esophagitis in New York City. J Pediatr Gastroenterol Nutr 2017;64(1):22–5.

4. Mishra A, Rothenberg ME. Intratracheal IL-13 induces eosinophilic esophagitis by an IL-5, eotaxin-1, and STAT6- dependent mechanism. Gastroenterology 2003;125:1419–27.

5. Rothenberg ME, Spergel JM, Sherrill JD, et al. Common variants at 5q22 associate with pediatric eosinophilic esophagitis. Nat Genet 2010;42(4):289–91.

6. Liacouras CA, Markowitz JE. Eosinophilic esophagitis: a subset of eosinophilic gastroenteritis. Curr Gastroenterol Rep 1999;1:253–8.

7. Aceves SS, Newbury RO, Dohil R, et al. Esophageal remodeling in pediatric eosinophilic esophagitis. J Allergy Clin Immunol 2007;119(1):206–12.

8. Orenstein SR, Shalaby TM, Di Lorenzo C, et al. The spectrum of pediatric eosinophilic esophagitis beyond infancy: a clinical series of 30 children. Am J Gastroenterol 2000;95:1422–30.

9. Fogg MI, Ruchelli E, Spergel JM. Pollen and eosinophilic esophagitis. J Allergy Clin Immunol 2003;112:796–7.

10. Ngo P, Furuta GT, Antonioli DA, et al. Eosinophils in the esophagus – peptic or allergic eosinophilic esophagitis? Case series of three patients with esophageal eosinophilia. Am J Gastroenterol 2006;101:1666–70.

11. Remedios M, Campbell C, Jones DM, et al. Eosinophilic esophagitis in adults: clinical, endoscopic, histologic findings, and response to treatment with fluticasone propionate. Gastrointest Endosc 2006;63:3–12.

12. Faubion WA Jr, Perrault J, Burgart LJ, et al. Treatment of eosinophilic esophagitis with inhaled corticosteroids. J Pediatr Gastroenterol Nutr 1998;27:90–3.

13. Arora AS, Perrault J, Smyrk TC. Topical corticosteroid treatment of dysphagia due to eosinophilic esophagitis in adults. Mayo Clin Proc 2003;78:830–5.

14. Noel RJ, Putnam PE, Collins MH, et al. Clinical and immunopathologic effects of swallowed fluticasone for eosinophilic esophagitis. Clin Gastroenterol Hepatol 2004;2:568–75.

15. Kelly KJ, Lazenby AJ, Rowe PC, et al. Eosinophilic esophagitis attributed to gastroesophageal reflux: improvement with an amino acid-based formula. Gastroenterology 1995;109:1503–12.

16. Liacouras CA, Spergel JM, Ruchelli E, et al. Eosinophilic Esophagitis: A 10-Year Experience in 381 Children. Clinical Gastroenterology and Hepatology 2005;3: 1198–206.

17. Kagalwalla AF, Shah , Li BU, et al. Identification of specific foods responsible for inflammation in children with eosinophilic esophagitis successfully treated with empiric elimination diet. J Pediatr Gastroenterol Nutr 2011;53(2):145–9.

18. Simoniuk U, Mcmanus C, Kiire C. Eosinophilic Gastroenteritis-a diagnostic enigma. BMJ Case Rep 2012.

19. Klein NC, Hargrove RL, Sleisenger MH, et al. Eosinophilic gastroenteritis. Medicine (Baltimore) 1970;49:299–319.

20. Spergel JM, Pawlowski NA. Food allergy. Mechanisms, diagnosis, and management in children. Pediatr Clin North Am 2002;49:73–96, vi.

21. Goldman H, Proujansky R. Allergic proctitis and gastroenteritis in children. Clinical and mucosal biopsy features in 53 cases. Am J Surg Pathol 1986;10:75–86.

22. Tsibouris P, Galeas T, Moussia M, et al. Two cases of eosinophilic gastroenteritis and malabsorption due to Enterobious vermicularis. Dig Dis Sci 2005;50: 2389–92.

23. Chira O, Badea R, Dumitrascu D, et al. Eosinophilic ascites in a patient with Toxocara canis infection. A case report. Rom J Gastroenterol 2005;14:397–400.

24. Van Laethem JL, Jacobs F, Braude P, et al. Toxocara canis infection presenting as eosinophilic ascites and gastroenteritis. Dig Dis Sci 1994;39:1370–2.

25. Papadopoulos AA, Tzathas C, Polymeros D, et al. Symptomatic eosinophilic gastritis cured with Helicobacter pylori eradication. Gut 2005;54:1822.

26. Montalto M, Miele L, Marcheggiano A, et al. Anisakis infestation: a case of acute abdomen mimicking Crohn's disease and eosinophilic gastroenteritis. Dig Liver Dis 2005;37:62–4.

27. Koga M, Fujiwara M, Hotta N, et al. Eosinophilic gastroenteritis associated with Epstein–Barr virus infection in a young boy. J Pediatr Gastroenterol Nutr 2001; 33:610–2.

28. Schwake L, Stremmel W, Sergi C. Eosinophilic enterocolitis in a patient with rheumatoid arthritis. J Clin Gastroenterol 2002;34:487–8.

29. Reese GE, Constantinides VA, Simillis C, et al. Diagnostic precision of anti-Saccharomyces cerevisiae antibodies and perinuclear antineutrophil cytoplasmic antibodies in inflammatory bowel disease. Am J Gastroenterol 2006; 101:2410–22.

30. Teele RL, Katz AJ, Goldman H, et al. Radiographic features of eosinophilic gastroenteritis (allergic gastroenteropathy) of childhood. Am J Roentgenol 1979;132:575–80.
31. Barak N, Hart J, Sitrin MD. Enalapril-induced eosinophilic gastroenteritis. J Clin Gastroenterol 2001;33:157–8.
32. Justinich C, Katz A, Gurbindo C, et al. Elemental diet improves steroid-dependent eosinophilic gastroenteritis and reverses growth failure. J Pediatr Gastroenterol Nutr 1996;23:81–5.
33. Chehade M, Magid MS, Mofidi S, et al. Allergic eosinophilic gastroenteritis with protein-losing enteropathy: intestinal pathology, clinical course, and long-term follow-up. J Pediatr Gastroenterol Nutr 2006;42:516–21.
34. Whitington PF, Whitington GL. Eosinophilic gastroenteropathy in childhood. J Pediatr Gastroenterol Nutr 1988;7:379–85.
35. Siewert E, Lammert F, Koppitz P, et al. Eosinophilic gastroenteritis with severe protein-losing enteropathy: successful treatment with budesonide. Dig Liver Dis 2006;38:55–9.
36. Di Gioacchino M, Pizzicannella G, Fini N, et al. Sodium cromoglycate in the treatment of eosinophilic gastroenteritis. Allergy 1990;45:161–6.
37. Tien FM, Wu JF, Jeng YM, et al. Clinical features and treatment responses of children with eosinophilic gastroenteritis. Pediatr Neonatol 2011;52(5):272–8.
38. Kerner JA Jr. Formula allergy and intolerance. Gastroenterol Clin North Am 1995; 24:1–25.
39. Simpser E. Gastrointestinal allergy. In: Altschuler SM, Liacouras CA, editors. Clinical pediatric gastroenterology. Philadelphia: Churchill Livingstone; 1998. p. 113–8.
40. Shannon WR. Demonstration of food proteins in human breast milk by anaphylactic experiments in guinea pig. Am J Dis Child 1921;22:223–5.
41. Donta ST, Myers MG. Clostridium difficile toxin in asymptomatic neonates. J Pediatr 1982;100:431–4.
42. Anveden-Hertzberg L, Finkel Y, Sandstedt B, et al. Proctocolitis in exclusively breast-fed infants. Eur J Pediatr 1996;155:464–7.
43. Odze RD, Bines J, Leichtner AM, et al. Allergic proctocolitis in infants: a prospective clinicopathologic biopsy study. Hum Pathol 1993;24:668–74.
44. Machida HM, Catto Smith AG, Gall DG, et al. Allergic colitis in infancy: clinical and pathologic aspects. J Pediatr Gastroenterol Nutr 1994;19:22–6.
45. Goldman H. Allergic disorders. In: Ming S-C, Goldman H, editors. Pathology of the gastrointestinal tract. Philadelphia: WB Saunders; 1992. p. 171–87.
46. Juvonen P, Mansson M, Jakobsson I. Does early diet have an effect on subsequent macromolecular absorption and serum IgE? J Pediatr Gastroenterol Nutr 1994;18:344–9.
47. Hill SM, Milla PJ. Colitis caused by food allergy in infants. Arch Dis Child 1990; 65:132.

Gastroesophageal Reflux Disease

Hayat Mousa, MD[a,b],*, Maheen Hassan, MD[a,b]

KEYWORDS

- Gastroesophageal reflux • Endoscopy • Impedance • Proton pump inhibitors
- Lifestyle changes • Extraesophageal symptoms • Pediatrics

KEY POINTS

- Gastroesophageal reflux is a normal physiologic process that does not require treatment.
- In infants, reducing feeding volumes, offering smaller, more frequent meals, thickening feeds, and positioning can reduce reflux episodes; these infants should not be placed on acid suppression.
- Gastroesophageal reflux disease (GERD) occurs when reflux of gastric contents causes troublesome symptoms or complications. First-line treatment in children and adolescents includes lifestyle modification and acid suppression.
- GERD can have atypical presentations, such as recurrent pneumonia, upper airway symptoms, nocturnal or difficult to control asthma, dental erosions, and Sandifer syndrome.
- Diagnosis of GERD is largely based upon history and physical, but endoscopy and pH impedance can be used to help support the diagnosis in atypical presentations.

INTRODUCTION

Gastroesophageal reflux (GER) is a normal physiologic process. It is defined as the involuntary flow of stomach content back into the esophagus.[1] Most episodes of reflux are into the distal esophagus, brief, and asymptomatic. GER disease (GERD) occurs when reflux causes troublesome symptoms or complications.[2]

PHYSIOLOGY

Multiple mechanisms are in place to protect from reflux: the antireflux barrier, esophageal clearance, and esophageal mucosal resistance. The antireflux barrier is composed of the lower esophageal sphincter (LES), the angle of His, the crural

Disclosure Statement: The authors have no commercial or financial conflicts of interest or any funding sources to disclose.
[a] University of California, San Diego, 3020 Children's Way, MOB 211, MC 5030, San Diego, CA 92123, USA; [b] Division of Pediatric Gastroenterology, Hepatology, and Nutrition, Rady Children's Hospital, 7960 Birmingham Way, Room 2110, MC 5030, San Diego, CA 92123, USA
* Corresponding author.
E-mail address: hmousa@ucsd.edu

Pediatr Clin N Am 64 (2017) 487–505
http://dx.doi.org/10.1016/j.pcl.2017.01.003
0031-3955/17/© 2017 Elsevier Inc. All rights reserved.

diaphragm, and the phrenoesophageal ligament.[3] The LES consists of tonically contracted circular smooth muscles, composed of the intrinsic muscles of the distal esophagus and the sling fibers of the proximal stomach.[4] The crural diaphragm forms the esophageal hiatus and encircles the proximal LES. The phrenoesophageal ligament anchors the distal esophagus to the crural diaphragm. A small portion of the LES, up to 2 cm in adults, is intraabdominal. The LES resting pressure is higher than the intraabdominal pressure, and this prevents reflux of gastric contents into the distal esophagus. The angle of His is an acute angle between the great curvature of the stomach and the esophagus, and acts as an antireflux barrier by functioning like a valve. Esophageal clearance limits the duration of contact between luminal contents and esophageal epithelium.[1] Gravity and esophageal peristalsis remove volume from the esophageal lumen, and salivary and esophageal secretions neutralize acid. Esophageal mucosal resistance comes into play when acid contact time is prolonged, and this is determined genetically.

MECHANISMS OF GASTROESOPHAGEAL REFLUX

Anything that interferes with these lines of defense can lead to GER. Inappropriate transient LES relaxation is among the most important causes of GERD in children.[5,6] Increased intraabdominal pressure relative to LES resting pressure permits the reflux of gastric contents into the distal esophagus.[6] Increased intraabdominal pressure can be caused by medications, the Valsalva maneuver, the Trendelenburg position, or lifting. Position and posture influence the angle of His, with esophageal acid exposure greater in the right side sleeping position than in the left position. Esophageal clearance is also delayed in the right position.[1] Although little is known about the angle of His in infants, it is hypothesized that this angle is less acute in young infants and becomes acute after 1 year of age; this would predispose their stomach to a more vertical lie and therefore increased ease of reflux.[1] In sliding hiatal hernias, there is a weakness of the phrenoesophageal ligament leading to an upward displacement of the LES into the lower mediastinum. As a result, the defense of the LES, angle of His, and the diaphragm are compromised.[3] The LES and crural diaphragm no longer overlap, and the LES length and pressure are reduced. Another proposed mechanism by which hiatal hernia leads to GER is by creating a hernia sac between the LES proximally and the crural diaphragm distally.[7] This sac has increased acid exposure and impaired clearance, and can reflux during subsequent swallow relaxations of the LES.[7]

DISTINGUISHING GASTROESOPHAGEAL REFLUX FROM GASTROESOPHAGEAL REFLUX DISEASE

Whereas GER is a normal physiologic process, GERD occurs when reflux of gastric contents causes troublesome symptoms or complications.[2] In infants, crying and fussiness are often attributed to GERD, but are nonspecific and difficult to distinguish from other causes. GERD can cause infants to associate feeding with pain, and as a result feeding aversion, anorexia, and failure to thrive can develop.[2] Respiratory complications are less common, but recurrent pneumonia and interstitial lung disease secondary to reflux can occur owing to aspiration of gastric contents.[8] Reflux worsening asthma symptoms has also been reported.[9,10] Histologic changes can also help distinguish the two, with esophageal biopsies in GERD typically showing findings of basal zone hyperplasia, papillary lengthening, and neutrophil infiltration.[11,12]

EPIDEMIOLOGY

There are few pediatric-specific data on GER and GERD epidemiology with incidence and prevalence based on questionnaires. The incidence of GERD in pediatrics was estimated to be 0.84 per 1000 person-years.[13] After 1 year of age, the incidence of GERD decreases with until age 12, and then reaches a maximum at age 16 to 17. The prevalence varies by study and age. It is estimated that 10% of all children have GER[14] and 1.8% to 8.2% have GERD.[14,15] The estimated prevalence of GERD in infants 0 to 23 months, children 2 to 11 years old, and adolescents 12 to 17 years old is 2.2% to 12.6%, 0.6% to 4.1%, and 0.8% to 7.6%, respectively.

PRESENTING SYMPTOMS
Infancy

Daily regurgitation in healthy infants is physiologic and common, with the prevalence being highest in the first 3 to 4 months of life, at between 41% and 73%.[16–18] A large proportion of these infants regurgitate more than 4 times a day. Prevalence decreases to 14% at 7 months of age,[17] and to less than 5% after 12 months of age.[16,18] GERD can be difficult to diagnose in infants because they present with nonspecific symptoms that can be difficult to distinguish from other conditions (**Box 1**).[19,20] These symptoms include choking, gagging, irritability, regurgitation, refusal to feed, and poor weight gain. Crying, irritability, and vomiting are often attributed to GERD,[18] but can be indistinguishable from milk protein allergy[21,22] and do not correlate well with reflux on pH impedance studies,[23,24] or improve after trials of proton pump inhibitors (PPIs).[25,26] A history and physical examination should be done to rule out warning signals that require further investigation (**Box 2**),[19] before attributing them to GERD.

Childhood

GERD is often diagnosed in adults based on a history of substernal, burning pain, with or without regurgitation.[2] The diagnosis of GERD can similarly be made in adolescents.[27] However, history is unreliable in children under the age of 12, and these children can also present with different symptoms. In addition to the aforementioned typical GERD symptoms, 21% of children reported nausea or vomiting.[13] Abdominal pain and cough are also reported frequently.[28] In children with erosive esophagitis, cough, anorexia, and feeding refusal were found to be more frequent and severe in children ages 1 to 5 years of age, as compared with older children, while heartburn was less severe. Symptoms have not been found to be predictive of mucosal damage.

Children with certain underlying disorders are at high risk for developing severe and chronic GERD (**Table 1**).[19]

Atypical Presentations

An association between asthma and reflux measured by pH or impedance has been reported,[29] although the etiology is not established. Proposed mechanisms of GERD contributing to asthma include aspiration of gastric acid resulting in airway inflammation and causing vagally mediated bronchial or laryngeal spasm.[30] Alternatively, asthma may contribute to GERD. Pulmonary hyperinflation occurs as a result of chronic asthma. This hyperinflation causes the diaphragm to flatten, displacing the LES into the thoracic cavity, which has a negative atmosphere pressure, and thereby reduces the LES resting pressure and eliminates the angle of His. Studies have shown that the majority of children with asthma have an abnormal pH impedance study[31]; however, the use of a PPI in unselected patients with wheezing or asthma is of

Box 1
Differential diagnosis for emesis is an infant or child

Gastrointestinal obstruction

- Esophageal web
- Esophageal stricture
- Tracheoesophageal fistula
- Pyloric stenosis
- Duodenal atresia
- Malrotation with intermittent volvulus
- Intestinal duplication
- Antral/duodenal web
- Hirschsprung disease
- Foreign body/bezoar
- Incarcerated hernia
- Imperforate anus

Other gastrointestinal disorders

- Celiac disease
- Milk/soy protein allergy
- Achalasia
- Gastroparesis
- Peptic ulcer
- Eosinophilic esophagitis/gastroenteritis
- Inflammatory bowel disease
- Appendicitis
- Pancreatitis
- Cholecystitis/choledocholithiasis

Neurologic

- Intracranial mass
- Hydrocephalus
- Subdural hematoma
- Intracranial hemorrhage
- Infant migraine
- Chiari malformation

Infectious

- Meningitis
- Gastroenteritis
- Sinusitis
- Urinary tract infection
- Pneumonia
- Otitis media

- Hepatitis
- Sepsis

Metabolic/endocrine

- Galactosemia
- Hereditary fructosemia
- Urea cycle defects
- Amino and organic acidemias
- Fatty acid oxidation disorders
- Lysosomal storage disorders
- Congenital adrenal hyperplasia
- Diabetic ketoacidosis

Renal

- Obstructive uropathy
- Nephrolithiasis
- Renal tubular acidosis
- Renal insufficiency

Other

- Self-induced vomiting
- Cyclic vomiting syndrome
- Rumination
- Overfeeding
- Autonomic dysfunction
- Munchausen syndrome by proxy
- Medication/vitamin/drug toxicity
- Child abuse

Adapted from Vandeplas Y, Rudolph CD, Di Lorenzo C, et al. Pediatric gastroesophageal reflux clinical practice guidelines: joint recommendations of the North American Society for Pediatric Gastroenterology, Hepatology, and Nutrition (NASPGHAN) and the European Society for Pediatric Gastroenterology, Hepatology, and Nutrition (ESPGHAN). J Pediatr Gastroenterol Nutr 2009;49(4):498–547; and Chandran L, Chitkara M. Vomiting in children: reassurance, red flag, or referral? Pediatr Rev 2008;29(6):183–92.

limited benefit.[32] Patients who may benefit from GERD treatment include those with heartburn, nocturnal asthma symptoms, or steroid-dependent and difficult-to-control asthma.[9,10]

Recurrent pneumonia and interstitial lung disease may be complications of GERD owing to aspiration of gastric contents.[8] Although an abnormal esophageal pH study may increase the probability of GERD causing recurrent aspirations, there is no definitive test that can prove GERD's causal role.[33]

Upper airway symptoms attributed to GERD include hoarseness, chronic cough, or a sensation of a lump in the throat,[34] although there are no strong data to support this claim.[35] Laryngoscopic findings attributed to reflux include erythema, edema, cobblestoning, and nodularity, although with low sensitivity and specificity[36,37] and poor correlation with pH probe studies.[38]

Box 2
Warning signals that require investigation in infants with vomiting

Bilious emesis

Gastrointestinal bleeding: hematemesis, coffee ground emesis, hematochezia

Choking, gagging, coughing with feeds

Forceful emesis

Onset of emesis after 6 months of life

Failure to thrive

Diarrhea/constipation

Fever

Lethargy

Hepatosplenomegaly

Bulging fontanelle

Microcephaly or macrocephaly

Seizures

Abdominal tenderness or distention

Suspected genetic syndrome

Studies revealed a cause and effect relationship between GERD and dental erosions,[39] with worse dental erosions when GERD symptoms are present. Other contributing factors to dental erosions include drinking juice, bulimia, racial and genetic factors affecting the characteristic of enamel and saliva, and children with neurologic impairment.

Table 1
Medical conditions at high risk for gastroesophageal reflux disease

Condition	Contributing Factors
Neurologic impairment	Decreased esophageal clearance • Supine position • Abnormal swallow • Abnormal muscle tone Increased reflux episodes • Heightened gag reflex • Delayed gastric emptying • Constipation • Skeletal abnormalities • Medication side effects
Obesity	
Esophageal atresia	Esophagus is congenitally dysmotile After surgery, a hiatal hernia is often present
Chronic respiratory disorders • Bronchopulmonary dysplasia • Cystic fibrosis • Idiopathic interstitial fibrosis	Unknown
Lung transplantation	Pneumonectomy contributes to esophageal and gastric motor dysfunction

Sandifer syndrome, in which there is spasmodic torsional dystonia with arching of the back and rigid opisthotonic posturing of the neck and back, is an uncommon but specific presentation of GERD.[2] It must be distinguished from seizures, dystonia, or infantile spasms.[40] When related to GERD, it improves with antireflux treatment.

An apparent life-threatening event (ALTE) was first defined in 1986 as an episode that is frightening to the observer and that is characterized by some combination of apnea, color change, marked change in muscle tone, choking, or gagging.[41] The term ALTE was recently replaced by the term "brief resolved unexplained event," which is characterized by a sudden, brief, and resolved episode occurring in an infant under 1 year of age that consists of one of more of the following: cyanosis or pallor; absent, decreased, or irregular breathing; marked change in tone; and altered level of responsiveness. Because the change was recently made, published studies have evaluated GERD association with the ALTE definition. The results are conflicting. Although most series fail to demonstrate a temporal relationship between the two,[29,42] multiple studies do show that there is an association.[43–45] If other causes have been ruled out and GER is suspected, the diagnosis can be better evaluated by recording synchronous symptoms on multichannel intraluminal impedance (MII)/pH esophageal monitoring in combination with cardiorespiratory monitoring. When using esophageal manometry in conjunction with cardiorespiratory monitoring, infants with ALTE were found to have swallowing as the most frequent esophageal event associated with spontaneous respiratory events. This suggests a dysfunctional regulation of the swallow–respiratory interactions, and needs to be investigated further.[46] When using polysomnography with esophageal pH and impedance monitoring, apnea was seldom associated with reflux. When it was, the predominant sequence of events was obstructive or mixed apnea followed by reflux, suggesting against reflux as a cause of apnea.[47]

Apnea and sleep quality have similarly been evaluated by a combination of polysomnography with esophageal pH and impedance monitoring. The data, again, are conflicting. In some, GER was found unlikely to be related to apneic events and rarely seemed to cause sleep awakening.[48,49] Instead, awakening and arousal was precipitating GER. Another group has shown that acid and non–acid reflux was associated with sleep interruption in infants,[50] and acid reflux was associated with sleep interruption in obese children.[51]

DIAGNOSIS

The diagnosis of GERD can largely be based on history and physical examination alone. There are several tools, however, to help make the diagnosis when there is an atypical presentation and to assess the severity and consequence of GERD.

Endoscopy

On endoscopy, visualizing endoscopic breaks in the mucosa is the most reliable evidence of reflux esophagitis.[19] The classic histologic findings of GERD are basal zone hyperplasia, papillary lengthening, and neutrophilic infiltration.[12] Although the histologic findings are not specific to GERD alone and have not correlated well with symptom severity of GERD in children,[52] they can help to support the diagnosis. The sensitivity of histology increases if multiple biopsies are taken, sampling in the mid and distal esophagus.[11,53] If using this method, the sensitivity of histology was 96% in patients with erosive esophagitis and 76% with nonerosive reflux disease.[53] The additional usefulness of pursuing endoscopy includes ruling out other disorders that can masquerade as GERD, such as eosinophilic esophagitis; identifying complications of reflux disease; and evaluating for empirical treatment failure.[54]

pH and Impedance

Twenty-four–hour esophageal pH monitoring measures the frequency and duration of acid esophageal reflux. This test can be performed by either placing a nasal catheter, or by clipping a wireless sensor to the esophageal mucosa via endoscopy. A decrease in the intraesophageal pH to less than 4 is considered acidic exposure. For criteria to diagnose acid reflux, please refer to the North American Society for Pediatric Gastro-enterology, Hepatology, and Nutrition–European Society for Pediatric Gastroenter-ology, Hepatology, and Nutrition consensus paper from 2009.[19] The main indications for pH monitoring include evaluating endoscopy-negative patients for abnormal esophageal acid exposure if they are being considered for antireflux proced-ures and evaluating patients who are refractory to PPI therapy.[55] There are limitations to standard pH monitoring. It is a poor detector of weakly acidic (pH of 4-7) reflux[56] and can also overestimate acid exposure by picking up "pH-only" episodes, in which there is no reflux.[57] In infants and children, weakly acidic GER is more prevalent than in adults,[57,58] which can explain why abnormal esophageal pH monitoring does not correlate with symptom severity in infants.[59] Abnormal esophageal pH is observed more frequently in adults and children with erosive esophagitis.[60,61]

MII uses change in impedance to measure the anterograde and retrograde move-ment of fluid, solids, and air in the esophagus. Dual pH-MII is able to detect reflux regardless of pH value, detect anterograde versus retrograde flow thereby distinguish-ing between swallows and GER, determine the height of refluxate, and differentiate between liquid, gas, or mixed refluxate.[62] Nonacid pH is defined as a pH of greater than 4 and the reflux index is defined as the percentage of time the pH drops to less than 4. **Tables 2** and **3** provide the reflux parameter definitions and normal values for reflux per 24 hours in infant and children. Normal values for infants and children with nonacid and acid reflux were determined by Mousa and colleagues[63] in a multi-center study evaluating multiple parameters of reflux via pH/MII in a very clean popu-lation. The infant and children selected had no evidence of acid reflux or symptoms associated with regurgitation. They were also off antireflux medications at the time of the procedure and did not have a fundoplication. Based on the study, in infants, more than 48 acid reflux episodes or more than 67 nonacid reflux episodes in 24 hours are considered pathologic. With children, more than 55 acid reflux episodes or more than 34 nonacid reflux episodes in 24 hours is considered pathologic.

In infants and children, pH-MII optimizes the yield of the GER–symptom associa-tion.[64] Indications for pH-MII include (1) evaluating the efficacy of antireflux therapy, (2) endoscopy-negative patients with symptoms concerning for reflux despite PPI therapy in whom documentation of nonacid reflux will alter clinical management,[55,62] (3) evaluating tube fed patients for reflux, because the majority of refluxate during tube feeding is nonacidic,[62] and (4) differentiating aerophagia from GER.

Motility Testing

Findings on esophageal manometry are not sensitive or specific enough to make the diagnosis of GERD, but can identify alternate motor disorders that may present similar to GERD.[19,54] Esophageal dysmotility is present in a proportion of patients with GERD,[65] with motor dysfunctions of both the LES and esophageal body being the ma-jor factors predicting medical refractoriness of reflux disease in children.[66] However, patients with gastroparesis are at increased risk for GERD,[67] and there are studies that show that infants and young children with delayed gastric emptying tend to be more symptomatic,[68] gastric emptying studies do not confirm the diagnosis of GERD[69] and are not recommended for its routine evaluation.

Table 2
Reflux parameters on pH-multichannel intraluminal impedance

Definitions	
Liquid reflux	Drop in impedance of $\leq$50% of baseline value with subsequent recovery, in $\geq$2 of the distal-most channels
Acid GER	pH decreases and remains <4 for $\geq$5 s; if pH was already <4, it decreases by $\geq$1 pH unit for $\geq$5 s; with or without a decrease in impedance of $\leq$50% of baseline value
Nonacid GER	pH increases, remains unchanged, or decreases by $\geq$1 pH unit while remaining $\geq$4, with a retrograde decrease in impedance of $\leq$50% of baseline value in $\geq$2 of the distal-most channels
Gas reflux	Simultaneous and rapid increases in impedance in $\geq$2 channels (>3000 Ohms) of the distal-most channels
Extent of reflux migration	
Localized to distal esophagus	Height of reflux is confined to the 2 most distal impedance channels (channels 5 and 6)
Proximal	Height of refluxate reaches either or both of the most proximal channels (channels 1 and/or 2)
Parameters of symptom association	
Reflux index	Percent of time pH is <4
Symptom index	Percent of symptoms episodes that are related to reflux ([no. of reflux-related symptom episodes ÷ total no. of symptom episodes] × 100) • Positive when >50%
Symptom sensitivity index	Percent of symptom associated reflux episodes ([no. of reflux-related symptom episodes ÷ total no. of reflux episodes] × 100) • positive when >10%
Symptoms associated probability	Statistical probability that symptoms and GER events are associated • Positive when >95%

Abbreviation: GER, gastroesophageal reflux.

Upper gastrointestinal studies

Although GERD is reported commonly on upper gastrointestinal studies, the correlation between reflux reported on upper gastrointestinal studies and 24-h pH monitoring is poor.[70,71] Therefore, upper gastrointestinal studies should be reserved for defining anatomic abnormalities and not reflux.

Diagnostic Trial of Acid Suppression

Because GERD is diagnosed primarily based on symptoms alone in older children and adolescents, responding to an empirical trial of PPI therapy helps to support, although it cannot confirm, a diagnosis of GERD.[72] In both children[73] and adolescent[27] patients with endoscopically proven GERD, a 4- to 8-week course of PPI improves symptoms significantly. There are limitations to performing a PPI trial to diagnose GERD. It does not control for placebo effect, spontaneous resolution of symptoms, and the possibility that other conditions may improve on PPI treatment. Additionally, it does not differentiate between healing esophagitis and reflux symptoms.[54] PPI therapy is more apt to resolve esophagitis than GERD symptoms, so a negative PPI trial does not exclude GERD as a diagnostic possibility. A trial of acid suppression in infants and young children is not warranted, because symptoms suggestive of GERD are less specific.[26]

Table 3
Normal values for acid and nonacid reflux on pH/multichannel intraluminal impedance per 24 hours in infants and children

	Infants		Children	
	Median (IQR)	95th Percentile	Median (IQR)	95th Percentile
Index of acid regurgitation (%)	0.6 (0.3–0.9)	1.4	0.4 (0.2–0.8)	1.3
No. of acid regurgitation episodes in 24 h	20 (11–26)	48	14 (11–15)	55
Index of nonacid regurgitation (%)	0.7 (0.5–1.2)	2.5	0.1 (0–0.3)	1.0
No. of nonacid regurgitation episodes in 24 h	32 (16–45)	67	6 (3–11)	34
Index of GER episodes (%)	1.4 (0.9–1.2)	2.9	0.6 (0.3–1.2)	2.4
No. of GER episodes in 24 h	54 (33–69)	93	21 (11–41)	71

Abbreviations: GER, gastroesophageal reflux; IQR, interquartile range.

Adapted from Mousa H, Machado R, Orsi M, et al. Combined multichannel intraluminal impedance-pH (MII-pH): multicenter report of normal values from 117 children. Curr Gastroenterol Rep 2014;16(8):400; and Vandenplas Y, Rudolph CD, Di Lorenzo C, et al. Pediatric gastroesophageal reflux clinical practice guidelines: joint recommendations of the North American Society for Pediatric Gastroenterology, Hepatology, and Nutrition (NASPGHAN) and the European Society for Pediatric Gastroenterology, Hepatology, and Nutrition (ESPGHAN). J Pediatr Gastroenterol Nutr 2009;49(4):498–547.

Bronchoalveolar Lavage and Pepsin (for Evidence of Microaspiration with Reflux or Swallowing Disorder)

Evaluating pulmonary aspirates for pepsin has been investigated as a biomarker for GERD. Although studies support the association of the 2 conditions,[74–76] problems with prior studies include pepsin assays not being specific to pepsin A, the isoform found exclusively in the stomach.[77] Other pepsin isoforms, mainly pepsin C, are also produced in the lungs, pancreas, and seminal vesicles, thereby limiting specificity. Prospective studies evaluating children with chronic cough, asthma,[78] and GERD[79] have found that lung pepsin does not predict pathologic esophageal reflux, nor does it correlate with extraesophageal symptoms or quality of life score. Lung pepsin did, however, correlate with lung inflammation, suggesting a role for pepsin as a biomarker for reflux-related lung disease.[78]

TREATMENT
Infant

Infant regurgitation is common and largely physiologic, peaking at 3 to 4 months of age, and resolving by 12 to 13 months of age.[18] In thriving infants in whom symptoms of regurgitation are likely secondary to physiologic GER, management should focus on parental education and support.[80] For formula-fed infants, reducing feeding volumes in overfed infants, or offering smaller, more frequent meals, can decrease reflux episodes.[19] Changing the infant's body position while awake can be effective. The prone and left side down positions are associated with fewer reflux episodes,[81,82] but should be recommended only in awake infants under the age of 1 to decrease the risk of sudden infant death syndrome. Thickening feeds helps to reduce the visual symptoms of GER,[83,84] although it does not esophageal reflux frequency, as shown by pH monitoring.[85,86]

PPI use has been increasing steadily in infants with the most common reasons for use being identified as GER (59%) and poor feeding (23%).[87] The mean age of use, between 4 and 8 months of age, correlates with the timing of physiologic reflux. The majority of infants who are being placed on antireflux drugs do not meet the criteria for GERD.[88] PPIs have not been shown to benefit infant symptoms attributed to GER over placebo,[25,26] and discontinuing antireflux medications in this age group has not shown to cause a significant difference in symptoms. Therefore, antireflux medications are not recommended for infants with GER.

Milk protein sensitivity can be difficult to differentiate from GER symptoms with no diagnostic tools to differentiate between the 2 entities.[89] A prospective study found that 85 of 204 patients with documented GER by pH impedance testing had milk protein sensitivity.[21] Therefore, infants with recurrent vomiting and persistent symptoms may benefit from a 2- to 4-week trial of an extensively hydrolyzed protein formula.[22,90]

Children and Adolescents

Lifestyle changes
Recommendations for lifestyle changes are derived from adult data. Although there is some physiologic evidence that various foods as well as alcohol and tobacco affect the pressure of the LES, targeted interventions have not shown any benefit in clinical trials.[91,92] Patients should avoid foods and beverages that trigger their personal GERD symptoms. The only beneficial measures documented are weight loss in obese patients,[93] avoidance of late night eating,[94] elevation of the head of the bed, and prone or left-sided sleeping position.[95]

Acid suppression
Histamine-2 receptor antagonists Parietal cells secrete acid in response to 3 stimuli: histamine at the H2 histamine receptor, acetylcholine, and gastrin. Histamine 2 receptor agonists (H2RAs) suppress gastric acid secretion by competitively inhibiting histamine at the parietal cell's H2 receptor. In adequate doses, H2RAs are effective in the treatment of peptic disease[96] and healing erosive esophagitis compared with placebo.[97,98] However, patients requiring more than occasional use can develop to rapid tachyphylaxis.[99] Dosage requirements vary by age, but children require a relative higher dose than adults.[96]

Proton pump inhibitors PPIs are the most potent acid suppressants. They work by blocking the final step in acid secretion: the gastric H^+/K^+-adenosine triphosphatase (ATPase), which causes resorption of K^+ ions and secretion of H^+ ions. Compared with H2RAs and placebo, PPIs provide faster and increased relief of symptoms and are more effective in healing erosive esophagitis.[97,100,101] After erosive esophagitis is healed, there is a low rate of relapse and recurrence of GERD symptoms.[102] Thus, prolonged courses of PPI are not recommended without continued diagnosis.

There is increasing evidence of side effects from prolonged acid suppression, resulting from hypochlorhydria. For this reason, the smallest effective dose of acid suppression for only the necessary period of time should be used.[54] Hypochlorhydria impairs vitamin B_{12}, calcium, and iron absorption. PPI therapy has been associated with fractures in adults with osteoporosis, as well as fractures in young adults.[103] This same association has not been seen in children younger than 18 years of age. Long-term acid suppression also has increased infectious risks. In neonates, H2RA therapy is associated with higher rates of necrotizing enterocolitis.[104] Long-term hypochlorhydria is hypothesized to alter the intraluminal environment, promoting the growth of small bowel bacteria.[105] This leads to small bowel bacterial overgrowth, a condition in which the bacteria cause excessive fermentation, resulting in symptoms of bloating, abdominal pain, and diarrhea. The reduction in gastric acid secretion allows pathogen colonization from the upper gastrointestinal tract. In PPI users, a significant positive dose–response relationship has been observed between PPI use and increased risk of community-acquired pneumonia.[106,107] There was a similar increased risk, although no dose–response relationship, seen with H2RA use. With both PPI and H2RA use, there is an increased risk of gastroenteritis[107] as well as community-acquired *Clostridium difficile* infection.[108] Gastric polyps and nodules can be noted after prolonged PPI therapy, but these changes are benign.[54]

Antacids Antacids are compounds containing different combinations, such as calcium carbonate, sodium bicarbonate, aluminum, and magnesium hydroxide. They provide rapid but short-term symptom relief by buffering gastric acid, and in high doses are as effective as H2RAs.[109,110] These drugs have no efficacy in healing erosive esophagitis.[111] Dosing of these medications is based on age and weight (**Table 4**).

SURGICAL MANAGEMENT

Fundoplication is an antireflux surgery that may benefit children with confirmed GERD who have failed optimal medical therapy, who are dependent on medical therapy over a long period of time, or who have life-threatening complications of GERD.[19] Although studies are needed to confirm which cohort of GERD patients are most likely to benefit from a fundoplication, it is suggested for those with respiratory complications, including asthma or recurrent aspiration related to GERD.

Despite its value in preventing GERD, fundoplication has other consequences including gas bloat syndrome, impaired gastric accommodation, gastric hypersensitivity, rapid gastric emptying, retching, or dysphagia.[112] Children with neurologic

Table 4		
Pharmacologic agents for the treatment of gastroesophageal reflux disease		
Medication	**Dose**	**Age**
Proton pump inhibitors		
Omeprazole	0.7–3.3 mg/kg/d, max 20 mg/d	≥2 y
Lansoprazole	0.7–3 mg/kg/d	≥1 y
Esomeprazole	<20 kg: 10 mg/d ≥20 kg: 10-20 mg/d	≥1 y
Pantoprazole	≥15 kg to <40 kg: 20 mg/d ≥40 kg: 40 mg/d	Pediatric indication for erosive esophagitis in ≥5 y
Histamine-2 receptor antagonists		
Famotidine	1 mg/kg/d divided in 2–3 doses, max 20 mg bid	≥1 mo
Ranitidine	5–10 mg/kg/d divided in 2–3 doses, max 300 mg/d	≥1 mo
Cimetidine	400 mg 4×/d	No pediatric indication
Antacids		
Calcium carbonate	2–5 yo: 375–400 mg PRN; max 1500 mg/d 6–11 yo: 750–800 mg PRN; max 3000 mg/d ≥12 yo: 500–3,000 mg PRN; max 7500 mg/d	≥2 y
Sucralfate		No pediatric indication for independent treatment of gastroesophageal reflux disease

Abbreviations: max, maximum; PRN, as needed; yo, years old.

impairments suffer from many conditions, such as scoliosis and epilepsy, which decrease the success rate of antireflux therapy. In this group of children, fundoplication is associated with an high recurrence rate and significant morbidity and mortality, with a 40% surgical failure rate, 12% to 30% rate of recurrent reflux, 59% experiencing postoperative complications, and a 1% to 3% mortality rate. Surgery done in early infancy also has a higher failure rate and greater risk for surgical mortality.[113]

Transpyloric feeds have been proposed as an alternative to fundoplication in patients with GERD who are medically complex. Reflux can still occur during transpyloric feeds, and is thought to be a result of increased transient LES relaxations when fat is instilled into the small bowel.[114] Despite this phenomenon, the number of reflux events and the percentage of full-column events during transpyloric feeds are lower when compared with gastric feeds. Studies comparing transpyloric feeds and fundoplication are few, but suggest that there is a trend toward more major complications with fundoplication compared with gastrojejunal feeds in neurologically impaired children.[115] The 2 therapies have comparable rates in decreasing aspiration pneumonia, although neither eliminates the risk completely.[116]

REFERENCES

1. Vandenplas Y, Hassall E. Mechanisms of gastroesophageal reflux and gastroesophageal reflux disease. J Pediatr Gastroenterol Nutr 2002;35(2):119–36.
2. Sherman PM, Hassall E, Fagundes-Neto U, et al. A global, evidence-based consensus on the definition of gastroesophageal reflux disease in the pediatric population. Am J Gastroenterol 2009;104(5):1278–95 [quiz: 1296].
3. Mikami DJ, Murayama KM. Physiology and pathogenesis of gastroesophageal reflux disease. Surg Clin North Am 2015;95(3):515–25.
4. Mittal RK, Balaban DH. The esophagogastric junction. N Engl J Med 1997; 336(13):924–32.
5. Kawahara H, Dent J, Davidson G. Mechanisms responsible for gastroesophageal reflux in children. Gastroenterology 1997;113(2):399–408.
6. Werlin SL, Dodds WJ, Hogan WJ, et al. Mechanisms of gastroesophageal reflux in children. J Pediatr 1980;97(2):244–9.
7. Herregods TV, Bredenoord AJ, Smout AJ. Pathophysiology of gastroesophageal reflux disease: new understanding in a new era. Neurogastroenterol Motil 2015; 27(9):1202–13.
8. Boesch RP, Daines C, Willging JP, et al. Advances in the diagnosis and management of chronic pulmonary aspiration in children. Eur Respir J 2006;28(4): 847–61.
9. Khoshoo V, Le T, Haydel RM Jr, et al. Role of gastroesophageal reflux in older children with persistent asthma. Chest 2003;123(4):1008–13.
10. Kiljander TO, Harding SM, Field SK, et al. Effects of esomeprazole 40 mg twice daily on asthma: a randomized placebo-controlled trial. Am J Respir Crit Care Med 2006;173(10):1091–7.
11. Schneider NI, Plieschnegger W, Geppert M, et al. Validation study of the Esohisto consensus guidelines for the recognition of microscopic esophagitis (histoGERD Trial). Hum Pathol 2014;45(5):994–1002.
12. Ismail-Beigi F, Horton PF, Pope CE 2nd. Histological consequences of gastroesophageal reflux in man. Gastroenterology 1970;58(2):163–74.
13. Ruigomez A, Wallander MA, Lundborg P, et al. Gastroesophageal reflux disease in children and adolescents in primary care. Scand J Gastroenterol 2010;45(2): 139–46.

14. Martigne L, Delaage PH, Thomas-Delecourt F, et al. Prevalence and manage-
    ment of gastroesophageal reflux disease in children and adolescents: a nation-
    wide cross-sectional observational study. Eur J Pediatr 2012;171(12):1767–73.
15. Nelson SP, Chen EH, Syniar GM, et al. Prevalence of symptoms of gastroesoph-
    ageal reflux during childhood: a pediatric practice-based survey. Pediatric
    Practice Research Group. Arch Pediatr Adolesc Med 2000;154(2):150–4.
16. Hegar B, Dewanti NR, Kadim M, et al. Natural evolution of regurgitation in
    healthy infants. Acta Paediatr 2009;98(7):1189–93.
17. Nelson SP, Chen EH, Syniar GM, et al. Prevalence of symptoms of gastroesoph-
    ageal reflux during infancy. A pediatric practice-based survey. Pediatric Prac-
    tice Research Group. Arch Pediatr Adolesc Med 1997;151(6):569–72.
18. Martin AJ, Pratt N, Kennedy JD, et al. Natural history and familial relationships of
    infant spilling to 9 years of age. Pediatrics 2002;109(6):1061–7.
19. Vandenplas Y, Rudolph CD, Di Lorenzo C, et al. Pediatric gastroesophageal re-
    flux clinical practice guidelines: joint recommendations of the North American
    Society for Pediatric Gastroenterology, Hepatology, and Nutrition (NASPGHAN)
    and the European Society for Pediatric Gastroenterology, Hepatology, and Nutri-
    tion (ESPGHAN). J Pediatr Gastroenterol Nutr 2009;49(4):498–547.
20. Chandran L, Chitkara M. Vomiting in children: reassurance, red flag, or referral?
    Pediatr Rev 2008;29(6):183–92.
21. Iacono G, Carroccio A, Cavataio F, et al. Gastroesophageal reflux and cow's
    milk allergy in infants: a prospective study. J Allergy Clin Immunol 1996;97(3):
    822–7.
22. Vandenplas Y, Gottrand F, Veereman-Wauters G, et al. Gastrointestinal manifes-
    tations of cow's milk protein allergy and gastrointestinal motility. Acta Paediatr
    2012;101(11):1105–9.
23. Funderburk A, Nawab U, Abraham S, et al. Temporal association between
    reflux-like behaviors and gastroesophageal reflux in preterm and term infants.
    J Pediatr Gastroenterol Nutr 2016;62(4):556–61.
24. Heine RG, Jordan B, Lubitz L, et al. Clinical predictors of pathological gastro-
    oesophageal reflux in infants with persistent distress. J Paediatr Child Health
    2006;42(3):134–9.
25. Moore DJ, Tao BS, Lines DR, et al. Double-blind placebo-controlled trial of
    omeprazole in irritable infants with gastroesophageal reflux. J Pediatr 2003;
    143(2):219–23.
26. Orenstein SR, Hassall E, Furmaga-Jablonska W, et al. Multicenter, double-blind,
    randomized, placebo-controlled trial assessing the efficacy and safety of proton
    pump inhibitor lansoprazole in infants with symptoms of gastroesophageal re-
    flux disease. J Pediatr 2009;154(4):514–20.e4.
27. Gold BD, Gunasekaran T, Tolia V, et al. Safety and symptom improvement with
    esomeprazole in adolescents with gastroesophageal reflux disease. J Pediatr
    Gastroenterol Nutr 2007;45(5):520–9.
28. Gupta SK, Hassall E, Chiu YL, et al. Presenting symptoms of nonerosive and
    erosive esophagitis in pediatric patients. Dig Dis Sci 2006;51(5):858–63.
29. Tolia V, Vandenplas Y. Systematic review: the extra-oesophageal symptoms of
    gastro-oesophageal reflux disease in children. Aliment Pharmacol Ther 2009;
    29(3):258–72.
30. Malfroot A, Dab I. Pathophysiology and mechanisms of gastroesophageal reflux
    in childhood asthma. Pediatr Pulmonol Suppl 1995;11:55–6.
31. Scarupa MD, Mori N, Canning BJ. Gastroesophageal reflux disease in children
    with asthma: treatment implications. Paediatr Drugs 2005;7(3):177–86.

32. Stordal K, Johannesdottir GB, Bentsen BS, et al. Acid suppression does not change respiratory symptoms in children with asthma and gastro-oesophageal reflux disease. Arch Dis Child 2005;90(9):956–60.

33. Cucchiara S, Santamaria F, Minella R, et al. Simultaneous prolonged recordings of proximal and distal intraesophageal pH in children with gastroesophageal reflux disease and respiratory symptoms. Am J Gastroenterol 1995;90(10): 1791–6.

34. Koufman JA. The otolaryngologic manifestations of gastroesophageal reflux disease (GERD): a clinical investigation of 225 patients using ambulatory 24-hour pH monitoring and an experimental investigation of the role of acid and pepsin in the development of laryngeal injury. Laryngoscope 1991;101(4 Pt 2 Suppl 53): 1–78.

35. Wo JM, Grist WJ, Gussack G, et al. Empiric trial of high-dose omeprazole in patients with posterior laryngitis: a prospective study. Am J Gastroenterol 1997; 92(12):2160–5.

36. Branski RC, Bhattacharyya N, Shapiro J. The reliability of the assessment of endoscopic laryngeal findings associated with laryngopharyngeal reflux disease. Laryngoscope 2002;112(6):1019–24.

37. Hicks DM, Ours TM, Abelson TI, et al. The prevalence of hypopharynx findings associated with gastroesophageal reflux in normal volunteers. J Voice 2002; 16(4):564–79.

38. McMurray JS, Gerber M, Stern Y, et al. Role of laryngoscopy, dual pH probe monitoring, and laryngeal mucosal biopsy in the diagnosis of pharyngoesophageal reflux. Ann Otol Rhinol Laryngol 2001;110(4):299–304.

39. Pace F, Pallotta S, Tonini M, et al. Systematic review: gastro-oesophageal reflux disease and dental lesions. Aliment Pharmacol Ther 2008;27(12):1179–86.

40. Kabakus N, Kurt A. Sandifer Syndrome: a continuing problem of misdiagnosis. Pediatr Int 2006;48(6):622–5.

41. National Institutes of Health consensus development conference on infantile apnea and home monitoring, Sept 29 to Oct 1, 1986. Pediatrics 1987;79(2):292–9.

42. Cendon RG, Jiménez MJ, Valdés JA, et al. Intraluminal impedance technique in the diagnosis of apparent life-threatening events (ALTE). Cir Pediatr 2008;21(1): 11–4 [in Spanish].

43. Newman LJ, Russe J, Glassman MS, et al. Patterns of gastroesophageal reflux (GER) in patients with apparent life-threatening events. J Pediatr Gastroenterol Nutr 1989;8(2):157–60.

44. Semeniuk J, Kaczmarski M, Wasilewska J, et al. Is acid gastroesophageal reflux in children with ALTE etiopathogenetic factor of life threatening symptoms? Adv Med Sci 2007;52:213–21.

45. Gorrotxategi P, Eizaguirre I, Saenz de Ugarte A, et al. Characteristics of continuous esophageal pH-metering in infants with gastroesophageal reflux and apparent life-threatening events. Eur J Pediatr Surg 1995;5(3):136–8.

46. Hasenstab KA, Jadcherla SR. Respiratory events in infants presenting with apparent life threatening events: is there an explanation from esophageal motility? J Pediatr 2014;165(2):250–5.e1.

47. Arad-Cohen N, Cohen A, Tirosh E. The relationship between gastroesophageal reflux and apnea in infants. J Pediatr 2000;137(3):321–6.

48. Jaimchariyatam N, Tantipornsinchai W, Desudchit T, et al. Association between respiratory events and nocturnal gastroesophageal reflux events in patients with coexisting obstructive sleep apnea and gastroesophageal reflux disease. Sleep Med 2016;22:33–8.

49. Qureshi A, Malkar M, Splaingard M, et al. The role of sleep in the modulation of gastroesophageal reflux and symptoms in NICU neonates. Pediatr Neurol 2015; 53(3):226–32.
50. Machado R, Woodley FW, Skaggs B, et al. Gastroesophageal reflux causing sleep interruptions in infants. J Pediatr Gastroenterol Nutr 2013;56(4):431–5.
51. Machado RS, Woodley FW, Skaggs B, et al. Gastroesophageal reflux affects sleep quality in snoring obese children. Pediatr Gastroenterol Hepatol Nutr 2016;19(1):12–9.
52. Quitadamo P, Woodley FW, Skaggs B, et al. Gastroesophageal reflux in young children and adolescents: is there a relation between symptom severity and esophageal histological grade? J Pediatr Gastroenterol Nutr 2015;60(3):318–21.
53. Zentilin P, Savarino V, Mastracci L, et al. Reassessment of the diagnostic value of histology in patients with GERD, using multiple biopsy sites and an appropriate control group. Am J Gastroenterol 2005;100(10):2299–306.
54. Kahrilas PJ, Shaheen NJ, Vaezi MF, et al. American Gastroenterological Association Medical Position Statement on the management of gastroesophageal reflux disease. Gastroenterology 2008;135(4):1383–91, 1391.e1–5.
55. Hirano I, Richter JE. ACG practice guidelines: esophageal reflux testing. Am J Gastroenterol 2007;102(3):668–85.
56. Rosen R, Lord C, Nurko S. The sensitivity of multichannel intraluminal impedance and the pH probe in the evaluation of gastroesophageal reflux in children. Clin Gastroenterol Hepatol 2006;4(2):167–72.
57. Woodley FW, Mousa H. Acid gastroesophageal reflux reports in infants: a comparison of esophageal pH monitoring and multichannel intraluminal impedance measurements. Dig Dis Sci 2006;51(11):1910–6.
58. Wenzl TG, Schenke S, Peschgens T, et al. Association of apnea and nonacid gastroesophageal reflux in infants: investigations with the intraluminal impedance technique. Pediatr Pulmonol 2001;31(2):144–9.
59. Salvatore S, Hauser B, Vandemaele K, et al. Gastroesophageal reflux disease in infants: how much is predictable with questionnaires, pH-metry, endoscopy and histology? J Pediatr Gastroenterol Nutr 2005;40(2):210–5.
60. Cucchiara S, Staiano A, Gobio Casali L, et al. Value of the 24 hour intraoesophageal pH monitoring in children. Gut 1990;31(2):129–33.
61. Vandenplas Y, Franckx-Goossens A, Pipeleers-Marichal M, et al. Area under pH 4: advantages of a new parameter in the interpretation of esophageal pH monitoring data in infants. J Pediatr Gastroenterol Nutr 1989;9(1):34–9.
62. Mousa HM, Rosen R, Woodley FW, et al. Esophageal impedance monitoring for gastroesophageal reflux. J Pediatr Gastroenterol Nutr 2011;52(2):129–39.
63. Mousa H, Machado R, Orsi M, et al. Combined multichannel intraluminal impedance-pH (MII-pH): multicenter report of normal values from 117 children. Curr Gastroenterol Rep 2014;16(8):400.
64. Loots CM, Benninga MA, Davidson GP, et al. Addition of pH-impedance monitoring to standard pH monitoring increases the yield of symptom association analysis in infants and children with gastroesophageal reflux. J Pediatr 2009; 154(2):248–52.
65. Patcharatrakul T, Gonlachanvit S. Gastroesophageal reflux symptoms in typical and atypical GERD: roles of gastroesophageal acid refluxes and esophageal motility. J Gastroenterol Hepatol 2014;29(2):284–90.
66. Cucchiara S, Campanozzi A, Greco L, et al. Predictive value of esophageal manometry and gastroesophageal pH monitoring for responsiveness of reflux disease to medical therapy in children. Am J Gastroenterol 1996;91(4):680–5.

67. Fass R, McCallum RW, Parkman HP. Treatment challenges in the management of gastroparesis-related GERD. Gastroenterol Hepatol (N Y) 2009;5(10 Suppl 18):4–16.

68. Argon M, Duygun U, Daglioz G, et al. Relationship between gastric emptying and gastroesophageal reflux in infants and children. Clin Nucl Med 2006; 31(5):262–5.

69. Knatten CK, Avitsland TL, Medhus AW, et al. Gastric emptying in children with gastroesophageal reflux and in healthy children. J Pediatr Surg 2013;48(9): 1856–61.

70. Serna-Gallegos D, Basseri B, Bairamian V, et al. Gastroesophageal reflux reported on esophagram does not correlate with pH monitoring and high-resolution esophageal manometry. Am Surg 2014;80(10):1026–9.

71. Aksglaede K, Pedersen JB, Lange A, et al. Gastro-esophageal reflux demonstrated by radiography in infants less than 1 year of age. Comparison with pH monitoring. Acta Radiol 2003;44(2):136–8.

72. Numans ME, Lau J, de Wit NJ, et al. Short-term treatment with proton-pump inhibitors as a test for gastroesophageal reflux disease: a meta-analysis of diagnostic test characteristics. Ann Intern Med 2004;140(7):518–27.

73. Tolia V, Bishop PR, Tsou VM, et al. Multicenter, randomized, double-blind study comparing 10, 20 and 40 mg pantoprazole in children (5-11 years) with symptomatic gastroesophageal reflux disease. J Pediatr Gastroenterol Nutr 2006; 42(4):384–91.

74. Reder NP, Davis CS, Kovacs EJ, et al. The diagnostic value of gastroesophageal reflux disease (GERD) symptoms and detection of pepsin and bile acids in bronchoalveolar lavage fluid and exhaled breath condensate for identifying lung transplantation patients with GERD-induced aspiration. Surg Endosc 2014;28(6):1794–800.

75. Starosta V, Kitz R, Hartl D, et al. Bronchoalveolar pepsin, bile acids, oxidation, and inflammation in children with gastroesophageal reflux disease. Chest 2007;132(5):1557–64.

76. Njere I, Stanton M, Davenport M. Identification of pepsin in bronchoalveolar fluid (BAL) as a new test for the detection of pulmonary aspiration associated with gastroesophageal reflux. J Pediatr Surg 2006;41(10):1787 [author reply: 1787–8].

77. Kia L, Pandolfino JE, Kahrilas PJ. Biomarkers of reflux disease. Clin Gastroenterol Hepatol 2016;14(6):790–7.

78. Rosen R, Johnston N, Hart K, et al. The presence of pepsin in the lung and its relationship to pathologic gastro-esophageal reflux. Neurogastroenterol Motil 2012;24(2):129–33, e84–5.

79. Dy F, Amirault J, Mitchell PD, et al. Salivary pepsin lacks sensitivity as a diagnostic tool to evaluate extraesophageal reflux disease. J Pediatr 2016;177:53–8.

80. Orenstein SR, McGowan JD. Efficacy of conservative therapy as taught in the primary care setting for symptoms suggesting infant gastroesophageal reflux. J Pediatr 2008;152(3):310–4.

81. Loots C, Kritas S, van Wijk M, et al. Body positioning and medical therapy for infantile gastroesophageal reflux symptoms. J Pediatr Gastroenterol Nutr 2014;59(2):237–43.

82. Corvaglia L, Rotatori R, Ferlini M, et al. The effect of body positioning on gastro-esophageal reflux in premature infants: evaluation by combined impedance and pH monitoring. J Pediatr 2007;151(6):591–6, 596.e1.

83. Craig WR, Hanlon-Dearman A, Sinclair C, et al. Metoclopramide, thickened feedings, and positioning for gastro-oesophageal reflux in children under two years. Cochrane Database Syst Rev 2004;(4):CD003502.

84. Moukarzel AA, Abdelnour H, Akatcherian C. Effects of a prethickened formula on esophageal pH and gastric emptying of infants with GER. J Clin Gastroenterol 2007;41(9):823–9.

85. Bailey DJ, Andres JM, Danek GD, et al. Lack of efficacy of thickened feeding as treatment for gastroesophageal reflux. J Pediatr 1987;110(2):187–9.

86. Khoshoo V, Ross G, Brown S, et al. Smaller volume, thickened formulas in the management of gastroesophageal reflux in thriving infants. J Pediatr Gastroenterol Nutr 2000;31(5):554–6.

87. Barron JJ, Tan H, Spalding J, et al. Proton pump inhibitor utilization patterns in infants. J Pediatr Gastroenterol Nutr 2007;45(4):421–7.

88. Khoshoo V, Edell D, Thompson A, et al. Are we overprescribing antireflux medications for infants with regurgitation? Pediatrics 2007;120(5):946–9.

89. Nielsen RG, Bindslev-Jensen C, Kruse-Andersen S, et al. Severe gastroesophageal reflux disease and cow milk hypersensitivity in infants and children: disease association and evaluation of a new challenge procedure. J Pediatr Gastroenterol Nutr 2004;39(4):383–91.

90. Vandenplas Y, De Greef E. Extensive protein hydrolysate formula effectively reduces regurgitation in infants with positive and negative challenge tests for cow's milk allergy. Acta Paediatr 2014;103(6):e243–50.

91. Eherer A. Management of gastroesophageal reflux disease: lifestyle modification and alternative approaches. Dig Dis 2014;32(1–2):149–51.

92. Meining A, Classen M. The role of diet and lifestyle measures in the pathogenesis and treatment of gastroesophageal reflux disease. Am J Gastroenterol 2000;95(10):2692–7.

93. Ness-Jensen E, Hveem K, El-Serag H, et al. Lifestyle intervention in gastroesophageal reflux disease. Clin Gastroenterol Hepatol 2016;14(2):175–82.e1-3.

94. Piesman M, Hwang I, Maydonovitch C, et al. Nocturnal reflux episodes following the administration of a standardized meal. Does timing matter? Am J Gastroenterol 2007;102(10):2128–34.

95. Kaltenbach T, Crockett S, Gerson LB. Are lifestyle measures effective in patients with gastroesophageal reflux disease? An evidence-based approach. Arch Intern Med 2006;166(9):965–71.

96. Kelly DA. Do H2 receptor antagonists have a therapeutic role in childhood? J Pediatr Gastroenterol Nutr 1994;19(3):270–6.

97. Khan M, Santana J, Donnellan C, et al. Medical treatments in the short term management of reflux oesophagitis. Cochrane Database Syst Rev 2007;(2):CD003244.

98. Sabesin SM, Berlin RG, Humphries TJ, et al. Famotidine relieves symptoms of gastroesophageal reflux disease and heals erosions and ulcerations. Results of a multicenter, placebo-controlled, dose-ranging study. USA Merck Gastroesophageal Reflux Disease Study Group. Arch Intern Med 1991;151(12):2394–400.

99. McRorie JW, Kirby JA, Miner PB. Histamine2-receptor antagonists: rapid development of tachyphylaxis with repeat dosing. World J Gastrointest Pharmacol Ther 2014;5(2):57–62.

100. Chiba N, De Gara CJ, Wilkinson JM, et al. Speed of healing and symptom relief in grade II to IV gastroesophageal reflux disease: a meta-analysis. Gastroenterology 1997;112(6):1798–810.

101. van Pinxteren B, Sigterman KE, Bonis P, et al. Short-term treatment with proton pump inhibitors, H2-receptor antagonists and prokinetics for gastro-oesophageal reflux disease-like symptoms and endoscopy negative reflux disease. Cochrane Database Syst Rev 2010;(11):CD002095.

102. Boccia G, Manguso F, Miele E, et al. Maintenance therapy for erosive esophagitis in children after healing by omeprazole: is it advisable? Am J Gastroenterol 2007;102(6):1291-7.

103. Freedberg DE, Haynes K, Denburg MR, et al. Use of proton pump inhibitors is associated with fractures in young adults: a population-based study. Osteoporos Int 2015;26(10):2501-7.

104. Guillet R, Stoll BJ, Cotten CM, et al. Association of H2-blocker therapy and higher incidence of necrotizing enterocolitis in very low birth weight infants. Pediatrics 2006;117(2):e137-42.

105. Hegar B, Hutapea EI, Advani N, et al. A double-blind placebo-controlled randomized trial on probiotics in small bowel bacterial overgrowth in children treated with omeprazole. J Pediatr (Rio J) 2013;89(4):381-7.

106. Laheij RJ, Sturkenboom MC, Hassing RJ, et al. Risk of community-acquired pneumonia and use of gastric acid-suppressive drugs. JAMA 2004;292(16): 1955-60.

107. Canani RB, Cirillo P, Roggero P, et al. Therapy with gastric acidity inhibitors increases the risk of acute gastroenteritis and community-acquired pneumonia in children. Pediatrics 2006;117(5):e817-20.

108. Dial S, Delaney JA, Barkun AN, et al. Use of gastric acid-suppressive agents and the risk of community-acquired Clostridium difficile-associated disease. JAMA 2005;294(23):2989-95.

109. Cucchiara S, Staiano A, Romaniello G, et al. Antacids and cimetidine treatment for gastro-oesophageal reflux and peptic oesophagitis. Arch Dis Child 1984; 59(9):842-7.

110. Iacono G, Carroccio A, Montalto G, et al. Magnesium hydroxide and aluminum hydroxide in the treatment of gastroesophageal reflux. Minerva Pediatr 1991; 43(12):797-800 [in Italian].

111. Behar J, Sheahan DG, Biancani P, et al. Medical and surgical management of reflux esophagitis. A 38-month report of a prospective clinical trial. N Engl J Med 1975;293(6):263-8.

112. Hauer JM. Does Nissen fundoplication decrease reflux-related problems including respiratory illness in children with neurological impairment? JAMA Pediatr 2014;168(2):188.

113. Kubiak R, Spitz L, Kiely EM, et al. Effectiveness of fundoplication in early infancy. J Pediatr Surg 1999;34(2):295-9.

114. Rosen R, Hart K, Warlaumont M. Incidence of gastroesophageal reflux during transpyloric feeds. J Pediatr Gastroenterol Nutr 2011;52(5):532-5.

115. Livingston MH, Shawyer AC, Rosenbaum PL, et al. Fundoplication and gastrostomy versus percutaneous gastrojejunostomy for gastroesophageal reflux in children with neurologic impairment: a systematic review and meta-analysis. J Pediatr Surg 2015;50(5):707-14.

116. Srivastava R, Downey EC, O'Gorman M, et al. Impact of fundoplication versus gastrojejunal feeding tubes on mortality and in preventing aspiration pneumonia in young children with neurologic impairment who have gastroesophageal reflux disease. Pediatrics 2009;123(1):338-45.

Caustic Ingestions and Foreign Bodies Ingestions in Pediatric Patients

Jacob A. Kurowski, MD*, Marsha Kay, MD

KEYWORDS

- Caustic ingestion • Foreign body • Coins • Button batteries • Magnets • Endoscopy
- Pediatric

KEY POINTS

- Caustic ingestions continue to cause significant morbidity in children, and review of proper household storage should be considered at well child visits.
- Major or fatal complications from button battery ingestions has significantly increased in the past 3 decades as they became increasingly commonplace in household devices, especially the 20-mm lithium button battery.
- Rare-earth metal magnets in toys were recalled, and production was banned by the Consumer Product Safety Commission in 2014. However, they are already present in many households and multiple magnets swallowed together can cause necrosis of any bowel that comes between the magnets.
- The introduction of laundry and dishwasher packets or "pods" has presented a new harm if ingested, causing respiratory distress, hospitalization, and possible intubation. These packets cannot be removed with an endoscope.

INTRODUCTION

Inherently, children unintentionally ingest objects or substances within reach, most commonly in the household. Interestingly, the first pediatric foreign body ingestion of record was of a shoe buckle in 1692 by 4-year-old Friedrich Wilhelm I. It has been previously cited that "Friedrich the Great" swallowed the shoe buckle, but he was not born until 1712, and it was his father, born in 1688 and known as the "Soldier King," who reportedly achieved this unique honor. Both caustic and foreign body ingestions result in significant morbidity, mortality, and health care utilization. It is our job as health care providers to prevent and manage these ingestions. This article reviews the incidence, assessment, management, and complications of caustic and foreign body ingestions in children.

Department of Pediatric Gastroenterology, Hepatology and Nutrition, Cleveland Clinic Foundation, 9500 Euclid Avenue, Dept A111, Cleveland, OH 44195-0001, USA
* Corresponding author.
E-mail address: kurowsj@ccf.org

pediatric.theclinics.com

CAUSTIC INGESTIONS

The 2014 annual report of the American Association of Poison Control Centers (AAPCC) documented more than 1 million documented substance exposures in children ≤5 years, which represent 50% of all exposures. Roughly 25% of these exposures were to cosmetics/personal care products or household cleaning substances.[1] More than 95% of the time, the exposure was due to a single substance. There is a male-to-female predominance of 1.3:1 in children ≤5 years of age. Of the 25 fatalities in children ≤5 years of age, only one was due to a caustic agent, sodium hypochlorite. As the ingestion in young children is accidental, the volume of the offending agent is typically low, resulting in low mortality as opposed to intentional ingestions in adolescents and adults, which are higher in volume. The AAPCC report does not have details of morbidity with respect to each ingested agent.

Caustic ingestions in young children more commonly occur once they are ambulating and have access to cabinets and shelves with common household products. Household laundry bleach is the most common caustic ingestion and traditionally contains sodium hypochlorite, an alkalotic chlorine solution. Household bleach typically contains sodium hypochlorite with a pH ≥11 and a low concentration of 5% to 12%, with the lower concentration making it less harmful. Sodium hypochlorite is also present in toilet bowl cleaner, drain cleaner, pool cleaner, and household sprays/wipes but at a much higher concentration than that found in household bleach, significantly increasing the risk of injury. Other sodium-based salts are often added to bleach at a low concentration to minimize splashing. Bleach alternatives or "stain removers" may contain hydrogen peroxide or boric acid. Lye is classically made of potassium or sodium hydroxide, which is also found in drain cleaner, homemade detergents/soaps, hair relaxers, and paint strippers. The original Liquid-Plumr on the market in 1967 contained 30% sodium hydroxide and resulted in numerous severe ingestions with subsequent esophageal necrosis requiring esophagectomy from exposure to even a few cubic centimeters. Within a few years, the concentration was reduced to 5%, where most of these products remain. Another problematic and often overlooked risk is the storage of harmful agents in improper containers, such as a reused food container that results in accidental ingestion by the unsuspecting child or adolescent. Detergent packets have also become a significant danger and are discussed later in the article.

In 26% of teenagers and 69% of adults, caustic ingestions are intentional, classified as suspected suicide, misuse, or abuse. Of the 1173 fatalities in the 2014 AAPCC report, 75% were intentional ingestions. Intentional ingestions are often characterized by ingestion of high-volume household agents with higher toxicity (higher concentration) due to the nature of the ingestion. Household bleach still accounts for 35% of the household cleaning substances ingested in teenagers and adults and 14% of ingestions in children ≤12 years of age.

There are caustic ingestion guidelines from both the pediatric and the adult literature, which are imperfect, but which serve as an excellent guide to the clinician managing the patient following ingestion.

Pathophysiology of Caustic Injury

The extent of mucosal injury from caustic ingestion depends on the concentration and pH of the substance in addition to the viscosity, location of contact, and contact time. Alkalis are typically colorless, odorless liquids posing an increased risk of a high-volume accidental ingestion.

Alkalis constitute most caustic ingestions, inducing liquefaction necrosis. Saponification of lipids allows deep penetration to submucosa and muscularis, resulting in thrombosis of vessels and fibrosis of tissue, even perforation. Alkalis often injure the proximal intestinal tract, including the mouth, pharynx, esophagus, and stomach, along with the trachea if aspirated. Alkali agents with pH ≤12 seldom cause significant injury unless they are of a high concentration. An agent with pH >12 will cause considerable injury regardless of the concentration. Although hair relaxer (without lye) is one of the most common causes of pediatric oropharyngeal injury with a pH of 11 to 12, it rarely causes esophageal injury and endoscopy is not always indicated.[2,3] **Table 1** contains a list of common household caustic agents.

Acids constituted less than 5% of all toxic ingestions in the 2014 AAPCC annual report. Strong acids with pH <2 result in coagulation necrosis as the result of ischemia and are less likely to penetrate or perforate.[4] Acidic liquids tend to have a bitter taste, decreasing their volume of ingestion with either accidental or intentional ingestions. Acids also have a lower viscosity with rapid esophageal clearance and increased gastric injury, often seen as hemorrhage in the antrum. Common household acids include hydrochloric acid (toilet bowl cleaner), sulfuric acid (stain removers, car battery), and phosphoric acid (hair dye).

Presentation

One of the earliest pediatric case series of caustic ingestions in 1983 by Gaudreault and colleagues[5] reviewed symptoms and associated esophageal lesions in 378 patients. They found that 82% of patients with symptoms had grade 0 or 1 esophageal injury on esophagoscopy versus 12% of asymptomatic patients who had a grade 2 lesion, providing the foundation of current management, which is that the clinical manifestations of caustic ingestion do not predict presence or severity of esophageal lesions in children (**Table 2**). In children with symptoms, the most common presenting symptoms are vomiting, dysphagia, excessive salivation, abdominal pain, refusal to drink, or an oropharyngeal burn. Oral burns include lip or tongue erythema and edema, leukoplakia, or ulceration. Rarely do patients present with airway symptoms, such as shortness of breath or hypoxia, and if present, these are associated with more significant injury. Symptoms of sepsis are indicative of esophageal perforation, which may require emergent surgical debridement and/or esophagectomy. A 2006 review of 473 pediatric patients admitted to the hospital with suspected significant caustic ingestion reported 80% had esophageal lesions, although only 40% of those with esophageal findings and 33% of the total group had significant lesions. In the same series, 17% of patients had gastric lesions at the time of first endoscopy. Oropharyngeal burns were not seen in 61% of patients with esophageal lesions.[6] The authors speculate that the high

---

Table 1
Common household caustic agents

Household Product	Type	Chemical
Bleach, drain cleaners, pool cleaners	Alkali	Sodium hypochlorite Sodium hydroxide
Dishwasher detergent	Alkali	Sodium hydroxide
Floor stripper, degreaser	Alkali	Potassium hydroxide
Toilet bowl cleaner	Acid	Hydrochloric acid
Car batteries, stain removers	Acid	Sulfuric acid
Hair dye	Acid	Phosphoric acid

From Contini S, Scarpignato C. Caustic injury of the upper gastrointestinal tract: a comprehensive review. World J Gastroenterol 2013;19(25):3919.

Table 2
Endoscopic grade of esophageal caustic injury

Grade 0	No identifiable injury
Grade 1	Erythema and edema of mucosa
Grade 2a	Noncircumferential and superficial ulceration with white plaques or hemorrhage
Grade 2b	Circumferential injury or deep ulcerations with features of 2a
Grade 3a	Small or patchy necrosis
Grade 3b	Extensive or circumferential necrosis
Grade 4	Perforation before or during endoscopy

Data from Kay M, Wyllie R. Caustic ingestions in children. Curr Opin Pediatr 2009;21(5):651–4.

frequency of lesions in this series may potentially relate to the availability of more caustic agents, that is, agents with a higher concentration and a higher or lower pH in Turkey compared with the United States, and as a result of different regulatory requirement and practices relating to nonoriginal container use.

Assessment and Management

Patients with a potential ingestion should be directed to the closest Emergency Department (ED) for evaluation if not already done. The parents should be instructed to bring the original bottle of the suspected caustic agent to the ED to facilitate evaluation. Household bleach being the most common caustic agent rarely causes significant injury from accidental ingestion, and patients can be safely observed if asymptomatic. If a patient has a questionable history of ingestion without oral lesions, is asymptomatic, and ingested a "low-risk" agent, a per os challenge of liquids can be considered with physician observation. Oral liquids are often tolerated even with minor burns and do not require treatment. For any patient whom is symptomatic, has oropharyngeal burns, or has significant history of ingestion, an upper endoscopy is recommended. Timing of endoscopy is important, ideally between 12 and 24 hours following the ingestion. An endoscopy done too early may not show the extent of the burns and an endoscopy done after 48 hours increases the risk of perforation if necrosis has occurred. Acid suppression is also given to prevent any further injury. Dysphagia can develop starting at 2 weeks and up to 6 weeks after the ingestion, at which point a radiographic esophagram followed by upper endoscopy can be performed to evaluate for esophageal stricture.[7] Intentional ingestions raise concern for a significant ingestion and injury and should be evaluated with endoscopy due to the risk of a high volume of intake and increased rate of gastric injury with brisk swallows that may spare the oropharynx from injury, or in the case of acid ingestions.[8]

Induction of emesis with syrup of ipecac after a caustic ingestion is strongly contraindicated because this may further expose the esophagus to the offending agent. The same goes for any liquids to dilute or neutralize the caustic agent, which may also lead to vomiting. Nasogastric tubes may be placed at time of endoscopy if circumferential burns are present to serve as a stent when there may be increased risk of stricture. Nasogastric tubes, however, should not be placed blindly because manipulation of a necrotic esophagus may lead to perforation.

Endoscopy

Endoscopy for caustic ingestion should ideally be performed in the operating room with anesthesia, a protected airway, and not as an elective procedure in an outpatient facility. The degree of esophageal injury is graded at time of the initial endoscopy and is the main reason endoscopy is performed. The grading system has been adapted and modified based on thermal burns of the skin with the addition of subclassification based on extent and depth of injury (see **Table 2**).[9] Between 50% and 90% of pediatric patients will have either grade 0 or 1 esophageal injury at endoscopy and can be fed and discharged safely.[5,6,10] For patients with grade 2 to 4 injury, there is limited published literature on the outcome in pediatrics; however, the risk of stricture formation requiring dilation at follow-up is higher with circumferential grade 2b or 3 lesions (**Fig. 1**).[10,11]

Most strictures will occur in the 1 to 2 months following a caustic ingestion at the site of injury. Thus, alkali agents result in esophageal strictures causing dysphagia, and acidic agents result in pyloric strictures causing gastric outlet obstruction. Up to 90% of ingestion patients will have noncircumferential esophageal injury (grade 0-2a) and are at low risk for stricture formation with further imaging or endoscopy done on an as-needed basis. For those with circumferential esophageal injury, 50% of patients with grade 2b injury and 75% with grade 3 injury develop strictures requiring endoscopic dilation.[6,10,11] Data on gastric injuries are limited, and although the number of pyloric strictures is low, they can occur after any degree of injury. Patients with grade 4 injury (perforation before or during endoscopy) have a high rate of sepsis and mortality, and endoscopy should not be performed if perforation is suspected.

Corticosteroids have been used to prevent stricture formation via reduction of fibroblast proliferation after caustic ingestion in patients with grade 2 or 3 injury in children or adults. However, corticosteroid administration has not shown any benefit in meta-analysis and has remained a controversial practice.[12,13] A recent prospective study in children with a mean age of 4.1 ± 2.63 years demonstrated a benefit to steroid administration as the group given intravenous methylprednisolone 1 g/1.73 m^2/d for 3 days required an endoscopic dilation of esophageal stricture in 9.5% (4/42) of cases versus 29.3% (12/41) in the control group with mean time to stricture of 4 to 5 weeks ($P = .038$).[14] All of the prospective studies assessing corticosteroids have a limited number of patients, variable treatment courses, and different criteria of esophageal injury for enrollment, thus limiting any recommendation for corticosteroid use in this setting. In addition, there are no prospective studies on the use of antibiotics after

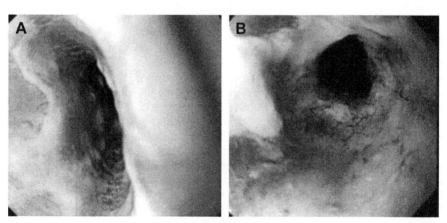

Fig. 1. A 3-year-old girl after ingestion of cuticle softener with sodium hydroxide. (*A*) Grade 2a injury with white plaques in mid-esophagus. (*B*) Grade 2B circumferential injury in distal esophagus. (*Courtesy of* Lee M. Bass, MD, Ann & Robert H. Lurie Children's Hospital of Chicago, Chicago, IL.)

caustic ingestion, although this has been used if a patient has evidence of deep ulcerations, necrosis, signs/symptoms of infection, or if steroids are administered.[15]

The incidence of either squamous cell carcinoma or adenocarcinoma of the esophagus is reported to be as high as 8% of all caustic ingestions, representing a 1000-fold increased risk in esophageal cancer compared with the general population.[16–18] The time to diagnosis of esophageal cancer after caustic ingestion has a wide spectrum from 1 to 71 years with most cases occurring 3 to 4 decades later. Many of the published series on esophageal cancer after caustic ingestion are more than 20 year old and do not account for other risk factors, including smoking or Barrett esophagus. Most of the cancers are diagnosed at the bifurcation of the trachea, an area where injury and stasis are more common, or site of stricture and are amenable to resection. Survival rates are reportedly 40% at 1 year and 13% at 5 years, although these data were published in 1989.[19] There are no formal recommendations for endoscopic dysplasia screening, including timing and interval, but is recommended by these investigators, especially for patients who had ingestion during childhood and now are adult aged.

Prevention

Prevention of caustic ingestion is 2-fold, identifying at-risk patients (young children and suicidal patients) and identifying chemicals to ensure proper storage. There has been significant government intervention starting with the Federal Caustic Poison Act in the United States enacted in 1927 to label substances identified as "poison," which included many of the chemicals in **Table 1**. Prevention has evolved under the US Occupational Safety and Health Administration with the creation of Safety Data Sheets for all hazardous chemicals to include identification, ingredients, first-aid measures, handling and storage, and so forth. It is also important for health care providers to inform patients and parents about proper storage of household agents, including keeping substances in their original container. Riffat and Cheng[10] reported 6 of 50 cases of caustic ingestion at a pediatric hospital in Australia were due to accidental ingestion of a caustic solution stored in containers normally used for drinking. Cakmak and colleagues[20] reported that children with a history of caustic ingestion had an increase in impulsive behavior as rated by their parents when compared with healthy controls. There are many opportunities to prevent caustic ingestions, and review of this topic should be considered at younger well-child visits.

FOREIGN BODIES

In the 1970s, the US Consumer Product Safety Commission (CPSC) developed a small parts cylinder that approximates the size of a child's trachea, banning the sale of any small objects less than 57.1 mm long by 31.7 mm wide for use by children less than 3 years of age in an attempt to decrease the incidence of foreign body ingestions. There were almost 128,000 foreign body ingestions in the 2014 annual report of the AAPCC, of which 69% were in children ≤5 years and 83% were ≤19 years of age. Foreign bodies included in this report are in the category of Foreign Bodies/Toys/Miscellaneous that includes coins and desiccants (78%), writing utensils (15%), and batteries (7%).[1] Sharp (needles, pins) and blunt objects along with food impaction are not delineated. At least 98% of the ingestions in children are accidental, far different than the rate in adults.[21] Intentional ingestions in older children and adults may be the result of psychiatric impairment (self-harm or suicidal ideation), intellectual disability, intoxication, or secondary gain seen in prisoners. Accidental ingestion of dental objects such as dental retainers or dentures in teenagers and older adults, respectively, are more common with increased exposure time to the oropharynx.[22]

Symptoms of foreign body ingestion depend on the type and size of foreign object, size of the patient, location of the object, and duration of the ingestion. Presentation may include dysphagia, drooling, choking, emesis, refusal to eat, odynophagia, chest pain, or respiratory distress. Foreign bodies may also be found incidentally in young children after obtaining radiographs to evaluate respiratory symptoms. Respiratory symptoms may be related to aspiration or external compression of the trachea. As a general rule, any child with a symptomatic foreign body should undergo urgent endoscopy for removal. Perforation of the esophagus into the mediastinum or erosion into the aorta, a rare occurrence, may result in sepsis and severe hemorrhage, which may be fatal. Luckily, more than 80% of foreign bodies will pass asymptomatically, even seen in the diaper as an unexpected finding on occasion.[23]

Coins and Blunt Objects

Coins are the most common evaluated foreign body ingested by children. In the United States from 1994 to 2003, Chen and colleagues[24] reported 252,000 coin ingestions treated in EDs in children ≤14 years of age with 20 fatalities, all in patients ≤4 years of age. The likelihood of esophageal impaction is inversely related to the size of the child and correlates with the size of the object. The smaller the child, the smaller the object that may become impacted.[25] A coin in the esophagus of an asymptomatic child can be monitored for passage a maximum of 24 hours before removal if the time of ingestion is known, but in the majority of cases, earlier endoscopic removal is ideal. Pennies make up 45% of ingested coins in the United States; however, larger coins such as nickels and quarters are more likely to become lodged in the esophagus or even obstruct the pylorus.[24] Objects can become lodged at 3 different points in the esophagus, with approximately 70% at the upper esophageal sphincter/thoracic inlet, 20% at aortic notch (mid-esophagus), and 10% at lower esophageal sphincter. On radiograph in most cases, the face of a coin projects anteriorly and the rim on lateral view projects parallel to the esophageal lumen (**Fig. 2**). Coins in the trachea will appear in the opposite configuration.

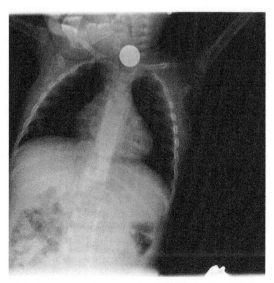

Fig. 2. A 12-month-old with a penny in the esophagus at the thoracic inlet demonstrated on AP chest radiograph. Coin was successfully removed with rat-toothed forceps.

Health care personnel should obtain both an anteroposterior (AP) and a lateral radiograph to identify the "step-off" or double halo seen with disc batteries, which require emergent removal. Objects lodged at the upper esophageal sphincter can often be removed with Magill forceps, whereas anything distal should be removed with an endoscope. Patients with a history of esophageal inflammation or stricture (ie, eosinophilic esophagitis, EoE), previous surgery (tracheoesophageal fistula, esophageal atresia, or fundoplication), or those who swallow multiple coins are at higher risk of retaining the coin in the esophagus. The assistance of a pediatric otolaryngologist may be needed for esophageal foreign bodies above the upper esophageal sphincter, those with history esophageal surgery, or foreign bodies lodged for more than 24 hours with possible erosion into the esophageal wall.

Coins or small blunt objects in the stomach can be monitored for much longer than the esophagus because most will pass through the pylorus and remaining intestinal tract uneventfully. Objects longer than 5 cm and 2 cm in width are less likely to pass through the pylorus of an adolescent, and size criteria need to be adjusted accordingly for smaller pediatric patients. An asymptomatic patient can have a follow-up radiograph 2 to 3 weeks after ingestion followed by another at 4 to 6 weeks. Elective endoscopic removal should be scheduled if the object remains at 4 to 6 weeks. A symptomatic patient with vomiting, abdominal pain, or hematemesis should have urgent endoscopic removal. Symptoms may occur if the object is obstructing the pylorus or is adhering to the mucosa, causing local erosion.

Batteries

The 2014 AAPCC annual report documented more than 9000 battery ingestions of which more than 50% were in patients ≤5 years of age. Just less than 50% of the battery ingestions were "disc" or "button" batteries, commonly composed of lithium or zinc as their negative electrode. Batteries are in countless household products, and button batteries are increasingly common in watches, keyless entry remotes, hearing aids, small flashlights, and many electronic toys. Both cylindrical and button batteries are commonly ingested; however, button batteries have significantly higher morbidity because of their shape and size and primarily are related to the mechanism by which they discharge electrical current. The button battery in the esophagus quickly allows discharge of electrical current when both faces are touched by opposing walls of the esophagus, generating hydroxide, followed by leakage of alkaline (nonlithium) or organic (lithium) electrolytes, and pressure necrosis. The lithium button batteries are typically 3 V, double what most zinc or nickel batteries are capable of. Damage to the esophagus occurs quickly with burns and stenosis resulting after just 2 hours. More severe complications reported include but are not limited to tracheoesophageal fistula, perforation, aortoesophageal fistula, vocal cord paralysis, mediastinitis, cardiac or respiratory arrest, pneumothorax, and pneumoperitoneum.[26]

If battery ingestion is suspected, a radiograph should be obtained immediately to evaluate the location. A battery in the esophagus prompts emergent endoscopic removal even if the patient is asymptomatic and is not nil per os and is ideally performed within 2 hours of ingestion (**Fig. 3**). A button battery in the esophagus on AP and lateral radiographs is similar appearing to a coin with the addition of a double halo or rims signifying the cathode (larger rim) and anode (smaller rim). The negative pole of the battery induces the most injury, and location of this pole relative to aorta or trachea is very helpful in identifying potential complications. The most common button batteries on the market are CR 2016, CR 2025, and CR 2032, all 20 mm in diameter, as the first 2 digits indicate with the difference in their depth or height (millimeters) indicated by the second 2 digits (**Fig. 4**). The largest analysis of battery ingestions

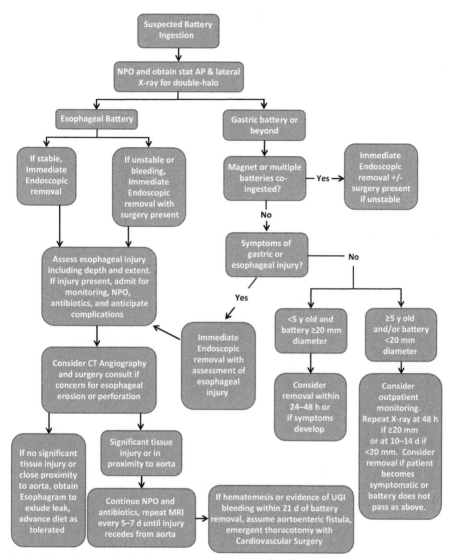

Fig. 3. Button battery ingestion management algorithm. CT, computed tomography; NPO, nil per os; UGI, upper gastrointestinal series. (*Adapted from* Kramer RE, Lerner DG, Lin T, et al. Management of ingested foreign bodies in children: a clinical report of the NASPGHAN endoscopy committee. J Pediatr Gastroenterol Nutr 2015;60(4):562–74.)

published by Litovitz and colleagues[26] reviewed 25 years of reports from the National Poison Data System receiving input from the AAPCCs and the National Battery Ingestion Hotline and found that since 2000 greater than 90% of major or fatal ingestions were due to ingestion of 20-mm lithium button batteries, which have increased in prevalence and utilization in the home over the same time period. There has also been an almost 7-fold increase in the proportion of major or fatal complications since 1985 due to the same factors. The National Capital Poison Center (NCPC) has published tips and guidelines online at www.poison/org/battery along with a 24-hour National Battery Ingestion Hotline 202-625-3333.

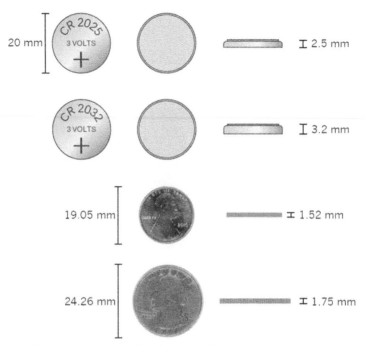

Fig. 4. Lithium button batteries used in digital watches, automotive remotes, digital clocks, and computers. "CR" represents a lithium battery. The 4-digit number signifies the diameter and width in millimeters. The front and larger rim is the positive pole and the back and smaller rim is the negative pole. For comparison, a US Lincoln penny and Washington quarter each with a rim equal in size.

There are limited data on removal of gastric batteries, and the guidelines differ between the NCPC and North American Society for Pediatric Gastroenterology, Hepatology, and Nutrition (NASPGHAN), depending on the size of the battery. The NCPC guidelines are derived from the Litovitz and colleagues[26] report in 2010, whereas the NASPGHAN guideline was updated in 2015. The NCPC guidelines recommend a radiograph and endoscopic removal if the battery is ≥15 mm in an asymptomatic child less than 6 years of age, whereas NASPGHAN recommends endoscopic removal within 24 to 48 hours if the battery is ≥20 mm and the child is less than 5 years of age.[27] A recent report from Lee and colleagues[28] describes moderate or major complications (erosions, ulcers) to gastric tissue in 4 children who ingested lithium button batteries, 3 of which were removed within 4 to 8 hours after ingestion. Given the increasing complication rate with lithium button batteries, earlier endoscopic removal from the stomach may be warranted, especially in at-risk situations, a smaller child, larger battery, prior surgery, or other factors that may delay gastric emptying.

Magnets

Magnets are more recently described ingested foreign bodies that possess significant injury risk when more than one is swallowed. The rare-earth metal magnets composed of neodymium, iron, and boron are 5 to 10 times stronger than the typical refrigerator magnets made of ferrite and have been increasingly used in toys. A single magnet is typically passed unnoticed; however, if rare-earth metal magnets are swallowed together or with another metallic object, sequelae are significant and can be life-threatening.

Magnets that are separated when passing through the intestinal tract have caused bowel perforation, intestinal fistula, obstruction and volvulus, sepsis, and death because of attraction across loops of bowel.[29–31]

As a result of the multiple injuries and emergency room visits, the CPSC settled in 2014 with the manufacturers of Buckyballs and Buckycubes that included a recall with a refund and officially banning production, sale, or distribution in the United States following a voluntary earlier action by the other manufacturers of these rare-earth magnets.[32] The CPSC has also released a performance standard that any new magnet from a set must not fit into a CPSC small parts cylinder or have a lower specified force, effective April 1, 2015.[33] For now, this has limited the sale of several rare-earth metal magnet products, but numerous sets of magnets are already in households in the United States and ingestions continue to occur regularly.

If magnet or magnets ingestion is suspected, a frontal supine radiograph should be first obtained to quantify the number and location of the magnets (**Fig. 5**). A lateral radiograph can assist in this evaluation. If more than 1 magnet was ingested and within endoscopic reach, urgent endoscopic removal is indicated to prevent sequelae as previously described. If beyond endoscopic reach, patients should be monitored in the hospital for progression with surgical consultation for removal if needed (**Fig. 6**). A single magnet in an asymptomatic patient can be monitored with serial radiographs and education to keep all nearby magnetic objects, including clothing, away from the patient. Consider administration of polyethylene glycol 3350 if beyond the stomach and progression is halted for either single or multiple magnets; in addition, surgical input is warranted if multiple magnets are present and are nonprogressive and/or if there are any symptoms or radiographic evidence of intestinal obstruction, perforation, or other potential complication.

Sharp Objects

Sharp objects comprise a smaller number of foreign body ingestions in children, and incident data are not readily available. Sharp objects include nails, screws, toothpicks, broken glass, and pins. These types of objects are also the frequent source of intentional ingestions by psychiatric or incarcerated patients. Increase in the use of disposable diapers that no longer use safety pins have also contributed to a decrease in sharp object ingestion in children; however, safety pin ingestion still occurs in young children in cultures where disposable diapers are not used as well as in groups that use safety pins to fasten jewelry or other objects to infants' and toddlers' clothing. Incidental sharp object ingestions in adults are frequently caused by animal bones, notably fish and chicken.

Ingestion of a single straight pin generally follows Jackson's axiom: "advancing points perforate and trailing points do not," moving through the intestinal tract uneventfully blunt end first.[34] However, ingestion of multiple pins and other sharp objects have a more than 30% incidence of complication, including gastric and intestinal perforation. Sharp objects in the esophagus often present with dysphagia, but objects more distal can be asymptomatic even for weeks. Sung and colleagues[35] reviewed the complications (ulcers, lacerations, erosions, and perforation) of 316 cases of esophageal foreign bodies and found an increased risk of complication if impaction was greater than 24 hours, was of fish or animal bones, or the object was ≥3 cm in size. The sharp object can penetrate a variety of points in the tract with the most common being in the region of the ileocecal valve, even piercing extraluminal structures.[36–39]

Any sharp object located in the esophagus should be emergently removed. Sharp objects in the oropharynx may be removed with Magill forceps.

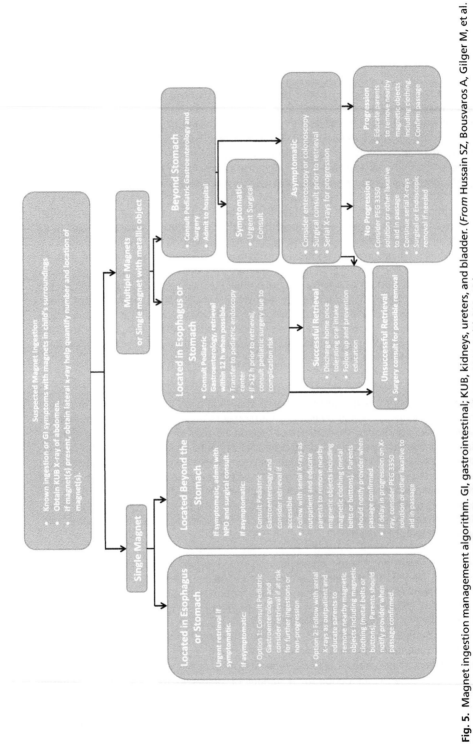

Fig. 5. Magnet ingestion management algorithm. GI, gastrointestinal; KUB, kidneys, ureters, and bladder. (*From* Hussain SZ, Bousvaros A, Gilger M, et al. Management of ingested magnets in children. J Pediatr Gastroenterol Nutr 2012;55(3):239–42.)

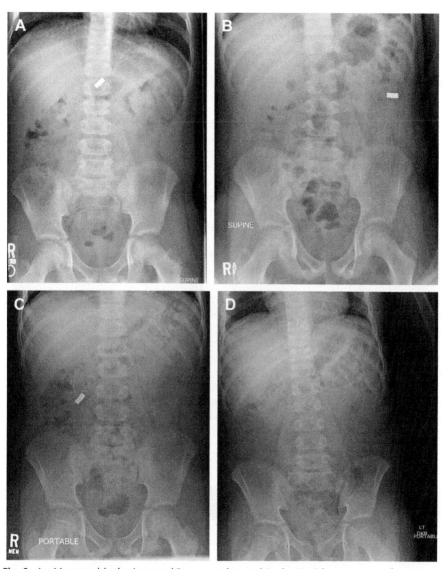

Fig. 6. An 11-year-old who ingested 3 rare-earth metal "cubes" with progression from stomach: (*A*) 1 hour after ingestion while at outside hospital to left upper quadrant presumed small bowel, (*B*) 4 hours later (after transfer to endoscopy center), to distal small bowel in right upper quadrant, (*C*) 10 hours later, and finally passed (*D*) at 22 hours. Patient remained asymptomatic for duration of monitoring.

Symptomatic patients with sharp objects in the esophagus or beyond should have urgent attempted endoscopic removal. Overtubes and endoscopic hoods can help reduce the incidence of mucosal damage during removal but are not often sized for pediatric patients. Asymptomatic patients with single straight pin ingestion in the stomach may be followed with serial radiographs. All others should be followed by Gastroenterology and Surgery in the event of a suspected perforation.

Food Impaction

Food impaction is the most common foreign body encountered in adolescents and adults.[40] Up to 90% patients will have underlying esophageal pathology predisposing to impaction, including EoE, proton-pump inhibitor therapy-responsive esophageal eosinophilia (PPI-REE), postesophageal atresia repair, postfundoplication, and erosive esophagitis ± peptic stricture (**Fig. 7**).[41,42] Less common causes in the pediatric population are esophageal motility disorders, including achalasia. EoE is the result of eosinophil-predominant chronic inflammation in the esophagus mediated by antigen exposure with subsequent esophageal dysfunction. It often has a macroscopic mucosal appearance of edema with loss of vascularity, linear furrows, white plaques or specks, and characteristic rings with an appearance similar to the trachea. It can be delineated from PPI-REE only after a patient has been on an adequate dose of PPI for 6 to 8 weeks before endoscopy, making it difficult to diagnose in patients with initial presentation of food impaction–required endoscopic removal. Up to 50% of patients will have resolution of esophageal eosinophilia on PPI therapy.[43–45]

As with any foreign body, a radiograph can be obtained to evaluate the location of impaction, although difficult with radiolucent objects. Contrast administration should be avoided in patients with suspected food impaction due to increased risk of aspiration if contrast pools above the impaction. A patient who is unable to handle secretions or has neck pain requires urgent endoscopic decompression. Otherwise, endoscopy can be performed ideally within 12 to 24 hours of presentation. The procedure should be done with endotracheal intubation to protect the airway. Multiple passes are often required to remove the food in piecemeal fashion. This method is usually preferred over advancing the bolus into the stomach to avoid esophageal perforation when trying to push the food bolus distally to the already present esophageal abnormality. Food that passes into the stomach does not require removal. Biopsies can then be taken once the obstructing food is removed to evaluate for inflammation.

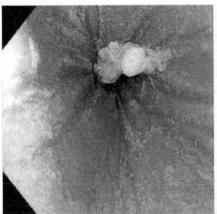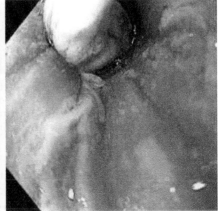

Fig. 7. Food bolus (meat) impaction at the lower esophageal sphincter in a teenage patient. The entire esophagus had findings concerning for EoE with edema, linear furrows, and white plaques at time of initial presentation. (*Courtesy of* Christine Pasquarella, MD, Cleveland Clinic Foundation, Cleveland, OH.)

Encapsulated Objects

Newer advances in packaging have led to new risks for foreign body ingestion in children. Although desiccant packets (silica) are one of the most commonly ingested objects in children, they do not pose any harm outside of a choking hazard.[1]

Several superabsorbent polymer-based children's toys, notably by Dunecraft Inc (Water Balz, Growing Skulls, and others), have been recalled by the CPSC. These toys quickly expand when exposed to water and have resulted in numerous bowel obstructions and deaths.[46,47] There have not been any reported cases of endoscopic removal of such objects.

Pediatric body packing of narcotics has been reported in children as young as 6 years of age.[48,49] Narcotics wrapped in waterproof material such as latex balloons, condoms, or gloves are swallowed or inserted into the rectum for smuggling. Complications arise when the packets rupture causing drug toxicity, or with intestinal obstruction, often pyloric, and may require surgical intervention. Endoscopic removal is contraindicated due to the high risk of rupturing the packages, which can cause an immediate fatal overdose. Patients should be monitored until passage. Consulting with local toxicology experts is recommended.

Detergent packets or "pods" for both laundry and dishwasher use have become a significant cause of toxic ingestion since their introduction and continues to increase. Exposure to the pods most commonly leads to vomiting, choking, ocular pain or conjunctivitis, and drowsiness or lethargy. In 2 separate evaluations of the National Poison Data System from 2012 to 2014, there were 3 deaths attributed to laundry detergent packet ingestion. Thus far, worse outcomes including hospitalization and intubation have resulted from laundry versus dishwasher detergent exposures.[50,51] These eye-catching packets with a water-soluble membrane pose significant health risk if ingested, and patient education is imperative. Endoscopic removal has not been recommended as the packets quickly dissolve and attempted removal may lead to further aspiration of aerosolized detergent.

SUMMARY

Children and adolescents inevitably swallow foreign material both accidentally and intentionally. Each type of ingestion carries its own set of risks and complications both short and long term, some requiring immediate attention while others close monitoring. In addition, new foreign body ingestion risks continue to arise with the advent of new technology. It is important to inform patients and families of these new risks, such as button batteries, rare-earth metal magnets, and detergent packets, that have all increased in prevalence in the home and may cause significant morbidity as well as anxiety if ingested. Consultation with a pediatric gastroenterologist and possibly the AAPCC at 1-800-222-1222 can help guide and evaluate when necessary.

REFERENCES

1. Mowry JB, Spyker DA, Brooks DE, et al. 2014 annual report of the American Association of Poison Control Centers' National Poison Data System (NPDS): 32nd annual report. Clin Toxicol (Phila) 2015;53(10):962–1147.

2. Aronow SP, Aronow HD, Blanchard T, et al. Hair relaxers: a benign caustic ingestion? J Pediatr Gastroenterol Nutr 2003;36(1):120–5.

3. Cowan D, Ho B, Sykes KJ, et al. Pediatric oral burns: a ten-year review of patient characteristics, etiologies and treatment outcomes. Int J Pediatr Otorhinolaryngol 2013;77(8):1325–8.

4. Haller JA Jr, Andrews HG, White JJ, et al. Pathophysiology and management of acute corrosive burns of the esophagus: results of treatment in 285 children. J Pediatr Surg 1971;6(5):578–84.
5. Gaudreault P, Parent M, McGuigan MA, et al. Predictability of esophageal injury from signs and symptoms: a study of caustic ingestion in 378 children. Pediatrics 1983;71(5):767–70.
6. Dogan Y, Erkan T, Cokugras FC, et al. Caustic gastroesophageal lesions in childhood: an analysis of 473 cases. Clin Pediatr (Phila) 2006;45(5):435–8.
7. Kay M, Wyllie R. Caustic ingestions in children. Curr Opin Pediatr 2009;21(5):651–4.
8. Ertekin C, Alimoglu O, Akyildiz H, et al. The results of caustic ingestions. Hepatogastroenterology 2004;51(59):1397–400.
9. Estrera A, Taylor W, Mills LJ, et al. Corrosive burns of the esophagus and stomach: a recommendation for an aggressive surgical approach. Ann Thorac Surg 1986;41(3):276–83.
10. Riffat F, Cheng A. Pediatric caustic ingestion: 50 consecutive cases and a review of the literature. Dis Esophagus 2009;22(1):89–94.
11. Betalli P, Falchetti D, Giuliani S, et al. Caustic ingestion in children: is endoscopy always indicated? The results of an Italian multicenter observational study. Gastrointest Endosc 2008;68(3):434–9.
12. Pelclova D, Navratil T. Do corticosteroids prevent oesophageal stricture after corrosive ingestion? Toxicol Rev 2005;24(2):125–9.
13. Fulton JA, Hoffman RS. Steroids in second degree caustic burns of the esophagus: a systematic pooled analysis of fifty years of human data: 1956-2006. Clin Toxicol (Phila) 2007;45(4):402–8.
14. Usta M, Erkan T, Cokugras FC, et al. High doses of methylprednisolone in the management of caustic esophageal burns. Pediatrics 2014;133(6):E1518–24.
15. Millar AJ, Cox SG. Caustic injury of the oesophagus. Pediatr Surg Int 2015;31(2):111–21.
16. Kiviranta UK. Corrosion carcinoma of the esophagus; 381 cases of corrosion and nine cases of corrosion carcinoma. Acta Otolaryngol 1952;42(1–2):89–95.
17. Appelqvist P, Salmo M. Lye corrosion carcinoma of the esophagus: a review of 63 cases. Cancer 1980;45(10):2655–8.
18. Ti TK. Oesophageal carcinoma associated with corrosive injury–prevention and treatment by oesophageal resection. Br J Surg 1983;70(4):223–5.
19. Isolauri J, Markkula H. Lye ingestion and carcinoma of the esophagus. Acta Chir Scand 1989;155(4–5):269–71.
20. Cakmak M, Gollu G, Boybeyi O, et al. Cognitive and behavioral characteristics of children with caustic ingestion. J Pediatr Surg 2015;50(4):540–2.
21. Kramer RE, Lerner DG, Lin T, et al. Management of ingested foreign bodies in children: a clinical report of the NASPGHAN endoscopy committee. J Pediatr Gastroenterol Nutr 2015;60(4):562–74.
22. Tiwana KK, Morton T, Tiwana PS. Aspiration and ingestion in dental practice: a 10-year institutional review. J Am Dent Assoc 2004;135(9):1287–91.
23. Kay M, Wyllie R. Pediatric foreign bodies and their management. Curr Gastroenterol Rep 2005;7(3):212–8.
24. Chen X, Milkovich S, Stool D, et al. Pediatric coin ingestion and aspiration. Int J Pediatr Otorhinolaryngol 2006;70(2):325–9.
25. Tander B, Yazici M, Rizalar R, et al. Coin ingestion in children: which size is more risky? J Laparoendosc Adv Surg Tech A 2009;19(2):241–3.

26. Litovitz T, Whitaker N, Clark L, et al. Emerging battery-ingestion hazard: clinical implications. Pediatrics 2010;125(6):1168–77.
27. Hussain SZ, Bousvaros A, Gilger M, et al. Management of ingested magnets in children. J Pediatr Gastroenterol Nutr 2012;55(3):239–42.
28. Lee JH, Lee JH, Shim JO, et al. Foreign body ingestion in children: should button batteries in the stomach be urgently removed? Pediatr Gastroenterol Hepatol Nutr 2016;19(1):20–8.
29. Liu S, Li J, Lv Y. Gastrointestinal damage caused by swallowing multiple magnets. Front Med 2012;6(3):280–7.
30. Naji H, Isacson D, Svensson JF, et al. Bowel injuries caused by ingestion of multiple magnets in children: a growing hazard. Pediatr Surg Int 2012;28(4):367–74.
31. Tavarez MM, Saladino RA, Gaines BA, et al. Prevalence, clinical features and management of pediatric magnetic foreign body ingestions. J Emerg Med 2013;44(1):261–8.
32. Buckyballs and buckycubes refunds now available through BuckyballsRecall.com; recall to refund will last until jan. 2015. 2014. Available at: http://www.cpsc.gov/Newsroom/News-Releases/2014/Buckyballs-and-Buckycubes-Refunds-Now-Available/. Accessed September 26, 2016.
33. CPSC approves strong federal safety standard for high-powered magnet sets to protect children and teenagers. 2014. Available at: http://www.cpsc.gov/en/Newsroom/News-Releases/2014/CPSC-Approves-Strong-Federal-Safety-Standard-for-High-Powered-Magnet-Sets-to-Protect-Children-and-Teenagers/. Accessed September 26, 2016.
34. Jackson C, Jackson CL. Diseases of the air and food passages of foreign body origin. Philadelphia: W. B. Saunders Company; 1937.
35. Sung SH, Jeon SW, Son HS, et al. Factors predictive of risk for complications in patients with oesophageal foreign bodies. Dig Liver Dis 2011;43(8):632–5.
36. Aktay AN, Werlin SL. Penetration of the stomach by an accidentally ingested straight pin. J Pediatr Gastroenterol Nutr 2002;34(1):81–2.
37. Goh BK, Chow PK, Quah HM, et al. Perforation of the gastrointestinal tract secondary to ingestion of foreign bodies. World J Surg 2006;30(3):372–7.
38. Mehran A, Podkameni D, Rosenthal R, et al. Gastric perforation secondary to ingestion of a sharp foreign body. JSLS 2005;9(1):91–3.
39. Palta R, Sahota A, Bemarki A, et al. Foreign-body ingestion: characteristics and outcomes in a lower socioeconomic population with predominantly intentional ingestion. Gastrointest Endosc 2009;69(3 Pt 1):426–33.
40. Eisen GM, Baron TH, Dominitz JA, et al. Guideline for the management of ingested foreign bodies. Gastrointest Endosc 2002;55(7):802–6.
41. Diniz LO, Towbin AJ. Causes of esophageal food bolus impaction in the pediatric population. Dig Dis Sci 2012;57(3):690–3.
42. Hiremath GS, Hameed F, Pacheco A, et al. Esophageal food impaction and eosinophilic esophagitis: a retrospective study, systematic review, and meta-analysis. Dig Dis Sci 2015;60(11):3181–93.
43. Dellon ES, Gonsalves N, Hirano I, et al. ACG clinical guideline: evidenced based approach to the diagnosis and management of esophageal eosinophilia and eosinophilic esophagitis (EoE). Am J Gastroenterol 2013;108(5):679–92 [quiz: 693].
44. Papadopoulou A, Koletzko S, Heuschkel R, et al. Management guidelines of eosinophilic esophagitis in childhood. J Pediatr Gastroenterol Nutr 2014;58(1):107–18.
45. Liacouras CA, Furuta GT, Hirano I, et al. Eosinophilic esophagitis: updated consensus recommendations for children and adults. J Allergy Clin Immunol 2011;128(1):3–20.e6 [quiz: 21–2].

46. Zamora IJ, Vu LT, Larimer EL, et al. Water-absorbing balls: a "growing" problem. Pediatrics 2012;130(4):e1011–4.

47. Dunecraft recalls water balz, skulls, orbs and flower toys due to serious ingestion hazard. 2012. Available at: http://www.cpsc.gov/en/Recalls/2013/Dunecraft-Recalls-Water-Balz-Skulls-Orbs-and-Flower-Toys-Due-to-Serious-Ingestion-Hazard-/. Accessed September 26, 2016.

48. Beno S, Calello D, Baluffi A, et al. Pediatric body packing: drug smuggling reaches a new low. Pediatr Emerg Care 2005;21(11):744–6.

49. Traub SJ, Kohn GL, Hoffman RS, et al. Pediatric "body packing". Arch Pediatr Adolesc Med 2003;157(2):174–7.

50. Valdez AL, Casavant MJ, Spiller HA, et al. Pediatric exposure to laundry detergent pods. Pediatrics 2014;134(6):1127–35.

51. Davis MG, Casavant MJ, Spiller HA, et al. Pediatric exposures to laundry and dishwasher detergents in the United States: 2013-2014. Pediatrics 2016;137(5).

Abdominal Pain in Children

From the Eternal City to the Examination Room

Donna K. Zeiter, MD

KEYWORDS

- Abdominal pain • Functional gastrointestinal disorders • Rome IV
- Visceral hypersensitivity

KEY POINTS

- Abdominal pain in children is a common entity.
- A majority of abdominal pain in children is classified as functional.
- The Rome Foundation and the Rome IV play a critical role in setting diagnostic criteria for research and practice as well as in educating the public and practitioners about functional gastrointestinal disorders (FGIDs).
- FGIDs are best understood using the biopsychosocial model of disease. Pain is a result of early life events, psychosocial factors, and physiologic factors.
- Physiologic factors leading to FGIDs include motility disturbance, visceral hypersensitivity, altered central nervous system (CNS) processing, altered mucosal and immune function, and altered gut microbiome.

Chronic abdominal pain continues to be one of the most common problems seen by pediatricians and pediatric gastroenterologists. Globally, irritable bowel syndrome (IBS) seems to affect 11% of the population, with 30% of these individuals presenting for medical care.[1] In a community-based study from 1996, 13% of middle school students and 17% of high school students experienced pain on a weekly basis.[2] A more recent study used online questionnaires and the ROME III criteria. In this study, parents of children living in the United States between the ages of 4 years and 18 years were asked to report on gastrointestinal symptoms[3]; 23.1% of children qualified for at least 1 FGID.[3] FGIDs account for approximately 50% of pediatric gastroenterology consultations.[4]

Disclosure: The author has nothing to disclose.
Department of Pediatrics, Division of Pediatric Gastroenterology, Hepatology and Nutrition, University of Maryland School of Medicine, 22 S. Greene St, Suite N5W68, Baltimore, MD 21201, USA
E-mail address: dzeiter@peds.umaryland.edu

Pediatr Clin N Am 64 (2017) 525–541
http://dx.doi.org/10.1016/j.pcl.2017.01.012
0031-3955/17/© 2017 Elsevier Inc. All rights reserved.
pediatric.theclinics.com

Abdominal pain continues to be a frustrating presenting symptom, putting strain on the current fast-paced health care environment. Diagnosis and treatment of a child with abdominal pain take time—time for listening, counseling, and education; time that is difficult to find in current practice settings. A vast majority of patients who present for evaluation of abdominal pain do not have organic disease in the classic sense and fall into a functional category.

Many providers still believe that children with chronic abdominal pain are anxious or stressed. According a survey by the American Academy of Pediatrics and the North American Society for Pediatric Gastroenterology, Hepatology and Nutrition, 16% of the 300 pediatricians surveyed thought that functional abdominal pain was a wastebasket diagnosis. Only 11% of these pediatricians thought that functional abdominal pain was a specific diagnosis based on clear criteria.[5] Any of these preconceptions has an impact on the physician-patient relationship and potentially affects future therapeutic interaction.

FGIDs have a significant impact on those effected. FGIDs lead to significant difficulties with long-term comorbidities, including depression anxiety, lifetime psychiatric disorders, social phobia, and somatic complaints.[4] The distinction between *organic disease* and *nonorganic disease* (FGIDs) is a spurious one. Research continues to support the understanding that these disorders are related to alterations in the enteric nervous system (ENS) and in the modulation between the ENS and the CNS, alterations that have an organic etiology through the modulation of neurotransmitters, receptors, and cellular processing pathways involved in the nervous system.

Abdominal pain is best understood within the framework of the biopsychosocial model of disease. The biopsychosocial model emphasizes the multifactorial nature of abdominal pain, including genetic, environmental, social, and psychological components. Treatment plans need to develop and adapt over time and be extremely individualized. As understanding of the pathophysiology of FGIDs increases, there will be a larger repertoire of therapies from which to select. This article reviews current understanding of pain-related FGIDS and the etiology, pathophysiology, and treatment modalities available.

ETIOLOGY

The possible causes of abdominal pain in children are numerous, ranging from benign disorders to life-threatening surgical emergencies. Abdominal pain may arise from disorders in multiple organ systems, including the pulmonary, gastrointestinal, urologic, and gynecologic systems. Infectious, neoplastic, metabolic, and anatomic mechanisms may all lead to the presenting symptom of abdominal pain (**Table 1**) Patients and families are left anxious. Providers are concerned that they may be missing a diagnosis. These concerns often lead to numerous referrals and ongoing potentially invasive testing. Fortunately, there are a several alarm symptoms that help practitioners differentiate those children with organic disease, who requiring further investigation from those with FGIDs (**Box 1**).[5] Without these symptoms, extensive testing is unlikely to uncover other disorders.

EVALUATION

The evaluation of a patient with abdominal pain begins with a detailed history and physical examination. Patients often describe their symptoms using "diagnoses," such as "I have been having problems with reflux." Providers must focus specifically on each symptom. How long has the pain been occurring? Has the pain gotten better or worse or remained stable? What is the pain's location? Is the pain associated with meals or sleep? Are there any specific triggers that worsen or alleviate the pain?

Table 1
Potential causes of abdominal pain in the pediatric patient

Functional	IBS
	FD
	Functional abdominal pain
	Functional constipation
	Cyclic vomiting syndrome
	Abdominal migraine
Gynecologic	Ovarian cyst
	Ovarian torsion
	Testicular torsion
Pulmonology	Pneumonia
Infectious	Viral
	Enterovirus, adenovirus
	Bacterial
	Salmonella, Shigella, Campylobacter, Yersinia, E coli
	Parasites
	Giardia, Entamoeba histolytica
Intestinal	Gastroesophageal reflux (esophagitis)
	Gastritis
	Ulcer (duodenal/peptic)
	Cholelithiasis, cholecystitis, choledochal cyst
	Pancreatitis (acute, chronic), pancreatic pseudocyst
	Hepatitis
	Inflammatory bowel disease (Crohn/ulcerative colitis)
	Eosinophilic disease (esophagitis, gastroenteritis)
	Carbohydrate malabsorption (lactose intolerance)
Metabolic	Diabetes mellitis
Neoplastic	Porphyria tumors
Structural/surgical	Malrotation
	Intussusception
	Polyp
	Foreign body
	Meckel diverticulum
	Volvulus
	Trauma
Urologic	Urinary tract infection
	Nephrolithiasis
	Urinary pelvic junction obstruction

History and physical examination should always include review of alarm symptoms, which may guide a provider to more specific testing (see **Box 1**). Clinical judgment should be used, however, in this evaluation and these alarm symptoms should be seen in the context of the entire history.[6] Finally, evaluation of the patient's functioning, although it often does not indicate the ultimate diagnosis, provides clues as to child and parent coping strategies.

At minimum, basic laboratory studies should include a complete blood cell count and urinalysis. Depending on the history, a complete metabolic panel, amylase, lipase, erythrocyte sedimentation rate, C-reactive protein, or thyroid function testing may be indicated.

In the appropriate clinical setting, the practitioner needs to evaluate for Infectious causes, such as *Giardia* and other parasitic, bacterial, and viral diseases.

Many patients with IBS present with diarrhea. In children, this may raise concerns for inflammatory bowel disease. Fecal calprotectin has become a more common

Box 1
Warning signs that suggest a higher risk of organic disease in children with chronic abdominal pain

Involuntary weight loss

Deceleration of linear growth

Gastrointestinal blood loss

Significant vomiting (bilious emesis, protracted vomiting)

Dysphagia

Odynophagia

Chronic severe diarrhea

Nighttime stooling

Pain awakening the child at night

Persistent right upper or right lower quadrant pain

Unexplained fever

Abnormal physical findings (clubbing, localized tenderness, mass, hepatomegaly, splenomegaly, perianal abnormalities, erythema nodosum)

Abnormal laboratory testing (elevated C-reactive protein/erythrocyte sedimentation rate, occult blood in stool)

Family history of inflammatory bowel disease

screening test for mucosal inflammation with values of less than 50 mg/g stool, suggesting that inflammation is unlikely.[7]

Although controversial, screening for celiac disease is recommended in the current Rome IV. In a prospective cohort study, the prevalence of celiac disease was 4 times higher in patients with IBS compared with the general population.[8]

Carbohydrate malabsorption may lead to abdominal pain, bloating, and diarrhea, symptoms that mimic IBS. The most common disaccharidase deficiency is primary lactase deficiency. Before more formal testing, a brief period of a lactose elimination diet should be considered in patients with compatible symptoms. Endoscopic biopsies may be sent for measured disaccharidase activity. Breath testing is a more functional test and is helpful in determining malabsorption of the tested disaccharide. Patients may be enzyme deficient or malabsorb carbohydrate; however, these abnormalities do not necessarily correlate with intolerance and symptoms.

Routine radiographic studies have minimal yield in patients with abdominal pain and no alarm symptoms. Abdominal radiographs may help define a pneumonia, demonstrate free air, and help evaluate intestinal air or access stool burden. Studies have indicated that without alarm symptoms, ultrasound has little utility in differentiating a patient with organic disease from functional causes. One study demonstrated that abdominal/pelvic ultrasound in patients with abdominal pain and no alarm symptoms only detected abnormalities in 1%.[9] Recent studies on cancer risks in children receiving CT have led to a move to limit its use as an investigational tool for abdominal pain.[10]

More invasive testing, such as endoscopy, remains controversial. Endoscopy in patients with chronic abdominal pain may find abnormalities 25% to 56% of the time; however, the presence of inflammation may not predict successful resolution of the problem.[11] There is little evidence that a normal endoscopy in patients without alarm symptoms provides benefit in the management of children with abdominal pain.[11] A recent study demonstrated that a negative endoscopy did not affect the persistence, frequency, or intensity of abdominal pain.[12] A negative endoscopy did not lead to improvement in school absenteeism or disruption of daily functioning.[12]

Fortunately, classification systems, such as ROME IV, exist to help physicians make a diagnosis of FGIDs in a proactive manner and not by exclusion.

ROME IV

Approximately 25 years ago, an international group of clinical practitioners and researchers met to establish a classification system for FGIDs, which would help in the diagnosis, the standardization of research, and dissemination of information on these common but poorly understood disorders. The symptoms-based classification was selected because it was thought the most relevant to clinical practice and less tied to a single pathophysiologic mechanism (ie, motility).[13] The process of consensus was used to revise these criteria in 1999, 2006, and most recently 2016 with the publication of *Rome IV*.[14] Rome IV now divides pediatric FGIDs into 3 forms[6]:

Nausea and vomiting disorders
Abdominal pain disorders
Defecation disorders

Pediatric FGIDs are outlined in chapters 15 and 16 of *Rome IV*.[6,15] **Boxes 2** and **3** outline those disorders. These criteria include all symptoms of FGIDs, not just the complaint of abdominal pain.

For the purposes of this article, however, functional abdominal pain, IBS, and functional dyspepsia (FD) are reviewed.

FUNCTIONAL ABDOMINAL PAIN DISORDERS (FAPDs) IN CHILDREN AND ADOLESCENTS

In Rome IV, the committee reevaluated the terminology used in describing pain-based FGIDs.

The term, *functional abdominal pain*, was not specific enough a descriptor for either clinical or research purposes. The terminology has been changed to FAPDs, which is inclusive of FD, IBS, functional abdominal pain–not otherwise specified (FAP-NOS), and abdominal migraine.[6] Each of these disorders has been carefully defined

---

Box 2
Childhood FGIDs, Neonate/toddler[10]

- Infant regurgitation

- Rumination syndrome

- Cyclic vomiting syndrome

- Infant colic

- Functional diarrhea

- Infant dyschezia

- Functional constipation

Data from Nurko S, Benninga M, Faure C, et al. Childhood functional gastrointestinal disorders, neonate/toddler. In: Drossman D, Chang L, Chey W, et al, editors. ROME IV, functional gastrointestinal disorders, disorders of gut-brain interaction. Raleigh (NC): The Rome Foundation; 2016. p. 1237–96.

Box 3
Childhood functional gastrointestinal disorders: child/adolescent

- Functional nausea and vomiting disorders
  - Cyclic vomiting syndrome
  - Functional nausea and functional vomiting
    - Functional nausea
    - Functional vomiting
  - Ruminations syndrome
  - Aerophagia

- FAPDs
  - FD
    - Postprandial distress syndrome
    - Epigastric pain syndrome
  - IBS
  - Abdominal migraine
  - FAP-NOS

- Functional defecation disorders
  - Functional constipation
  - Nonretentive fecal incontinence

Data from DiLorenzo C, Hyams J, Saps M, et al. Childhood functional gastrointestinal disorders, child/adolescent. In: Drossman D, Chang L, Chey W, et al, editors. ROME IV, functional gastrointestinal disorders, disorders of gut-brain interaction. Raleigh (NC): The Rome Foundation; 2016. p. 1297–371.

---

by the committee. The last phrase of each definition was altered to ensure that FAPD did not become a diagnosis of exclusion and mandates an appropriate, selective evaluation.

FD is defined as

- Bothersome symptoms at least 4 times a month for at least 2 months, which include
- Postprandial fullness
- Early satiation
- Epigastric pain or burning not associated with stooling
- After appropriate evaluation, symptoms that cannot be fully explained by another medical condition

IBS is defined as

Abdominal pain at least 4 days per month over at least 2 months associated with
1 or more of the following:
Related to defecation
A change in stool frequency
A change in stool form

In children with abdominal pain and constipation, the pain does not resolve with resolution of the constipation and, after appropriate evaluation, the symptoms cannot be fully explained by another medical condition.

IBS has been divided into 4 subtypes based on the Bristol Stool Form Scale[6]:

IBS-C — constipation predominate
IBS-D — diarrhea predominate
IBS-M — mixed stool types
IBS-U — unsubtyped

Subtyping of IBS has been important in directing therapy. Many current therapies are being targeted to treat and approved for use with specific subtypes.[6]

FAP-NOS is defined as abdominal pain occurring at least 4 times a month and all of the following:

- Episodic or continuous abdominal pain that does not occur solely during physiologic events
- Insufficient criteria for IBS, functional dyspepsia, or abdominal migraine—after appropriate evaluation, the symptoms cannot be fully explained by another medical condition.[6]

PATHOPHYSIOLOGY

FGIDs are the result of a complex interplay of factors that affect the individual and combine to produce disease. This paradigm is the biopsychosocial conceptual model. This model defines FGIDs as gastrointestinal symptoms resulting from a combination of

- Early life events, which may include
  - Genetics
  - Environmental factors (trauma, infections, parental behaviors)
- Psychosocial factors
  - Life stress
  - Personality traits
  - Psychological state
  - Coping
  - Social support
- Physiologic factors
  - Motility disturbance
  - Visceral hypersensitivity
  - Altered CNS processing
  - Altered mucosal and immune function
  - Altered gut microbiota[13]

Early Life Events

Early life pain or stress seems able to lead to chronic abdominal pain later in life through the development of visceral hypersensitivity. The abdominal pain may be the result of

- Increased sensitization of central neurons
- Sensitization of primary sensory neurons
- Impaired stress response through alterations in the hypothalamic-pituitary-adrenal axis (HPA) axis altered descending inhibition of sensory stimulation[16]

The development of CNS changes has been studied in neonatal rats[16] as well as human infants. Exposure to colonic irritation in neonatal rats results in permanent alteration in spinal neurons, which leads to visceral hypersensitivity, a decreased pain threshold, when they become adults.[16] Also in rats, somatic pain experienced in the neonatal period can increase sensitization of spinal neurons and lead to visceral hypersensitivity in adult rats.[16] Infants with prior surgical history have been shown to have increased need for anesthesia during procedures as well as higher pain control postoperatively.[17]

The sensory neurons of the ENS also seem to have a lower sensory threshold and increased signaling to the CNS in individuals with FAPD. Animal studies have shown that colonic irritation sensitizes the sensory neuron in the lumbosacral region, leading to increased signaling in response to colorectal distension.[18]

Stress seems to be 1 trigger for FGIDs in children. Animal studies have demonstrated the development of visceral hypersensitivity after stress events.[16] Stress events have also been shown to increase corticotropin-releasing factor (CRF) expression in the periventricular nucleus, locus coeruleus, and amygdala of adult rats.[19] This action alters the set point of the CRF system and may affect an organism's response to stress and pain later in life.

Pain signals sent by the ENS undergo processing in the spinal cord by inhibitory or excitatory neurons from the CNS. Studies evaluating the effect of fentanyl in response to rectal stimulation demonstrate an improved response in patients with IBS compared with controls. This suggests an alteration in the pain modulatory opioid system.[16]

Genetics

The clustering of FGIDs in families suggest a possible genetic cause of chronic abdominal pain, although this finding could be explained by common environmental factors. Twin studies have not been consistent; however, several studies from the United States, Australia, and Norway have shown increasing concordance for IBS in twins.[20]

Evidence supporting the role of early life events in the etiology of FGIDs has led to research into candidate genes. Studies have identified numerous genes and gene products, which may lead to altered visceral sensitivity and pain processing, including; α_2-adrenergic receptors, serotonin receptors, serotonin and norepinephrine transporters, interleukin (IL)-10, tumor necrosis factor (TNF)-α, TNF superfamily member 15, G proteins (involved in intracellular signaling and ion channels [SCN5A]).[21]

Using genome-wide association studies and data from the Screening Across the Lifespan Twin Study, a locus on 7p22.1 consistently showed increase genetic risk for IBS.[22] This area maps to 2 genes, KDEL receptor 2 gene (*KDELR2*) expressed in all tissues and glutamate receptor-ionotropic-delta 2 interacting protein (*GRID2IP*) localized expression in the brain. KELR2 seems to play a role in vesicle trafficking and transport to the endoplasmic reticulum. The gene seems more highly expressed in the rectum of patients with IBS. GRID2IP encodes a protein, delphilin, which plays a role in glutamatergic neurotransmission.[22]

Psychosocial Factors

Studies have demonstrated an increase rate of stress, anxiety, and depression in patients with FGIDs.[6] There do not seem to be any differences in psychosocial profiles among patients with different abdominal pain–based FGIDs.[23] Children with FAP have a decreased quality of life, frequent school avoidance, school absences, and social difficulties.[24] These pain syndromes are not short lived. In 25% to 45% of patients, these pain symptoms persist for 5 years.[24] Children with extraintestinal somatic symptoms, such as dizziness, back pain, headache, and depression, are more likely to have FGIDs, which extend into young adulthood.[25] It is important to know, however, that 50% of children with FGIDs have no emotional, behavioral, or social functioning problems.[26]

Each individual approaches stress differently. This approach depends on how a child perceives an event and the available coping strategies. Children who feel threatened by a pain event and use passive coping strategies do not have as good an outcome. Children who are more accepting of the pain and have accommodating coping strategies tend to have better function.[27]

In addition to individual strategies, a child's social network provides potential support for coping with chronic abdominal pain, in both positive and negative ways. Families and friends can facilitate wellness or promote disability.

Physiologic Factors

The network of communication between the gut and the brain includes the CNS (brain and spinal cord), the autonomic nervous system, the ENS, and the HPA axis.[28]

Sensations from the gastrointestinal tract are the result of signaling from mechanoreceptors located in the afferent terminal of spinal afferent nerves. These nerves have cell bodies in the vagal nodose ganglia and dorsal root spinal ganglia. The signals are then sent via vagal sensory afferents to the brainstem via the nodose ganglia and nucleus tractus solitarius. Serotonin is an important neurotransmitter in pain signaling, mainly through the 5-HT3 receptor.[29] Increased secretion of serotonin or decreased uptake of serotonin leads to increased pain signaling.[29]

In patients with visceral hypersensitivity, afferent sensory receptors seem to have a lower threshold for stimulation. These receptors continue to send pain signals after the stimulus has already passed.[30] This increased sensitivity may be triggered by intestinal inflammation related to inflammatory bowel disease, allergy, or infection.

The role of pain signal processing in the cerebral cortex has been investigated in humans using both functional MRI and PET. These imaging studies have demonstrated that pain signaling from the secondary somatosensory cortex projects to the limbic and paralimbic regions. These are areas of the brain that are important in an individual's mood, motivation, and cognition, all important components in the experience of visceral pain.[29] Functional MRI has demonstrated that patients with IBS have increased activation of the midcingulate cortex in response to rectal distention.[31] The cingulate cortex is believed an integrative center for emotional experience and pain information.[29]

The HPA axis is vital in coordinating the organism's response to stress. The HPA is part of the limbic system of the brain that is involved with memory and emotional response. Stress activates release of CRF from the hypothalamus, which then stimulates secretion of corticotropin from the pituitary. Corticotropin then stimulates the secretion of cortisol from the adrenal glands.

Both neural and hormonal mechanisms allow the brain to influence many cell functions in the intestine, including immune cells, epithelial cells, neurons, smooth muscle cells, interstitial cells of Cajal, and enterochromaffin cells.[28]

INFLAMMATION

There is evidence to suggest that an imbalance in proinflammatory and anti-inflammatory cytokines may play a role in the development of IBS.[6] Children with IBS seem to have a lower secretion of an anti-inflammatory cytokine (IL-10), which suggests altered immune regulation in this disease process. These changes are subtle and may be induced by prior infections.[6]

MICROBIOME

Studies have demonstrated differences in the microbiome of children with IBS. These children have a higher proportion of Proteobacteria than healthy children.[32] There seems to be bidirectional influence between the gut microbiome and the gut-brain axis via neural, endocrine, immune, and humoral mechanisms.[28]

In the CNS, studies using germ-free mice have demonstrated that the microbiome can effect stress reactivity as well as modulate the serotonergic system.[28,33] In these same germ-free mice, addition of probiotics has led to changes in gut-brain axis mRNA expression in the brain, reduced stress-induced release of cortisol, and reduced anxiety and depression behaviors.[28]

Peripherally, the microbiome may interact with the GBA by modulating afferent sensory nerves, producing molecules that act as local neurotransmitters, and through the production of short chain fatty acids, which can stimulate the sympathetic nervous system.[28]

The CNS also interacts in direct ways with the gut microbiome. For reasons not fully understood, bacteria in the colon contain binding sites for enteric neurotransmitters, the same neurotransmitters used in signaling by the ENS and CNS. The CNS directly controls the environment in which the microbiome resides by modulating intestinal motility; the secretion of acid, bicarbonate, and mucus; intestinal fluid handling and the mucosal immune system. These studies point to the microbiome as a compelling area of research and possible therapeutic target in the treatment of FGIDs.

THERAPY IN PAIN-RELATED FUNCTIONAL GASTROINTESTINAL DISORDERS

The development of a treatment plan for the patient with FGIDs is an individualized process. Therapeutic outcomes depend on a plan that directs treatment to many aspects of the disorder. The arms of therapy include

Dietary therapy
Pharmacologic therapy
Psychosocial support
Complementary/alternative interventions[34]

Simple reassurance in the setting of a strong clinical therapeutic relationship can be helpful in enabling children with FD to resume normal activity. Placebo response rates in patients with FGIDs range from 20% to 60%.[35]

Dietary Therapy

If FGIDs are understood as the result of visceral hypersensitivity, foods that increase abdominal distention, and therefore pain signaling, may complicate symptoms. Recently, studies have evaluated food triggers and have suggested a role of nonabsorbable carbohydrates, nonceliac gluten sensitivity, and food chemical sensitivity.[36]

More specifically, fermentable oligosaccharides, disaccharides and monosaccharides, and polyols (FODMAPs) are a group of poorly digestible carbohydrates that seem to participate in causing symptoms.[36] These carbohydrates include fructose, lactose, sorbitol, fructo-oligosaccharides, gluco- oligosaccharides, and mannitol. FODMAPs are believed to lead to symptoms through several mechanisms, including increase osmotic load and intestinal distention, altered intestinal motility, direct injury to colonic epithelium with increased permeability, and interaction with the intestinal microbiome and the varied metabolism of those organisms.[36]

There are few current tables of FODMAPs in foods and no validated FODMAP cutoff levels to help determine whether a food is truly high FODMAP. Recommendations are to attempt to keep FODMAPs below 3 g a day, however, to benefit IBS patients.[36] On a strict restriction, studies out of Australia have demonstrated a 74% response rate with durability linked directly to dietary compliance.[37]

Probiotics

Intestinal bacteria play a complex role in multiple processes, including effects on bowel motility, pain signaling, immune response, nutrient processing. Manipulation of this microbiome is a potential therapeutic target.

In a recent meta-analysis of placebo-controlled randomized studies,[38] *Lactobacillus rhamnosus* GG, *Lactobacillus reuteri* DSM 17938, and VSL#3 were all shown to increase treatment success with abdominal pain type FGIDs, especially in those patients with IBS. LGG and *L reuteri* DSM 17938 significantly decreases the intensity of the pain. The data for VSL#3 demonstrated that the intensity of pain and bloating was significantly lower than placebo; however, pain frequency was unchanged.[38] More research is needed to determine the exact strain, dosage, or combination that is the most effective.

Pharmacotherapy

Medications for the treatment of FGIDs target multiple points along the pain transmission pathway — from the peripheral receptor, the spinal cord, and also the cortex. Controlled trials in pediatrics continue to be rare.

Antibiotics

With the understanding that the microbiome plays an important role in the etiology of FGIDs, the use of antibiotics in therapy seems a logical step. TARGET-1 and TARGET-2 were 2 double-blind, placebo-controlled studies comparing rifaximin to placebo in the treatment of IBS without constipation.[39] These 2 large-scale trials, enrolling 1260 patients, demonstrated that a 14-day course of rifaximin, at a dose of 550 mg 3 times a day for 14 days, was superior to placebo in improving IBS symptoms with no increased risk of side effects.[39] The Food and Drug Administration–approved rifaximin for treatment of IBS-D in May 2015.

Antispasmodics

Although commonly used in treating patients with pain FGIDs, the anticholinergic hyoscyamine (Levsin) has not been studied in a controlled fashion.[40] Dicyclomine (Bentyl) has been studied in IBS-C and was found to improve overall IBS symptoms.[40]

Antidepressants

Antidepressants affect both the central and peripheral nervous system through multiple pathways, including anticholinergic effects, leading to decreased gastrointestinal transit, improved sleep, treatment of comorbid depression, and analgesia through receptor binding throughout the pain transmission pathway.[41] In a pediatric study, citalopram improved function and decreased pain in 84% of patients with FGIDs.[42]

Serotonin

Serotonin is a critical neurotransmitter in the pain pathway and is an attractive target for potential therapy. Two serotonin type 3 compounds have been developed and studied in adults, alosetron and cilansetron. Complications with these medications, including severe constipation and ischemic colitis, have restricted their use.[41]

Tegaserod, a serotonin type 4 antagonist, is used in constipation predominate IBS.

Psychosocial Support

One of the most important aspects of therapy in these patients is the development of a supportive doctor-patient relationship in which the patient is an active participant in developing to plan of care. Drossman,[13] in *Rome IV*, outlines 12 steps to enhance this relationship.

These steps include:

- Learning to engage the patient in the visit
- Being nonjudgmental and patient centered while taking the history

- Determining the immediate need for the patient visit
- Conducting a careful physical examination and cost-efficient investigation
- Determining patients' understanding of their illness and focus on their concerns
- Eliciting patient understanding of symptoms and provide education
- Responding to patient expectations
- Associating stress and symptoms in a way that is consistent with patient beliefs
- Setting limits
- Involving the patient in treatment
- Making recommendations consistent with patient interests
- Establishing an ongoing relationship[13]

Cognitive Behavioral Therapy

Psychological therapies are effective in the treatment of FGIDs and include parent training, family support, psychotherapy/cognitive behavioral therapy (CBT), relaxation, distraction, hypnotherapy, and biofeedback.[43]

Multiple studies have demonstrated that psychological therapy, such as hypnotherapy and CBT, are effective in the treatment of FGIDs.[44,45]

Family therapy and parent training help address acceptance of a rehabilitation approach to therapy. These interventions are also helpful in changing behaviors in the family that may promote disability or catastrophizing; ongoing behavioral plans should promote independence and functioning.

CBT is a psychotherapeutic approach focused on changing unhelpful cognitions, assumptions, beliefs, and behaviors.[43] During this therapy, patients learn a more biopsychosocial framework of disease. They may keep a diary of symptoms and events to help identify triggers or outcomes that can be targeted for intervention. Patients learn to question their thoughts, assumptions and beliefs that may not be helpful and formulate a new approach.[43]

Hypnotherapy helps patients focus away from the pain, alter sensory experience, decrease stress, promote relaxation, and provide a way to reconsider painful stimuli. In patients with FGIDs, there are gut-specific techniques that may be used.[43]

Complementary Medicine

Complementary medicine techniques may include acupuncture, Ayurveda medicine, chiropractic, homeopathy, and mind-body medicine. Modalities include herbal supplementation, massage therapy, acupuncture, and hypnotherapy.[46]

Peppermint oil is a common and studied herbal often used in patients with FGIDs. In 1 study in children, there was a 76% improvement in symptoms compared with a 19% placebo response.[47] Ginger has been shown helpful in patients with nausea and seems to have a prokinetic function.[46]

The use of massage therapy remains controversial. The underlying theory is that massage may reduce visceral hypersensitivity and alter gastrointestinal tone and motility. Although promising, more studies are needed to confirm its efficacy.

Acupuncture has been shown to effect acid secretion, gastrointestinal motility, and visceral pain in animals. Studies at this time, however, have not demonstrated efficacy for FGIDs.

Gut-directed hypnotherapy has been shown effective in both adults and children in the management of FGIDs. One study demonstrated that hypnotherapy was superior to standard medical therapy. Most interestingly, at 1-year follow-up, symptoms were successfully treated in 85% of the cases.

FUNCTIONAL DYSPEPSIA

Although FAP-NOS and IBS refer to more generalized abdominal pain, functional dyspepsia (FD) refers to symptoms that seem to refer to the gastroduodenal region. These symptoms may include abdominal bloating, epigastric pain, early satiety, belching, epigastric burning, nausea, and vomiting. In Rome IV, FD in children has been divided into 2 subtypes, postprandial distress syndrome and epigastric pain syndrome.[6,48] There is some controversy around this separation. A recent study demonstrated that in a significant number of patients, no clinical distinction was possible and 43% of children switched subtypes, suggesting a common pathophysiology.[49] In another study, however, 29% of patients fit into the postprandial distress syndrome, 24% met criteria for epigastric pain syndrome, 26% met criteria for both, and 21% did not fulfill either diagnosis.[50] The clinical distinction, when present, may provide an alternative to overuse of empiric acid-blocking therapy as well as alternatives to immediate endoscopy or subspecialty referral.[51]

FD is defined as symptoms occurring at least 4 times a month for at least 2 months, including

1. Postprandial fullness
2. Early satiety
3. Epigastric pain or burning not associated with stooling
4. After appropriate evaluation, symptoms that cannot be fully explained by another medical condition[6]

Postprandial distress syndrome is defined as bothersome postprandial fullness or early satiation that prevents finishing a meal. These sensations may include upper abdominal bloating, postprandial nausea, or excessive belching.[6]

Epigastric pain syndrome includes pain or burning located in epigastrium, a burning quality pain that may be induced or relieved by ingestion of a meal.[6]

The major pathophysiologic mechanisms of other FGIDs are also thought to lead to FD, including motility abnormalities, abnormalities of accommodation, and visceral hypersensitivity.[51]

A direct link between motor abnormalities and resultant symptoms is not firmly established.[52] Changes in gastric motor patterns may be the result of abnormalities of the vasovagal reflex, the intrinsic inhibitory innervation, or altered smooth muscle.[51] Approximately two-thirds of adults with FD have abnormal gastroduodenal motility, leading to postprandial fullness, nausea, and vomiting.[51]

Gastric accommodation is a motor event in which the gastric fundus seems to relax in an attempt to accept an incoming meal, without increasing gastric pressure. In patients with abnormal gastric accommodation, the food bolus seems to localize to the distal stomach. Abnormal gastric accommodation has been demonstrated in 40% of adult patient with FD, leading to early satiety or postprandial pain.[51]

Visceral hypersensitivity may occur at many levels in the upper gastrointestinal tract. Adults with FD have increased sensitivity to acid within the duodenum, leading to nausea in a subset of patients. Adults with FD have also been found more sensitive to gastric balloon distention, with increased brain signaling.[52]

Recent studies in adults have also demonstrated a link between prior infections, such as *Salmonella*, *Eshcherichia coli* 0157, *Campylobacter jejuni*, *Giardia lamblia*, and norovirus, and the development of FD.[53]

Work-up of Functional Dyspepsia

In the upper tract, alarm symptoms include vomiting, dysphagia, odynophagia, weight loss, hematemesis, and abnormal laboratory studies, such as anemia. In the setting of alarm symptoms, endoscopy is the most sensitive and specific test for the evaluation of other inflammatory causes of upper gastrointestinal symptoms. Gastric emptying scans may also be helpful in demonstrating motor dysfunction and delayed gastric emptying. Anatomic studies, such as an upper gastrointestinal radiograph, help define normal anatomy and evaluate for malrotation, hiatal hernia, rings, or webs. Upper gastrointestinal radiography does not establish the diagnosis of gastroesophageal reflux disease in any meaningful way.

Endoscopy continues to be controversial in pediatric FD. Adult Rome criteria have required an esophagogastroduodenoscopy; in pediatrics, esophagogastroduodenoscopy is not a requirement in the diagnosis of FD.[6] In a study from Hong Kong, 80 consecutive children with FD were evaluated.[54] Alarm symptoms included gastrointestinal blood loss, dysphagia, vomiting and right upper quadrant pain, nocturnal pain, family history of peptic ulcer disease, and weight loss. Endoscopic mucosal abnormalities were noted in 3 of 9 patients with alarm symptoms and 2 of 71 children without alarm symptoms.[54] If no alarm symptoms are present, a therapeutic trial of acid blockade, prokinetic agents, or other motility agents, such as cyproheptadine, may lead to symptomatic improvement.

Therapy

There are few randomized studies on the treatment of FD, especially in children. Acid suppression was shown helpful in a study comparing cimetidine, ranitidine, famotidine, and omeprazole in the treatment of children with FD. This study demonstrated a 53.8% symptom relief with omeprazole after 4 weeks of therapy, 44.4% for famotidine.[55] The study supported the use of proton pump inhibitors over H_2-receptor antagonists in the treatment of FD.

There are few data in children supporting the use of prokinetics in children for the treatment of FD. Pharmacotherapy has focused on agents that stimulate gastric emptying by targeting serotonin receptors (serotonin type 2 antagonists and serotonin type 4 agonists), dopamine, and motilin receptors.[51] Unfortunately, most of these agents, such as cisapride, domperidone, and reglan, are either ineffective or carry significant cardiac or neurologic risk.

Cyproheptadine, an antagonist of serotonin, histamine H_1, and muscarinic receptors, seems to improve gastric accommodation and has been shown to improve symptoms in children with FD. In a retrospective, open-label study, there was a 55% improvement in dyspeptic symptoms in pediatric patients.[56] There was also a 30% incidence of side effects; however, all were mild and self-limited. Only 2 of 80 children stopped therapy.[56]

As in the treatment of other FGIDs, antidepressant medications, such as tricyclic antidepressants and selective serotonin reuptake inhibitors, may also be helpful in treating FD. These medications may act by improving gut motility or modulations of visceral hypersensitivity.[51]

Abdominal pain continues to be a common and concerning symptom in children. Abdominal pain leads to frequent physician visits and often extensive testing. Rome IV has helped to define FGIDs, and promote education and research into these disorders. A fascinating, intricate web of neurologic signaling, hormonal signaling, commensal organisms, stress, anxiety, social support, and genetics seems involved in the ultimate manifestation of FGIDs. Further research is needed to more specifically define this interplay and effects. Therapeutic interventions need to address these multiple pathophysiologic mechanisms in the setting of individual experience of disease.

REFERENCES

1. Canavan C, West J, Card T. The epidemiology of irritable bowel syndrome. Clin Epidemiol 2014;6:71–80.
2. Hyams JS, Burke G, Davis P, et al. Abdominal pain and irritable bowel syndrome in adolescents: a community- based study. J Pediatr 1996;129:220–6.
3. Lewis ML, Palsson OS, Whitehead WE, et al. Prevalence of functional gastrointestinal disorders in children and adolescents. J Pediatr 2016;177:39–43.e3.
4. Nurko S, Di Lorenzo C. Functional abdominal pain: time to get together and move forward. J Pediatr Gastroenterol Nutr 2008;47:679–80.
5. Di Lorenzo C, Colletti RB, Lehmann HP, et al. Chronic abdominal pain in children: a clinical report of the American Academy of Pediatrics and the North American Society for Pediatric Gastroenterology, Hepatology and Nutrition. J Pediatr Gastroenterol Nutr 2005;40:245–8.
6. DiLorenzo C, Hyams J, Saps M, et al. Childhood functional gastrointestinal disorders, child/adolescent. In: Drossman D, Chang L, Chey W, et al, editors. ROME IV, functional gastrointestinal disorders, disorders of gut-brain interaction. Raleigh (NC): The Rome Foundation; 2016. p. 1297–371.
7. Henderson P, Anderson NH, Wilson DC. The diagnostic accuracy of fecal calprotectin during the investigation of suspected pediatric inflammatory bowel disease: a systematic review and meta-analysis. Am J Gastroenterol 2013;109(5):637–45.
8. Cristofori F, Fontana C, Magistà A, et al. Increased prevalence of celiac disease among pediatric patients with irritable bowel syndrome a 6-year prospective cohort study. JAMA Pediatr 2014;168(6):555–60.
9. Yip W, Ho T, Yip Y, et al. value of abdominal sonography in the assessment of children with abdominal pain. J Clin Ultrasound 1998;26:397–400.
10. Pearce MS, Salotti JA, Little MP, et al. Radiation exposure from CT scans in childhood and subsequent risk of leukaemia and brain tumours: a retrospective cohort study. Lancet 2012;380:499–505.
11. Di Lorenzo C, Colletti RB, Lehmann HP, et al. Chronic abdominal pain in children: a technical report of the American Academy of Pediatrics and the North American Society for Pediatric Gastroenterology, Hepatology and Nutrition: AAP Subcommittee and NASPGHAN Committee on Chronic Abdominal Pain. J Pediatr Gastroenterol Nutr 2005;40:249–61.
12. Bonilla S, Wang D, Saps M. The prognostic value of obtaining a negative endoscopy in children with functional gastrointestinal disorders. Clin Pediatr (Phila) 2011;50:396–401.
13. Drossman D. Functional gastrointestinal disorders and the Rome IV Process. In: Drossman D, Chang L, Chey W, et al, editors. ROME IV, functional gastrointestinal disorders, disorders of gut-brain interaction. Raleigh (NC): The Rome Foundation; 2016. p. 1–32.
14. Drossman D, Chang L, Chey W, et al. ROME IV, functional gastrointestinal disorders, disorders of gut-brain interaction. Fourth. Raleigh (NC): The Rome Foundation; 2016.
15. Nurko S, Benninga M, Faure C, et al. Childhood functional gastrointestinal disorders, neonate/toddler. In: Drossman D, Chang L, Chey W, et al, editors. ROME IV, functional gastrointestinal disorders, disorders of gut-brain interaction. Raleigh (NC): The Rome Foundation; 2016. p. 1237–96.
16. Miranda A. Early life events and the development of visceral hyperalgesia. J Pediatr Gastroenterol Nutr 2008;47:682–4.

17. Peters J, Schouw R, Anand K, et al. Doesneonatal surgery lead to increased pain sensitivity in later childhood? Pain 2005;114:444–54.
18. Lin C, Al-Chaer ED. Long-term sensitization of primary afferents in adult rats exposed to neonatal colon pain. Brain Res 2003;971:73–82.
19. Plotsky PM, Thrivikraman KV, Nemeroff CB, et al. Long-term consequences of neonatal rearing on central corticotropin-releasing factor systems in adult male rat offspring. Neuropsychopharmacology 2005;30:2192–204.
20. Talley N. Genetics and functional bowel disease. J Pediatr Gastroenterol Nutr 2008;47:680–2.
21. Saito Y, Talley N. Genetics of irritable bowel syndrome. Am J Gastroenterol 2008; 103:2100–4.
22. Ek WE, Reznichenko A, Ripke S, et al. Exploring the genetics of irritable bowel syndrome: a GWA study in the general population and replication in multinational case-control cohorts. Gut 2015;64:1774–82.
23. Rutten JMTM, Benninga MA, Vlieger AM. IBS and faps in children. J Pediatr Gastroenterol Nutr 2014;59:493–9.
24. Cunningham NR, Lynch-Jordan A, Mezoff AG, et al. Importance of addressing anxiety in youth with functional abdominal pain: suggested guidelines for physicians. J Pediatr Gastroenterol Nutr 2013;56(5):469–74.
25. Horst S, Shelby G, Anderson J, et al. Predicting persistence of functional abdominal pain from childhood into young adulthood. Clin Gastroenterol Hepatol 2014; 12(12):2026–32.
26. Schurman JV, Danda CE, Friesen CA, et al. Variations in psychological profile among children with recurrent abdominal pain. J Clin Psychol Med Settings 2008;15:241–51.
27. Walker LS, Smith CA, Garber J, et al. Testing a model of pain appraisal and coping in children with chronic abdominal pain. Health Psychol 2005;24:364–74.
28. Carabotti M, Scirocco A, Maselli MA, et al. The gut-brain axis: interactions between enteric microbiota, central and enteric nervous systems. Ann Gastroenterol 2015;28:203–9.
29. Wood JD. Functional abdominal pain: the basic science. J Pediatr Gastroenterol Nutr 2008;47:688–93.
30. DiLorenzo C, Youssef N, Sigurdsson L, et al. Visceral hyperalgesia in children with functional abdominal pain. J Pediatr 2001;139:838–43.
31. Naliboff B, Derbyshire S, Munakate J, et al. Cerebral activation in patients with irritable bowel syndrome and control subjects during rectosigmoid stimulation. Psychosom Med 2001;63:365–75.
32. Saulnier DM, Riehle K, Mistretta T-A, et al. Gastrointestinal microbiome signatures of pediatric patients with irritable bowel syndrome. Gastroenterology 2011;141(5): 1782–91.
33. Heijtz RD, Wang S, Anuar F, et al. Normal gut microbiota modulates brain development and behavior. Proc Natl Acad Sci U S A 2011;108:3047–52.
34. Giannetti E, Staiano A. Probiotics for irritable bowel syndrome: clinical data in children. J Pediatr Gastroenterol Nutr 2016;63:25–6.
35. Benninga MA, Mayer EA. The power of placebo in pediatric functional gastrointestinal disease. Gastroenterology 2009;137:1207–10.
36. Mansueto P, Seidita A, D'Alcamo A, et al. Role of FODMAPs in patients with irritable bowel syndrome. Nutr Clin Pract 2015;30:665–82.
37. Shepherd S, Gibson P. Fructoe malabsorption and symptoms of irritable bowel syndrome: guidelines for effective dietary management. J Am Diet Assoc 2006; 106:1631–9.

38. Korterink JJ, Ockeloen L, Benninga MA, et al. Probiotics for childhood functional gastrointestinal disorders: a systematic review and meta-analysis. Acta Paediatr 2014;103:365–72.
39. Pimentel M, Lembo A, Chey WD, et al. Rifaximin therapy for patients with irritable bowel syndrome without constipation. N Engl J Med 2016;364:22–32.
40. Trinkley KE, Nahata MC. Treatment of irritable bowel syndrome. J Clin Pharm Ther 2011;36:275–82.
41. Lebel A. Pharmacology. J Pediatr Gastroenterol Nutr 2008;47:703–6.
42. Campo J, Perel J, Lucas A, et al. Citalopram treatment of pediatric recurrent abdominal pain and comorbid internalizing disorders: an exploratory study. J Am Acad Child Adolesc Psychiatry 2004;43:1234–42.
43. Bursch B. Psychological/cognitive behavioral treatment of childhood functional abdominal pain and irritable bowel syndrome. J Pediatr Gastroenterol Nutr 2008;47:706–7.
44. Whitehead W. Hypnosis for irritable bowel syndrome: the empirical evidence of therapeutic effects. Int J Clin Exp Hypn 2006;54:7–20.
45. Duarte MA, Penna FJ, Andrade EMG, et al. Treatment of nonorganic recurrent abdominal pain: cognitive-behavioral family intervention. J Pediatr Gastroenterol Nutr 2006;43:59–64.
46. Vlieger A, Benninga M. Complementary Therapies for pediatric functional gastrointestinal disorders. J Pediatr Gastroenterol Nutr 2008;47:707–9.
47. Kline RM, Kline JJ, Di Palma J, et al. Enteric-coated, pH-dependent peppermint oil capsules for the treatment of irritable bowel syndrome in children. J Pediatr 2001;138:125–8.
48. Tilburg M, van, Hyams J, Leiby A. Functional dyspepsia in children: can we distinguish epigastric pain and postprandrial distress? Gastroenterology 2014;146:S143.
49. Turco R, Russo M, Martinelli M, et al. No Titdo distinct Functional Dyspepsia Subtypes Exist in Children? J Pediatr Gastroenterol Nutr 2016;62:387–92.
50. Schurman JV, Singh M, Singh V, et al. Symptoms and subtypes in pediatric functional dyspepsia: relation to mucosal inflammation and psychological functioning. J Pediatr Gastroenterol Nutr 2010;51:298–303.
51. Romano C, Valenti S, Benninga M. Functional dyspepsia: an enigma in a conundrum. J Pediatr Gastroenterol Nutr 2016;63(6):579–84.
52. Tack J, Talley N, Camilleri M, et al. Functional gastroduodenal disorders. Gastroenterology 2006;130:1466–79.
53. Futagami S, Itoh T, Sakamoto C. Systematic review with meta-analysis: post-infectious functional dyspepsia. Aliment Pharmacol Ther 2015;41:177–88.
54. Tam YH, Chan KW, To KF, et al. Impact of pediatric Rome III criteria of functional dyspepsia on the diagnostic yield of upper endoscopy and predictors for a positive endoscopic finding. J Pediatr Gastroenterol Nutr 2011;52:387–91.
55. Dehghani S, Imanieh M, Haghighat M. The comparative study of the effectiveness of cimetidine, ranitidine, famotidine, and omeprazole in the treatmtne of children with dyspepsia. ISRN Pediatr 2011;2011:219287.
56. Rodriguez L, Diaz J, Nurko S. Safety and efficacy of cyproheptadine for treating dyspeptic symptoms in children. J Pediatr 2013;163:261–7.

Gastrointestinal Bleeding and Management

Anita K. Pai, MD, Victor L. Fox, MD*

KEYWORDS

- Hematemesis • Hematochezia • Melena • Peptic ulcer • Varices
- Vascular anomaly • Endoscopy

KEY POINTS

- There is a broad clinical spectrum of gastrointestinal hemorrhage.
- Obtaining an accurate history and conducting a thorough physical examination can provide important clues about the location, severity, and likely etiology of gastrointestinal bleeding.
- There are blood tests, radiologic tools, and endoscopic methods to identify a bleeding source.
- Early consultation with a gastroenterologist is recommended, as endoscopy is often required for evaluation and may be needed to control hemorrhage.

INTRODUCTION

The presentation of gastrointestinal bleeding in children can vary from subtle findings of pallor and iron-deficiency anemia to obvious episodes of vomiting frank blood. Children present with this chief complaint in a variety of clinical settings, but there is a paucity of literature capturing the epidemiology of pediatric gastrointestinal hemorrhage. Gastrointestinal bleeding can manifest in several ways. Hematemesis is the expulsion of bright red or "coffee-ground" colored material from the mouth. This usually indicates bleeding proximal to the Ligament of Treitz, as fresh red blood exposed to an acidic environment turns brown.[1] Melena typically correlates with an esophageal, gastric, or proximal small intestinal bleeding source and leads to passage of black, tarry stool per rectum. This appearance can be attributed to oxidization by intestinal bacteria that convert hemoglobin to hematin.[2] In contrast, hematochezia is bright red or maroon-colored material that passes from the rectum. Although

Disclosure Statement: Dr V.L. Fox has received consulting fees as a member of the Clinical Advisory Board on Nutritional Insufficiency for Medtronic. Dr A.K. Pai has no financial disclosures or conflicts of interest to report.
Division of Gastroenterology, Hepatology, and Nutrition, Boston Children's Hospital, Harvard Medical School, 300 Longwood Avenue, Boston, MA 02115, USA
* Corresponding author.
E-mail address: victor.fox@childrens.harvard.edu

hematochezia most often occurs with lower small intestinal or colonic bleeding sources, a brisk upper gastrointestinal bleed may present as bright red blood per rectum, with blood in the intestinal lumen acting as a cathartic agent and accelerating transit. Obscure gastrointestinal bleeding is blood loss that is not identified by upper endoscopy, colonoscopy, and radiologic evaluation of the small intestine.[3] It can be further classified into obscure overt and obscure occult bleeding, based on extent of clinically obvious bleeding.[4] There are many exhaustive reviews of etiologies of pediatric gastrointestinal bleeding.[1,2,5–9] Our goal is to provide a framework for evaluation of patients with gastrointestinal bleeding and to review management principles.

DISCUSSION
Historical Report

A careful history may shed light on the source of bleeding and rate of blood loss. It is important to inquire about the color, quantity, and location of bleeding. The temporal association of the bleeding episode to other signs and symptoms, including abdominal pain, vomiting, and fevers should be characterized. Eliciting this history in an emergency scenario with distraught patients or unwitnessed events can be challenging. For instance, hemoptysis can be mistaken for hematemesis.[10] However, unveiling key historical details may provide critical clues to localize the bleeding source. A history of recent tonsillectomy, dental procedure, epistaxis, or nasogastric tube placement may indicate nasopharyngeal or oropharyngeal bleeding. An underlying anxiety disorder may be accompanied by chronic cheek chewing (morsicatio buccarum) with bleeding from the mouth or vomiting swallowed blood. Ingestion of a button battery or sharp foreign body may cause mucosal tears, ulcerations, or even life-threatening aortoenteric fistulae.[11] Discovery of prior intestinal operation could heighten concern for a bleeding ulcer from a surgical anastomosis (**Fig. 1**). A thorough medication history may reveal use of aspirin or other nonsteroidal anti-inflammatory drugs (NSAIDs) that could increase bleeding risk. Many substances can give the false

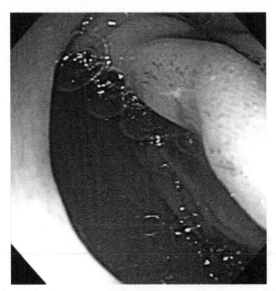

Fig. 1. Ulcer at jejunocolonic anastomosis in young girl with a history of jejunal atresia and multiple bowel resections as a neonate.

appearance of red blood (beets, food coloring, gelatin, candy[12]) or black, tarry stool (iron supplements, bismuth). Cefdinir, a third-generation cephalosporin, has been reported to cause maroon or red discoloration to stool in pediatric patients due to formation of a precipitate with iron-containing supplements.[13] Additional historical clues and corresponding etiologic sources in children and adolescents are summarized in **Table 1**.

Special Considerations in Neonates and Infants

There are unique etiologies of gastrointestinal bleeding in neonates and infants younger than 12 months. Common causes of gastrointestinal bleeding in an otherwise healthy infant are anal fissures and swallowed maternal blood (from delivery or from fissured nipples). To distinguish between fetal and maternal origin of blood, the Apt-Downey test can be applied, which capitalizes on the different denaturing properties of fetal and maternal hemoglobin in the presence of sodium hydroxide.[14] Occult gastrointestinal bleeding, hematochezia, or hematemesis may be presenting signs of cow's milk protein allergy in an infant.[15–17] Gastrointestinal bleeding can be a presenting symptom of an underlying coagulopathy. Vitamin K deficiency bleeding should be considered in neonates, particularly those with maternal exposure to antiepileptic medications that affect vitamin K, dysbiosis from antibiotic exposure, cholestasis, short bowel syndrome, or failure to receive perinatal vitamin K prophylaxis (eg, home delivery).[18,19] Clinically unstable, premature, or very low birth weight infants should be evaluated for necrotizing enterocolitis.[20] Bilious emesis warrants consideration of intestinal malrotation, as midgut volvulus can progress quickly to intestinal ischemia, sepsis, and death.[21] Hematochezia is a late clinical sign in many surgical emergencies, from volvulus to intussusception, and can herald compromise of vascular supply.[21]

Clinical Assessment

The clinician's physical examination serves to stratify the patient's illness severity and localize the source of bleeding. It is important to identify a patient who is ill-appearing, in pain, or has an altered sensorium. Assessment of the vital signs is an important early step. Children are known to have increased physiologic reserve compared with elderly patients and may maintain normal vital signs after an acute blood loss. Studies in pediatric trauma patients have demonstrated that hypotension may not be present until up to 25% of the circulating blood volume (80 mL/kg in children) has been compromised.[22] Therefore, heart rate, capillary refill, and pulse pressure may be more sensitive markers of hemodynamic instability than blood pressure soon after an acute blood loss. Careful consideration of the patient's other comorbidities prevents clinicians from being falsely reassured by normal vital signs. For instance, tachycardia may not be a reliable marker of hemodynamic decompensation in a patient on beta-blocker therapy.

The head and neck examination should screen for scleral icterus, conjunctival pallor, dental trauma, active bleeding in the oral cavity, epistaxis, or abnormal pigmentation of lips or buccal mucosa. The abdominal examination should evaluate for distension, tenderness to palpation, enlarged liver or spleen, and other stigmata of chronic liver disease (eg, ascites, prominent abdominal veins). A rectal examination may reveal perianal skin tags suspicious for Crohn disease, a palpable polyp in the rectal vault, fissures, hemorrhoids, or an anorectal vascular anomaly (**Fig. 2**). There also may be subtle clues to the chronicity of an illness. In addition to jaundice, bruising, and rashes, skin findings such as telangiectasias, blue nodules, hemangiomas, or pigmented macules (lentigines) could also raise suspicion for multisystem vascular

Table 1
Using historical clues to identify sources of bleeding

Site of Suspected Bleed	Historical Clues and Physical Examination Findings (*Potential Etiology in Italics*)
No gastrointestinal bleeding source	• Consumption of beets, food coloring, licorice, other candy[12] (*substances that can give appearance of hematemesis or melanotic stools*) • Use of cefdinir,[13] iron, bismuth (*medications that can discolor stool*)[8] • Menstruation, hematuria, hemoptysis[10] (*extra-intestinal bleeding sources*) • Recent consumption of horseradish, turnip, tomatoes, red cherries, meat (*false-positive guaiac test*)[8] • Recent tonsillectomy, adenoidectomy, dental procedure, epistaxis, habitual chewing of buccal mucosa (*oropharyngeal or nasopharyngeal bleeding source*) • Breastfeeding infant's mother with cracked nipples (*swallowed blood*) • Unexplained bleeding, discordant clinical picture and workup (*Munchausen syndrome by proxy*[38])
Esophageal mucosal injury	• Odynophagia after ingestion of doxycycline, alendronate, iron, potassium chloride (*medication-induced esophageal erosions or ulcers*)[39] • Symptoms of gastroesophageal reflux (*erosive esophagitis due to gastroesophageal reflux disease*) • Esophageal foreign body or nasogastric tube trauma[40] (*mucosal erosion, ulceration, bleeding*) • Vomiting, retching, bulimia, or alcohol intoxication (*Mallory-Weiss tear*)[41] • Retrosternal chest pain, odynophagia, dysphagia, especially in immunocompromised patient (*herpes esophagitis or other infectious esophagitis*)[42]
Esophageal/gastric variceal disease or portal gastropathy	• Ascites, jaundice, splenomegaly, palmar erythema, prominent abdominal vessels, skin excoriations due to pruritus (*portal hypertension or chronic liver disease*)
Gastric or duodenal mucosal injury	• Epigastric abdominal pain, *Helicobacter pylori*, nonsteroidal anti-inflammatory drug use, critically ill patient, burns, sepsis, mechanical ventilation (*stress gastritis and peptic ulcer disease*)[43]
Iatrogenic causes	• Prior intestinal operation (*anastomotic ulcer*)[44,45] • Surgical diversion of fecal stream (*diversion colitis*)[46] • History of recent endoscopy (*duodenal hematoma, mucosal tear from stricture dilation, post-sphincterotomy or post-polypectomy bleeding*)[47] • Recent liver biopsy, endoscopic retrograde cholangiopancreatography, or percutaneous cholangiogram (*hemobilia*)[48]
Vascular issue	• Sudden massive hematemesis, melena, hemodynamic instability (*Dieulafoy lesion*)[49,50] • Button battery ingestion, torrential bleeding episode (*aortoenteric fistula*)[11] • Multifocal cutaneous vascular malformations (*blue rubber bleb nevus syndrome*)[51] • Limb hypertrophy, hematochezia (*Klippel-Trenaunay syndrome with vascular malformation*)[52]

(continued on next page)

Table 1 (continued)	
Site of Suspected Bleed	**Historical Clues and Physical Examination Findings (*Potential Etiology in Italics*)**
	• Cutaneous hemangiomas and rectal bleeding (*infantile visceral hemangiomas*)[53]
	• Epistaxis, multiple telangiectases, positive family history (*Osler-Weber-Rendu or hereditary hemorrhagic telangiectasia*)[54]
	• Abdominal pain, purpuric rash, arthritis, hematuria (*vasculitis-Henoch-Schönlein purpura*)[55,56]
	• Turner syndrome, intermittent melena or hematochezia (*telangiectasia, venous ectasia*)[57,58]
	• Translucent skin, thin face, pinched nose, visible veins on chest, epigastric pain, melena (*type IV [vascular subtype] Ehlers-Danlos syndrome with mucosal fragility, ulcer disease, delicate vessels*)[59]
	• Congenital red-brown skin macules with thrombocytopenia and gastrointestinal bleeding (*cutaneovisceral angiomatosis with thrombocytopenia*)[60]
	• Other gastrointestinal venous or arteriovenous malformation
Polyps and tumors	• Painless intermittent rectal bleeding with normal stooling pattern in young child (*juvenile polyp*)
	• Phosphate and tensin homologue deleted on chromosome ten hamartoma tumor syndrome or Bannayan-Riley-Ruvalcaba syndrome with macrocephaly, autism spectrum, pigmented macules on penis (*juvenile polyposis syndrome*)
	• Pigmented macules on lips or buccal mucosa, intussusception (*Peutz-Jeghers syndrome with associated hamartomatous polyps*)
	• Family history of early-onset colorectal cancer (*familial adenomatous polyposis*)
	• Gastrointestinal stromal tumor
Infectious and inflammatory conditions	• Infantile cow milk protein allergy (*allergic proctocolitis*)
	• Antibiotic use, recent travel to endemic areas, consumption of undercooked meats, or immunocompromised state (*salmonella, shigella, Yersinia enterocolitica, Campylobacter jejuni, Escherichia coli, Cytomegalovirus, Clostridium difficile, Entamoeba histolytica*)
	• Family history of inflammatory bowel disease or other autoimmune diseases, chronic abdominal pain, growth issues, or bloody diarrhea with urgency, frequency, tenesmus, nighttime symptoms, abdominal pain (*ulcerative colitis or Crohn disease*)
	• Abdominal distension, vomiting, pain, fever, explosive diarrhea, rectal bleeding in infant with history of delayed meconium passage (*Hirschsprung-associated enterocolitis*)[61,62]
Intestinal ischemia	• History of drug use (*cocaine-induced intestinal ischemia*)[63]
	• Congenital heart disease (*mesenteric ischemia of childhood in hypoplastic left heart syndrome*)[64]
	• Prematurity, very low birth weight (*necrotizing enterocolitis*)[20]
	• Complicated intussusception (*Meckel diverticulum,[65] intestinal duplication*)
	• Bilious emesis (*malrotation with midgut volvulus*)[21]
	• Mesenteric vein thrombosis

(continued on next page)

Table 1 (continued)	
Site of Suspected Bleed	**Historical Clues and Physical Examination Findings (*Potential Etiology in Italics*)**
Mucosal injury in immunosuppressed state	• History of bone marrow transplantation (*graft-versus-host disease,*[66] *infectious colitis*) • Abdominal pain, neutropenia, fever, bloody stool (*neutropenic enterocolitis*) • Radiation enteritis • Chemotherapy exposure (*mycophenolate-induced colitis*)[67]
Anorectal bleeding source[9]	• Bowel movements with bright red blood coating hard stool (*fissure, hemorrhoids*) • Rectal foreign body, physical or sexual abuse[68]

This table summarizes potential site of gastrointestinal bleeding in children based on historical clues. Potential etiologies to explain the historical clues are noted in italics and parentheses.

disorders such as hereditary hemorrhagic telangiectasia, blue rubber bleb nevus syndrome, and cutaneovisceral angiomatosis with thrombocytopenia, or polyposis disorders, such as Peutz-Jeghers syndrome and juvenile polyposis syndrome (**Fig. 3**).

Management Principles

Risk-stratification of patients is based on the clinical history, vital signs, and initial laboratory tests. Hemodynamically stable, otherwise healthy children with minor bleeding (either small amounts of bright red blood per rectum, occasional episodes of hematochezia, or pink-tinged emesis) and normal blood tests may be candidates for hospital discharge with close follow-up. However, the patients and their families should be counseled on return precautions. If there are psychosocial stressors that compromise reliability of return to the hospital and urgent follow-up, hospital admission may be prudent. Patients who have had an acute, large-volume blood loss, have unstable vital signs, or have other serious comorbidities may benefit from monitoring in an intensive-care unit (ICU). Patients with a clinically significant bleeding episode who are hemodynamically stable may be admitted to a standard hospital bed.

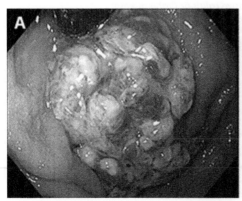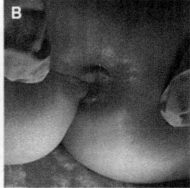

Fig. 2. Polypoid solitary rectal ulcer/mucosal prolapse lesion in distal rectum (*A*). Anal hemorrhoidal engorgement associated with rectal venous malformation (*B*).

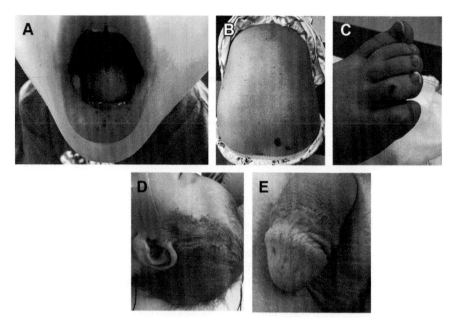

Fig. 3. Oral lentigines or pigmented macules in patient with Peutz-Jeghers syndrome (*A*). Multiple reddish-brown vascular skin lesions in child with cutaneovisceral angiomatosis with thrombocytopenia (*B*). Nodular blue cutaneous venous malformations in a boy with blue rubber bleb nevus syndrome (*C*). Regional face and scalp hemangioma in a female infant with PHACES syndrome (Posterior fossa malformations, Hemangiomas, Arterial anomalies, Cardiac defects and coarctation of the aorta, Eye abnormalities, and Sternal abnormalities or ventral developmental defects) (*D*). Pigmented macules on glans of penis in boy with phosphate and tensin homologue deleted on chromosome ten hamartoma tumor syndrome and juvenile polyposis (*E*).

Basic supportive measures include ensuring a stable airway and oxygenation, maintaining adequate blood volume, and correcting any underlying coagulopathy. For ICU patients, establishing secure intravenous (IV) access should be prioritized (preferably with 2 large-bore IV lines). Patients should be resuscitated with normal saline or lactated Ringers. Transfusion parameters depend on the clinical circumstances and the patient's other comorbidities. Based on the volume and acuity of blood loss, a blood transfusion also may be necessary to improve the oxygen carrying capacity of the circulating blood volume. However, there is some evidence that restrictive transfusion strategies may improve outcomes in adult patients with acute upper gastrointestinal bleeding.[23] In cases of portal hypertension and variceal bleeding, aggressive blood transfusion may raise the portal pressure, increasing the risk of subsequent bleeding episodes, and aggressive fluid resuscitation with saline solutions may exacerbate ascites burden. It is important to establish vigilant cardiorespiratory monitoring and to optimize hemodynamic conditions before therapeutic interventions. Coagulopathy due to defects in platelet number or function or other clotting factors should be corrected whenever possible.

The patient should be instructed to be nil per os (NPO) until further consultation with a pediatric gastroenterologist and determination of timing for endoscopic evaluation. For patients reporting unwitnessed bright red or coffee-ground emesis, nasogastric tube lavage may help confirm the diagnosis; however, the results can be deceptive.

Traumatic insertion of the nasogastric tube can give a bloody tinge to the lavaged fluid and be mistaken for an active bleed. Also, a negative nasogastric aspirate does not exclude the possibility of a major upper gastrointestinal bleeding source.[24,25] In cases of witnessed hematemesis episodes, nasogastric lavage may not have diagnostic utility, but it could reduce the gastric fluid burden to improve endoscopic visualization and decrease the chance of aspiration.[26] Passage of a nasogastric tube is very uncomfortable for patients. Some gastroenterologists defer nasogastric tube drainage in favor of draining the gastric contents under direct endoscopic visualization.

Diagnostic Testing

A proposed list of useful serologic laboratory tests is summarized in **Table 2** to assess the magnitude of the bleeding episode and evaluate for other comorbidities. The complete blood count (CBC) and red blood cell (RBC) indices can shed light on the severity and chronicity of bleeding. The chemistry profile may reveal hepatic or renal issues, and the coagulation panel and albumin are used to interrogate the liver synthetic function. A rise in the blood urea nitrogen (BUN) may be related to the catabolism of amino acids during intestinal digestion of RBCs. Additional tests can be guided by the clinical history, such as inflammatory markers for investigation of Crohn disease or ulcerative colitis. For well-appearing patients with suspected nonemergent bleeding presentations, this preliminary laboratory workup may be adequate. In cases of severe bleeding, changes in serial CBCs and clotting factors can portend a deteriorating clinical course and need for therapeutic interventions. In addition to blood tests, stool analysis for infectious agents may be pursued based on clinical risk factors (eg, antibiotic exposure, immunocompromised state, recent travel) in patients with lower intestinal bleeding and colitis symptoms.

There are also chemical tests that can confirm the presence of blood in stool or vomitus. Guaiac testing uses a peroxidase-like property of heme to facilitate the oxidation of guaiac (a phenolic compound), with the resultant blue color change indicating presence of blood. There are several conditions that lead to false-positive guaiac tests, if other substances with peroxidase activity are present (see **Table 1**).[8] False-negative guaiac tests can occur with expired guaiac cards and reagents, prolonged storage of specimens before testing, and recent consumption of vitamin C. Newer guaiac kits have improved specificity. Immunohistochemical tests for detection of occult blood have been used for colon cancer screening, with decreased

Table 2
Suggested laboratory workup

Blood Testing	Stool Studies	Other
Type and Screen	Salmonella	Gastroccult
Complete blood count	Shigella	
Inflammatory markers (erythrocyte sedimentation rate, C-reactive protein)	*Clostridium difficile* toxins A and B	
	Yersinia	
	Campylobacter	
Prothrombin time, international normalized ratio, partial thromboplastin time	*Escherichia coli*	
	Ova and parasite smear	
	Cytomegalovirus (if immunocompromised patient)	
Electrolyte panel, including blood urea nitrogen, creatinine	Entamoeba histolytica (if supported by geographic history)	
Liver chemistry panel	Stool guaiac test	
Fibrinogen	Fecal lactoferrin or calprotectin	

confounding by external factors. Despite high sensitivity and specificity, these results should be interpreted with caution, as even trace amounts of blood may be detected by immunohistochemical methods and potentially lead to unwarranted additional testing.[2]

Gastrointestinal endoscopy is the most important modality due to its superior diagnostic sensitivity and specificity, as well as therapeutic capability (**Fig. 4**). Emergent endoscopy is needed only if there is ongoing bleeding with hemodynamic instability that is not responsive to blood product transfusions. There is an increased risk of complications in emergent endoscopy compared with standard endoscopic procedures. This risk profile is attributed to the anesthetic challenges for a hemodynamically unstable patient, other comorbidities in a patient with active bleeding, the hazard of aspirating bloody gastric contents, and inadequate patient preparation.[27] For standard endoscopic procedures, deep sedation is adequate; however, for safe and technically successful therapeutic endoscopy in a patient with high-risk or active bleeding, general anesthesia with endotracheal tube placement is preferable, for improved airway protection. Emergent colonoscopy is less commonly indicated in children. A "rapid purge" administration of bowel preparation electrolyte solution via a nasogastric tube may improve the diagnostic yield.

Video capsule endoscopy (VCE) should be considered for the evaluation of a suspected small bowel source of gastrointestinal bleeding[28] because most of the small bowel is not visualized with standard upper endoscopy and colonoscopy (**Fig. 5**). The capsule passes through the intestine passively and without distention of the bowel lumen, so the mucosa is visualized in a more natural state. Although this modality does not allow for direct tissue sampling or use of therapeutic interventions, it is a noninvasive test that produces high-resolution images of this difficult to reach section of the gastrointestinal tract without need for anesthesia.[29] Limitations of VCE include inability to precisely localize a lesion, potential for missed lesions and false-positive findings, risk of incomplete study (based on a patient's inherent motility and battery life of the capsule), and possibility of capsule retention requiring surgical removal.[4] If the child is unable to swallow the wireless capsule device, it can be deployed endoscopically preferably beyond the stomach to avoid prolonged gastric retention.

Although plain radiography has little if any role in the diagnostic evaluation of gastrointestinal bleeding, more specialized radiologic testing can be useful. A Tc-99m pertechnetate scan is used to diagnose a Meckel diverticulum, a potential source of obscure gastrointestinal bleeding (**Fig. 6**). The reported sensitivity, specificity, and positive predictive value of this test are quite variable in the literature, with false-negative and false-positive results reported. One of the most common

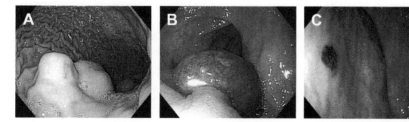

Fig. 4. Gastric GIST (gastrointestinal stromal tumor) discovered in preadolescent boy with unexplained abdominal pain and anemia (*A*). Colonic juvenile polyp in young child with intermittent painless rectal bleeding (*B*). Gastric venous malformation, characteristic for blue rubber bleb nevus syndrome (*C*).

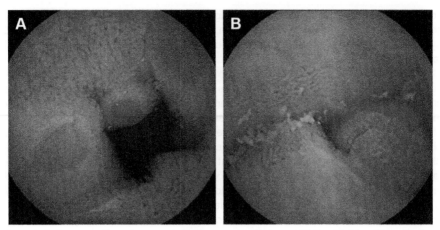

Fig. 5. Wireless capsule endoscopy revealing an occult source of chronic blood loss presenting with iron deficiency anemia and guaiac-positive stool in 2 young children. Multifocal erosions limited to proximal small bowel in 2-year-old boy (*A*). Solitary hamartomatous polyp in the jejunum of a 3-year-old girl (*B*).

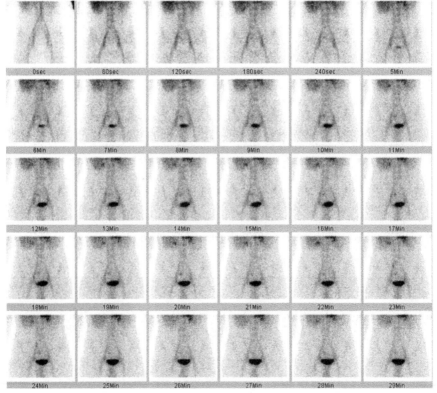

Fig. 6. A Tc-99m-pertechnetate scan demonstrating faint abnormal focus of tracer uptake in the right lower quadrant of the abdomen in an adolescent boy presenting with massive hematochezia. A Meckel diverticulum with marginal ulceration was removed and contained extensive gastric heterotopia.

etiologies of a false-positive scan is a gastrointestinal duplication, which also can contain heterotopic gastric mucosa and demonstrate intense uptake of tracer. Vascular lesions, arteriovenous malformations, gastrointestinal bleeding unrelated to heterotopic gastric mucosa, uterine blush, and retained tracer in the urinary collecting system also can be mistakenly diagnosed as a Meckel diverticulum.[30,31] False-negative scintigraphy scans are often due to the small amount of heterotopic gastric mucosa or technical elements (eg, obscuration by residual contrast from prior tests).[31] It is also important to remember that not all Meckel diverticula contain heterotopic gastric tissue, which is required to induce ulceration and bleeding. Some studies have advocated for the administration of an H2-receptor antagonist in the 1 to 2 days before the scan to inhibit acid secretion, reduce washout, and improve retention of the radiotracer in the gastric glands for enhanced visualization of heterotopic gastric mucosa.[31]

If an obscure overt bleeding source is suspected, a bleeding scan with technetium-99m-labeled RBCs may indicate the general location of bleeding within the gastrointestinal tract[32] (**Fig. 7**). This bleeding scan can detect hemorrhage if the bleeding rate is greater than 0.1 to 0.4 mL/min. Additional delayed images, 12 to 24 hours after the start of the study, may improve the sensitivity of the test.[33] However, localization of the bleeding source may be less reliable. If there is a high suspicion for a vascular anomaly not detected by the other modalities, computed tomography angiography or magnetic resonance angiography may identify the lesion (**Fig. 8**). Alternatively, direct angiography could confirm the diagnosis.[34] This strategy requires sedation, stable renal function, and the expertise of an interventional radiologist. Angiography is most effective when the bleeding rate is higher than 0.5 mL/min (higher than for labeled RBC scans).[35] However, angiography also offers the opportunity for embolization of involved vessels in ulcers or vascular anomalies.

Therapeutic Options

Medical therapy
Noninvasive pharmacologic strategies for management of gastrointestinal bleeding are summarized in **Table 3**. One objective of medical therapy is to decrease the risk of rebleeding, which may require consultation with other specialties. For instance, a multidisciplinary discussion may be needed to assess the risk profile of discontinuing prophylactic anticoagulation therapy in a cardiac patient with vulnerable shunt and concurrent gastrointestinal bleed. Acid-suppressing agents, such as Histamine2-receptor blockers and proton pump inhibitors may stabilize clot formation and promote ulcer healing. Children with gastroduodenal ulceration associated with *Helicobacter pylori* should undergo eradication with combination therapy (see **Table 3**). Octreotide has been demonstrated to be safe and effective in nonarterial severe gastrointestinal bleeding in children.[36] It is a synthetic somatostatin analogue that works by decreasing splanchnic blood flow, but it carries a small risk of bowel ischemia and hyperglycemia. Nonselective beta-blockers (eg, propranolol) have been used to decrease variceal bleeding in portal hypertension, but they have not been rigorously studied in pediatric populations.[37] Titration of propranolol dosing is also complicated by the variability of basal heart rates in different pediatric age groups and the challenges of measuring vital signs accurately in young children.

Endoscopic therapy
Therapeutic endoscopy is used in cases of active bleeding and with identification of other high-risk stigmata. High-risk lesions include ulcers with a nonbleeding visible vessel and oozing blood from an ulcer with an overlying clot (see **Fig. 7**). Identification

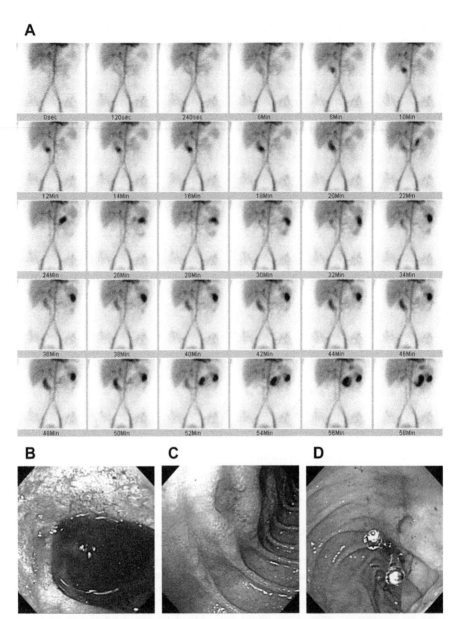

Fig. 7. A Tc-99m–labeled RBC scan localizing active bleeding in the proximal small bowel in a patient with cancer who presented with severe hematochezia (A). Upper gastrointestinal endoscopy revealing a fresh clot overlying a duodenal ulcer (B). Protruding vessel in base of ulcer after clot removal (C). Hemostatic metal clips applied to prevent recurrent bleeding (D).

of high-risk features and interventions to address these lesions is critical, as they carry an estimated 50% chance of recurrent bleeding after the first bleeding episode.[27] The proximity of deep ulcers to the large blood vessels affects bleeding risk and is another important consideration in therapeutic endoscopy. If high-risk features are noted during surveillance, it is prudent to confirm surgical backup, in the event that massive bleeding ensues during endoscopic manipulation.

Dedicated therapeutic endoscopes have large operating channels or 2 channels, one for interventional tools and the other channel for suction and irrigation functions. These therapeutic endoscopes have a larger diameter than standard endoscopes and are difficult to use in small children. The use of single-channel conventional endoscopes for therapeutic procedures in smaller children can be technically challenging but is generally effective. The most common endoscopic techniques and tools used to control acute, severe bleeding include injection, thermal coagulation, and mechanical hemostatic clips and ligation devices. The principle behind injection therapy is to achieve hemostasis by targeting visible vessels with epinephrine or a sclerosant alone or in combination (**Fig. 9**). This treatment is postulated to cause a hemostatic plug by vasoconstriction, local mechanical tamponade, and cytochemical reactions. Risks of this strategy include bowel ischemia with subsequent perforation and systemic side effects due to epinephrine absorption. Thermal coagulation can be applied by direct contact and noncontact modalities. Bipolar electrocoagulation probes may be used to contact tissue directly and coagulate oozing surface vessels. When pressed firmly against small arteries, bipolar probes are used to perform coaptive thermal coagulation or a welded closure of the bleeding vessel. Argon plasma coagulation (APC) is a noncontact modality in which a probe directs a stream of argon plasma to deliver

Table 3
Pharmacotherapy in pediatric patients with gastrointestinal bleeding

Agent	Dosing
Acid reduction	
Ranitidine (H2-receptor antagonist)	Oral: 4–8 mg/kg per day per os (PO) divided twice daily (maximum daily dose: 300 mg/d) Parenteral: 3–6 mg/kg per day intravenous (IV) divided every 6 h (maximum daily dose: 300 mg/d)
Omeprazole, esomeprazole, pantoprazole (proton pump inhibitor)	Oral: ≥15 kg to <40 kg: 20 mg PO daily ≥40 kg: 40 mg PO daily or 1 to 2 mg/kg/day Parenteral (limited pediatric data available) 0.8–1.6 mg/kg per day IV (maximum dose: 80 mg)
Cytoprotection	
Sucralfate	40–80 mg/kg per day PO (in 4 divided doses)
Vasoconstriction	
Octreotide	Continuous IV infusion (limited pediatric data available) 1 μg/kg IV bolus (max: 50 μg) followed by 1–2 μg/kg per hour continuous infusion. Once bleeding is controlled, decrease dose by 50% every 12 h
Vasopressin	Continuous IV infusion (limited pediatric data available): Initial: 2–5 mU/kg per minute, titrate dose as needed with maximum dose: 10 mU/kg per minute
Antibiotics for *Helicobacter pylori*	
Amoxicillin	25 mg/kg per dose PO twice daily (maximum dose: 1000 mg/dose)
Clarithromycin	10 mg/kg per dose PO twice daily (maximum dose: 500 mg/dose)
Metronidazole	10 mg/kg per dose PO twice daily (maximum dose: 500 mg/dose)

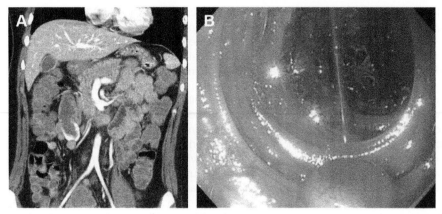

Fig. 8. CT angiography in a 16-year-old girl presenting with massive gastrointeestinal bleeding reveals contrast within loop of proximal small bowel during arterial phase (*A*). Pulsatile bleeding from Dieulafoy lesion found in jejunum during intraoperative enteroscopy (*B*).

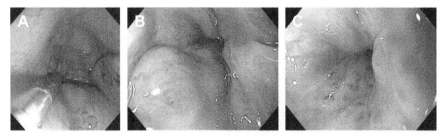

Fig. 9. Variceal sclerotherapy in infant with portal hypertension due to cirrhotic liver disease. Catheter with needle for injection (*A*). Varix before and immediately after injection (*B, C*).

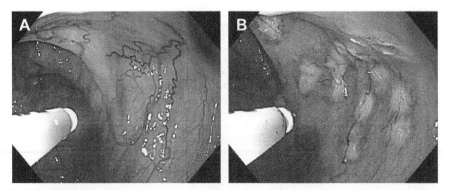

Fig. 10. APC therapy. Reticular venous malformation before and immediately after treatment (*A, B*).

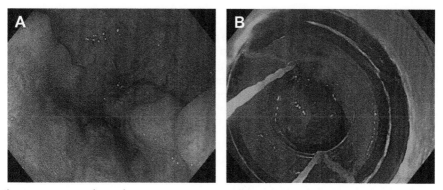

Fig. 11. Large esophageal varices in a patient with portal vein thrombosis (*A*). Band ligated varix viewed through endoscopic ligation adaptor (*B*).

thermal energy to nearby lesions. APC is most effective for treating superficial oozing from multiple lesions or a large surface area (**Fig. 10**). Hemostatic clips are highly effective for treating focal lesions (see **Fig. 7**). In cases of variceal disease, endoscopic band ligation and injection of sclerotherapeutic agents can arrest variceal hemorrhage. Variceal band ligation has been shown to be more effective than sclerotherapy in eliminating varices with lower rebleeding rates, but is not an option for infants due to the relatively large diameter of the band ligation adaptor (**Fig. 11**). Nearly all polyps in children can be safely and effectively removed endoscopically, avoiding unnecessary surgical intervention (**Fig. 12**).

Other therapy
Operative or interventional radiologic interventions should be pursued if bleeding cannot be controlled by medical or endoscopic interventions. Angiography may be useful to localize a source of obscure bleeding. In some situations, angiographic embolization may be preferred to operative intervention. However, duodenal ulcers may lead to brisk arterial bleeds or perforations that require urgent surgical control. There also are surgical strategies for creation of portosystemic shunts to manage gastroesophageal varices due to refractory portal hypertension.

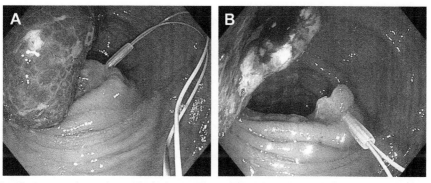

Fig. 12. Large colon polyp with thick vascular pedicle (*A*). Endoloop ligature applied to prevent postpolypectomy bleeding (*B*).

SUMMARY

Gastrointestinal bleeding can have variable presentations based on the location of the bleeding source, severity of the bleed, and age of the patient. A detailed history and physical examination provide clues about the underlying etiology. Careful monitoring of the patient's hemodynamic status and consideration of other comorbidities also will guide management decisions. Collaboration of gastroenterologists, interventional radiologists, and surgeons is encouraged to efficiently identify the source and effectively control the bleeding.

REFERENCES

1. Wyllie R, Hyams JS, Kay M. Pediatric gastrointestinal and liver disease. Philadelphia: Elsevier Health Sciences; 2015.
2. Boyle JT. Gastrointestinal bleeding in infants and children. Pediatr Rev 2008; 29(2):39–52.
3. Raju GS, Gerson L, Das A, et al. American Gastroenterological Association (AGA) Institute Technical Review on obscure gastrointestinal bleeding. Gastroenterology 2007;133(5):1697–717.
4. Fisher L, Lee Krinsky M, Anderson MA, et al. The role of endoscopy in the management of obscure GI bleeding. Gastrointest Endosc 2010;72(3):471–9.
5. Fox VL. Gastrointestinal bleeding in infancy and childhood. Gastroenterol Clin North Am 2000;29(1):37–66, v.
6. Chawla S, Seth D, Mahajan P, et al. Upper gastrointestinal bleeding in children. Clin Pediatr 2007;46(1):16–21.
7. Lane VA, Sugarman ID. Investigation of rectal bleeding in children. Paediatrics Child Health 2010;20(10):465–72.
8. Squires RH. Gastrointestinal bleeding. Pediatr Rev 1999;20(3):95–101.
9. Teach SJ, Fleisher GR. Rectal bleeding in the pediatric emergency department. Ann Emerg Med 1994;23(6):1252–8.
10. Pianosi P, Al-sadoon H. Hemoptysis in children. Pediatr Rev 1996;17(10):344–8.
11. Kramer RE, Lerner DG, Lin T, et al. Management of ingested foreign bodies in children: a clinical report of the NASPGHAN Endoscopy Committee. J Pediatr Gastroenterol Nutr 2015;60(4):562–74.
12. Ng YYR, Ong HL, Sim SW, et al. Candy crush: a confounding presentation of blood per rectum in a child. BMJ Case Rep 2015;2015 [pii:bcr2015211634].
13. Graves R, Weaver SP. Cefdinir-associated "bloody stools" in an infant. J Am Board Fam Med 2008;21(3):246–8.
14. Apt L, Downey WS. "Melena" neonatorum: the swallowed blood syndrome. J Pediatr 1955;47(1):6–12.
15. Coello-Ramirez P, Larrosa-Haro A. Gastrointestinal occult hemorrhage and gastroduodenitis in cow's milk protein intolerance. J Pediatr Gastroenterol Nutr 1984;3(2):215–8.
16. El Mouzan MI, Al Quorain AA, Anim JT. Cow's-milk-induced erosive gastritis in an infant. J Pediatr Gastroenterol Nutr 1990;10(1):111–3.
17. Kravis LP, Donsky G, Lecks HI. Upper and lower gastrointestinal tract bleeding induced by whole cow's milk in an atopic infant. Pediatrics 1967;40(4):661–5.
18. Shearer MJ. Vitamin K deficiency bleeding (VKDB) in early infancy. Blood Rev 2009;23(2):49–59.
19. Krzyżanowska P, Książyk J, Kocielińska-Kłos M, et al. Vitamin K status in patients with short bowel syndrome. Clin Nutr 2012;31(6):1015–7.

20. Sharma R, Hudak ML. A clinical perspective of necrotizing enterocolitis: past, present, and future. Clin Perinatol 2013;40(1):27–51.
21. Lee HC, Pickard SS, Sridhar S, et al. Intestinal malrotation and catastrophic volvulus in infancy. J Emerg Med 2012;43(1):e49–51.
22. Oldham KT, Brown B, LaPlante MM, et al. Principles and practice of pediatric surgery. 2nd edition. Available at: http://site.ebrary.com/lib/vanderbilt/Doc?id=10865287. Accessed February 24, 2017.
23. Villanueva C, Colomo A, Bosch A, et al. Transfusion strategies for acute upper gastrointestinal bleeding. N Engl J Med 2013;368(1):11–21.
24. Cuellar RE, Gavaler JS, Alexander JA, et al. Gastrointestinal tract hemorrhage: the value of a nasogastric aspirate. Arch Intern Med 1990;150(7):1381–4.
25. Silverstein FE, Gilbert DA, Tedesco FJ, et al. The national ASGE survey on upper gastrointestinal bleeding. Gastrointest Endosc 1981;27(2):94–102.
26. Feldman M, Friedman LS, Brandt LJ. Sleisenger and Fordtran's gastrointestinal and liver disease : pathophysiology/diagnosis/management. 10th edition. Available at: https://www.clinicalkey.com/dura/browse/bookChapter/3-s2.0-C20121000197; http://alltitles.ebrary.com/Doc?id=11045491. Accessed February 24, 2017.
27. Kay MH, Wyllie R. Therapeutic endoscopy for nonvariceal gastrointestinal bleeding. J Pediatr Gastroenterol Nutr 2007;45(2):157–71.
28. Iddan G, Meron G, Glukhovsky A, et al. Wireless capsule endoscopy. Nature 2000;405(6785):417.
29. El-Matary W. Wireless capsule endoscopy: indications, limitations, and future challenges. J Pediatr Gastroenterol Nutr 2008;46(1):4–12.
30. Kumar R, Tripathi M, Chandrashekar N, et al. Diagnosis of ectopic gastric mucosa using 99Tcm-pertechnetate: spectrum of scintigraphic findings. Br J Radiol 2005;78(932):714–20.
31. Kiratli PO, Aksoy T, Bozkurt MF, et al. Detection of ectopic gastric mucosa using 99mTc pertechnetate: review of the literature. Ann Nucl Med 2009;23(2):97–105.
32. Concha R, Amaro R, Barkin JS. Obscure gastrointestinal bleeding: diagnostic and therapeutic approach. J Clin Gastroenterol 2007;41(3):242–51.
33. Zettinig G, Staudenherz A, Leitha T. The importance of delayed images in gastrointestinal bleeding scintigraphy. Nucl Med Commun 2002;23(8):803–8.
34. Rollins E, Picus D, Hicks M, et al. Angiography is useful in detecting the source of chronic gastrointestinal bleeding of obscure origin. AJR Am J Roentgenol 1991; 156(2):385–8.
35. Zuckerman GR, Prakash C. Acute lower intestinal bleeding. Part I: clinical presentation and diagnosis. Gastrointest Endosc 1998;48(6):606–16.
36. Siafakas C, Fox VL, Nurko S. Use of octreotide for the treatment of severe gastrointestinal bleeding in children. J Pediatr Gastroenterol Nutr 1998;26(3):356–9.
37. Shneider BL. Portal hypertension in pediatrics: controversies and challenges 2015 report. In: de Franchis R, editor. Portal hypertension VI: proceedings of the sixth Baveno Consensus Workshop: stratifying risk and individualizing care. Cham (Switzerland): Springer International Publishing; 2016. p. 289–300.
38. Mills R, Burke S. Gastrointestinal bleeding in a 15 month old male: a presentation of Munchausen's syndrome by proxy. Clin Pediatr 1990;29(8):474–7.
39. Parfitt JR, Driman DK. Pathological effects of drugs on the gastrointestinal tract: a review. Hum Pathol 2007;38(4):527–36.
40. Prabhakaran S, Doraiswamy VA, Nagaraja V, et al. Nasoenteric tube complications. Scand J Surg 2012;101(3):147–55.
41. Bak-Romaniszyn L, Małecka-Panas E, Czkwianianc E, et al. Mallory-Weiss syndrome in children. Dis Esophagus 1999;12(1):65–7.

42. McBane RD, Gross JB. Herpes esophagitis: clinical syndrome, endoscopic appearance, and diagnosis in 23 patients. Gastrointest Endosc 1991;37(6): 600–3.

43. Brown K, Lundborg P, Levinson J, et al. Incidence of peptic ulcer bleeding in the US pediatric population. J Pediatr Gastroenterol Nutr 2012;54(6):733–6.

44. Marshall JM. Gastrojejunal ulcers in children. AMA Arch Surg 1953;67(3):490–2.

45. Sondheimer JM, Sokol RJ, Narkewicz MR, et al. Anastomotic ulceration: a late complication of ileocolonic anastomosis. J Pediatr 1995;127(2):225–30.

46. Harig JM, Soergel KH, Komorowski RA, et al. Treatment of diversion colitis with short-chain-fatty acid irrigation. N Engl J Med 1989;320(1):23–8.

47. Tringali A, Balassone V, De Angelis P, et al. Complications in pediatric endoscopy. Best Pract Res Clin Gastroenterol 2016;30(5):825–39.

48. Baillie J. Hemobilia. Gastroenterol Hepatol 2012;8(4):270–2.

49. Stockwell JA, Werner HA, Marsano LS. Dieulafoy's lesion in an infant: a rare cause of massive gastrointestinal bleeding. J Pediatr Gastroenterol Nutr 2000;31(1): 68–70.

50. Itani M, Alsaied T, Charafeddine L, et al. Dieulafoy's lesion in children. J Pediatr Gastroenterol Nutr 2010;51(5):672–4.

51. Fishman SJ, Smithers CJ, Folkman J, et al. Blue rubber bleb nevus syndrome: surgical eradication of gastrointestinal bleeding. Ann Surg 2005;241(3):523–8.

52. Azizkhan RG. Life-threatening hematochezia from a rectosigmoid vascular malformation in Klippel-Trenaunay syndrome: long-term palliation using an argon laser. J Pediatr Surg 1991;26(9):1125–8.

53. Soukoulis IW, Liang MG, Fox VL, et al. Gastrointestinal infantile hemangioma: presentation and management. J Pediatr Gastroenterol Nutr 2015;61(4):415–20.

54. Shovlin CL, Guttmacher AE, Buscarini E, et al. Diagnostic criteria for hereditary hemorrhagic telangiectasia (Rendu-Osler-Weber syndrome). Am J Med Genet 2000;91(1):66–7.

55. Chang WL, Yang YH, Lin YT, et al. Gastrointestinal manifestations in Henoch-Schönlein purpura: a review of 261 patients. Acta Paediatr 2004;93(11):1427–31.

56. Choong CK, Beasley SW. Intra-abdominal manifestations of Henoch-Schönlein purpura. J Paediatr Child Health 1998;34(5):405–9.

57. Eroglu Y, Emerick KM, Chou PM, et al. Gastrointestinal bleeding in Turner's syndrome: a case report and literature review. J Pediatr Gastroenterol Nutr 2002; 35(1):84–7.

58. Burge D, Middleton A, Kamath R, et al. Intestinal haemorrhage in Turner's syndrome. Arch Dis Child 1981;56(7):557–8.

59. Zakko L. Ehlers–Danlos syndrome type IV (vascular): gastrointestinal features. In: Wu GY, Selsky N, Grant-Kels JM, editors. Atlas of dermatological manifestations of gastrointestinal disease. New York: Springer New York; 2013. p. 73–4.

60. Prasad V, Fishman SJ, Mulliken JB, et al. Cutaneovisceral angiomatosis with thrombocytopenia. Pediatr Dev Pathol 2005;8(4):407–19.

61. Frykman PK, Short SS. Hirschsprung-associated enterocolitis: prevention and therapy. Semin Pediatr Surg 2012;21(4):328–35.

62. Rossi V, Avanzini S, Mosconi M, et al. Hirschsprung associated enterocolitis. J Gastrointest Dig Syst 2014;4:170.

63. Mizrahi S, Laor D, Stamler B. Intestinal ischemia induced by cocaine abuse. Arch Surg 1988;123(3):394.

64. Hebra A, Brown MF, Hirschl RB, et al. Mesenteric ischemia in hypoplastic left heart syndrome. J Pediatr Surg 1993;28(4):606–11.

65. St-Vil D, Brandt ML, Panic S, et al. Meckel's diverticulum in children: a 20-year review. J Pediatr Surg 1991;26(11):1289–92.
66. Lee KJ, Choi SJ, Yang HR, et al. Stepwise endoscopy based on sigmoidoscopy in evaluating pediatric graft-versus-host disease. Pediatr Gastroenterol Hepatol Nutr 2016;19(1):29–37.
67. Calmet FH, Yarur AJ, Pukazhendhi G, et al. Endoscopic and histological features of mycophenolate mofetil colitis in patients after solid organ transplantation. Ann Gastroenterol 2015;28(3):366–73.
68. Jenny C, Crawford-Jakubiak JE, Jenny C, et al. The evaluation of children in the primary care setting when sexual abuse is suspected. Pediatrics 2013;132(2):e558–67.

Celiac Disease and Nonceliac Gluten Sensitivity

Runa D. Watkins, MD*, Shamila Zawahir, MD

KEYWORDS

- Celiac disease • Gluten-free diet • Tissue transglutaminase • Autoimmune
- Children • Wheat allergy • Nonceliac gluten sensitivity

KEY POINTS

- Celiac disease is found in genetically susceptible individuals who carry the HLA DQ2 or DQ8 gene.
- Celiac serology testing is a good screening tool.
- The gold standard for diagnosis is still an upper endoscopy to acquire small bowel biopsies.
- Currently the only available treatment is gluten-free diet.
- NCGS can be considered in those without evidence of celiac disease and wheat allergy who have clinical improvement on a gluten-free diet.

INTRODUCTION

Celiac disease (CD) is an autoimmune enteropathy that causes damage to the small intestinal mucosa when gluten, found in wheat, barley, and rye, is ingested, which only occurs in genetically susceptible individuals. Innate gluten sensitivity, adaptive gluten sensitivity, and autoimmunity are essential in the development of CD.[1]

The prevalence of CD has been increasing worldwide, most likely because of greater awareness and better testing. Gluten has a high concentration of glutamine and proline residues referred to as prolamines, which are specifically found in wheat, barley, and rye. It is thought that under stressful situations, such as infection or surgery, the gliadin protein enters the lamina propria where it is deaminated by the enzyme tissue transglutaminase (tTG) and then it becomes attached to it to form a

Disclosure Statement: The authors have no commercial or financial disclosures.
Pediatric Gastroenterology & Nutrition, University of Maryland, 22 South Greene Street, N5W68, Baltimore, MD 21201, USA
* Corresponding author:
E-mail address: rwatkins@peds.umaryland.edu

complex. This specific complex is then presented to the antigen-presenting cell resulting in secretion of proinflammatory mediators.[2] This process ultimately produces intestinal inflammation resulting in crypt hyperplasia and villous atrophy. CD should also be considered in certain populations with an increased prevalence of CD, such as those with selective IgA deficiency, first-degree relatives of patients with CD, autoimmune thyroiditis, type I diabetes, Down syndrome, Turner syndrome, and Williams syndrome.[3]

EPIDEMIOLOGY

CD occurs in genetically susceptible individuals, but the pattern of genetic inheritance is still somewhat obscure. The prevalence of CD is about 1% within the United States and Europe, and this may be even higher in certain Northern European countries.[4] It is now becoming a common disorder in North Africa, the Middle East, and India. However, the diagnostic rates are low in these regions because of low availability of diagnostic facilities and poor disease awareness.[5] It is thought that the increase in prevalence is also attributed to the adaptation of Western gluten-rich dietary patterns. Many new diagnoses are also being made through screening individuals who are at risk because of family history of CD.

SYMPTOMS

The range of symptoms present in CD is a wide spectrum. Individuals may have the classic symptoms of abdominal pain with diarrhea or constipation, neurologic manifestations, or be completely asymptomatic. Symptoms are described as typical, atypical, and latent. **Table 1** lists the specific symptoms according to their categories. The classic, or typical symptoms, usually emerge in the pediatric age and consist of diarrhea, abdominal pain, and weight loss, and poor growth. The atypical presentations include osteoporosis, dermatitis herpetiformis, peripheral neuropathy, short stature, delayed puberty, dental enamel hypoplasia, and anemia. A mild elevation of serum liver enzymes is well described as an initial presentation of CD in pediatric patients. Headaches, seizures, and psychiatric symptoms are also associated with CD.

The latent form of CD is defined as having a predisposing gene, normal biopsy findings, and weakly positive serologies.[6] It is thought that environmental factors affect the disease's clinical presentation, the time at presentation, and the characteristics of the disease.[7] Theories are now emerging in regards to infectious agents playing a role, at least on the timing of the presentation.[8]

Table 1		
Signs and symptoms of celiac disease		
Typical	**Atypical**	**Latent**
Diarrhea	Osteoporosis/fractures	Gene positive
Abdominal pain	Dermatitis herpetiformis	Weakly positive serologies
Bloating	Nonspecific transaminitis	Normal biopsies
Gassy	Fatigue	
Constipation	Anemia	
Alternating diarrhea and	Migraines	
constipation	Peripheral neuropathy	
Failure to thrive/weight loss	Dental enamel hypoplasia	
Vomiting	Short stature/delayed puberty	

DIAGNOSIS OF CELIAC DISEASE

Until the 1950s, CD was a clinical diagnosis based on observations focused on malabsorptive features.[9] Now, the first step in determining if a patient has CD is to obtain serologies. The sensitivity and specificity of detecting CD is now close to 95% or greater, despite its checkered past. The antigliadin antibodies were first developed in the 1980s, but showed a sensitivity and specificity between 80% and 90%. The endomysial antibody (EMA) was developed next in the mid-1980s, which was found to be highly accurate, but difficult to standardize. This assay requires monkey esophagus or human tissue as a substrate, and an individual reading the sample, adding to interobserver variability. Despite the disadvantages, the sensitivity and specificity of EMA is found to be greater than 90%.[10] In the late 1990s, tTG was identified as a CD autoantigen and it has now become the test of choice not only for diagnosis, but also for monitoring CD, given its sensitivity of 99%.[11] The accuracy of deaminated gliadins is controversial. It seems to be the most sensitive and specific in those younger than 3 year old.[12] It is important to remember that a total IgA level should always be ordered to assess for selective IgA deficiency, because it is the most common immune deficiency in children If this is truly present, it will lead to false-negative results. Of note, low levels of IgA that are not deficient will not affect the test specificity. However, if an individual truly has selective IgA deficiency, serologic testing offers little advantage over directly proceeding to intestinal biopsy to establish the diagnosis. **Table 2** lists the antibody tests available and their associated sensitivities and specificities.

HLA testing should also be considered during a work-up for CD. It is known that 95% of those with CD are HLA DQ2 positive and the rest are HLA DQ8 positive. However, about 40% of the general population also carries one of these genes, making genetic testing poorly specific.[13] This test may be of benefit in those who are asymptomatic with negative serologies, but belong to an at-risk group. The high negative predictive value of genetic testing allows one to eliminate the possibility of ever developing the disease.

The gold standard for diagnosis is still with a small intestinal biopsy when an individual is consuming gluten, to document duodenal damage, mainly villous atrophy. Gross findings during an upper endoscopy include scalloping of the duodenal mucosa

Table 2 Serologic test comparison		
	Sensitivity %	Specificity %
AGA IgA	69–85	73–90
AGA IgG	75–90	82–95
DGP IgA	74–99	90–99
DGP IgG	63–95	90–99
EMA (IgA)	85–98	97–100
tTG IgA	90–99	94–99
tTG IgG	45–95	94–97

AGA IgA and AGA IgG tests are no longer recommended as initial testing because of the inferior accuracy.

Abbreviations: AGA, antigliadin antibody; DGP, deaminted gliadin peptide.

From Hill ID, Dirks MH, Liptak GS, et al. Guideline for the diagnosis and treatment of celiac disease in children: recommendations of the North American Society for Pediatric Gastroenterology, Hepatology and Nutrition. J Pediatr Gastroenterol Nutr 2005:40;1–19.

(**Fig. 1**). However, if this is not present, it does not exclude a diagnosis, because the microscopic changes are mainly consistent with a diagnosis. The characteristic histologic features include infiltration of lymphocytes in the epithelium (>25 lymphocytes per 100 epithelial cells), increased density and depth of crypts, and varying degrees of villous atrophy. This progression was first described by Marsh in 1992, and his scoring system, from stage 0 (normal) to stage 3 (villous blunting) subsequently modified by Oberhuber and colleagues,[14] is now widely used by pathologists (**Table 3** for Marsh classification).[15,16] Biopsy findings are not necessarily pathognomonic and are seen in other conditions. **Box 1** provides a list of other causes of villous atrophy occurring in the duodenum. It is the constellation of clinical, histologic, and serologic findings, and response to therapy, that ultimately provide a confirmation of a CD diagnosis (**Figs. 2–4**).

In 2012, the European Society of Gastroenterology, Hepatology and Nutrition published their guidelines for CD and suggested that a nonbiopsy diagnosis of CD could be considered in a certain patient population who has 10 times the elevation of tTg IgA, a positive EMA-IgA, and the presence of the HLA DQ2/8 haploytpe. The subsequent resolution of symptoms and normalization of the tTG titer on a gluten-free diet (GFD) confirms the diagnosis.[17] Although a nonbiopsy diagnosis of CD is desirable, there are potential risks of avoiding biopsy. Currently, there is no standardization of serologic tests for CD in the United States, because there are marked variations in antibody levels between commercial assays. There is also a possible risk of a false diagnosis of CD without the biopsy and placing a patient on a lifelong GFD. The North American Society for Pediatric Gastroenterology, Hepatology and Nutrition clinical practice guidelines differ in that they recommend a duodenal biopsy for the diagnosis of CD.[3]

There is a group of patients who has positive serology and normal histology. They can be grouped in the latent form, but one needs to make sure that they are exposed to adequate amounts of gluten before biopsy. One also needs to determine if an adequate number of biopsies were taken from the bulb and second portion of the duodenum and their histologic orientation is correct. Capsule endoscopy is helpful in this group of patients to look for mucosal scalloping. Abnormal capsule endoscopy can be followed by push enteroscopy to obtain biopsy. In this subgroup of patients, HLA

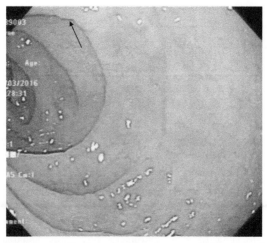

Fig. 1. Arrow pointing to gross finding of scallped mucosa in the second portion of the duodenum on endoscopy.

Table 3
Histologic features and grading of celiac disease

Marsh 0	Marsh 1	Marsh 2	Marsh 3A	Marsh 3B	Marsh 3C
No histologic changes	Increased IEL	Increased IEL with crypt hyperplasia	Increased IEL, crypt hyperplasia, partial villous atrophy	Increased IEL, crypt hyperplasia, subtotal villous atrophy	Increased IEL, crypt hyperplasia, total villous atrophy

Abbreviation: IEL, intraepithelial lymphocytosis.

typing is useful. If HLA DQ2 and DQ8 are negative, CD is unlikely. If positive, they can have potential CD-latent form and the next step is decided depending on each individual patient. If they are symptomatic, they can be placed on a GFD and the clinician would follow symptoms and serologies and consider rechallenging with a gluten-containing diet in the future. If they are asymptomatic, patients can stay on regular diet with close follow-up of their serology testing with potential rebiopsy in the future.

TREATMENT OF CELIAC DISEASE

Currently, the only available treatment of CD is a lifelong GFD. Treatment should only be started after diagnosis is confirmed by intestinal biopsy.

The goals of treatment are resolution of symptoms, maintenance of normal growth, and development and improvement of histology. Persistent villous atrophy and inflammation has been associated with increased morbidity and increased risk of malignancy. Adherence to the diet allows an individual to achieve a goal of histologic remission of their CD, which should occur within 1 to 2 years of strict diet adherence.[18] Studies show that about 45% to 80% of children are adherent to GFD. There are times where diet adherence may be difficult, especially during adolescent years. The common complaints of the diet are that foods are less tasty and more expensive. There is also associated anxiety and a negative social effect leading to decreased quality of life, because one is constantly needing to be vigilant to avoid gluten contamination.[19] Because of this, adolescents are in need of more psychosocial support and physician-dietician involvement with their daily routine and school life. But, a progressive decline

Box 1
Other causes of villous atrophy in the duodenum

Marasmus

Crohn disease

Giardiasis

Autoimmune enteropathy

Drug induced (ie, olmesartan)

Graft-versus-host disease

AIDS-associated enteropathy

Intestinal lymphoma

Tropical sprue

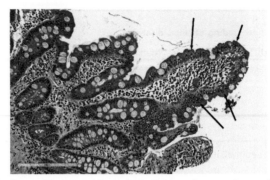

Fig. 2. Marsh 1 findings of increased intraepithelial lymphocytes (*arrows*), but architectural preservation of villi is present.

and eventual normalization of serology over 12 to 24 months of GFD is a good indicator of compliance with GFD.

Foods that are allowed in a GFD include beans; nuts; fresh eggs; fresh meats, fish, and poultry; fruits; vegetables; and most dairy products. Meats should not be breaded, batter coated, or marinated. It is important to make sure foods are not processed or mixed with gluten-containing grains, additives, or preservatives. There are many grains and starches that are part of a GFD, including almond meal flour, corn, cornmeal, coconut flour, quinoa, pea flour, potato flour, sorghum, soy, and tapioca. Patients should always avoid all foods and drinks that contain rye and barley. Barley is found in such products as malt, malt flavoring, and malt vinegar. Patients should also avoid triticale, which is a cross between wheat and rye that was first bred in laboratories during the late nineteenth century in Scotland and Germany.[20] Unless labeled gluten free, patients should avoid beer, candies, salad dressings, sauces, or soup bases. There are breads made with corn, rice, or soy that also contain gluten. Patients should avoid oats unless it is specified as gluten free, and currently, 50 g of gluten-free oats is considered safe.

Cross-contamination is also another important topic to discuss with families. It occurs when gluten-free foods come into contact with foods that contain gluten. It can happen during the manufacturing process, such as when the same equipment is used to make a variety of products. If a product carries a gluten-free label, the Food and Drug Administration requires that the product contain less than 20 parts per

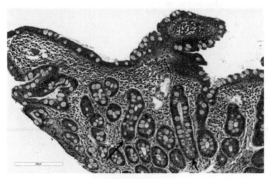

Fig. 3. Marsh 2 findings of crypt hyperplasia (*arrows*).

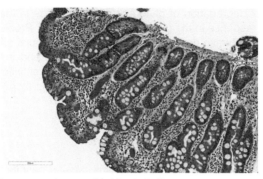

Fig. 4. Blunted villi seen, consistent with Marsh 3 disease.

million of gluten. However, the threshold of gluten in gluten-free products is under debate, because the consumption of even these trace amounts of gluten allowed by the Food and Drug Administration may be responsible for continuing symptoms seen by some patients with CD. In a study done by Faulkner-Hogg and coworkers,[21] most patients with CD with persistent symptoms who switched to a no detectable gluten diet had either partial or complete resolution of symptoms. Therefore, it is important to provide patients with extensive nutrition counseling, because patients need to be aware that products labeled "wheat-free" may still contain gluten.

POTENTIAL RESEARCH TREATMENTS

Currently the GFD includes flour from rice, corn, soybean, and other less popular crops, which are poor in B vitamins and essential nutrients. They are also often devoid of flavor. Because of this, genetically modified gluten has been proposed, which thus far has shown to have a decreased immunogenicity in those with CD.[22] Zonulin is extensively being studied, because it is an endogenous modulator of epithelial tight junctions. It is known that gliadin causes increased zonulin secretion leading to increased intestinal permeability, allowing the transport of gluten, which then triggers an inflammatory process.[22] Larazotide acetate is being trialed because it has shown to decrease tight junction permeability by inhibiting zonulin receptors, which leads to stabilization of the protein connections of the intestinal epithelium. It has also shown a blunted response of tTG antibodies when exposed to gluten contamination.[23] In a study by Paterson and colleagues,[24] there was a 70% increase in intestinal permeability following a gluten ingestion in the placebo group, compared with those who received 12 mg of larazotide acetate. Although it is unlikely to be a cure and does not provide a free pass to continue eating gluten, it may well be considered maintenance therapy to improve symptoms and quality of life, while still in conjunction with a GFD.

Therapeutic vaccines have also been considered with the aim of modifying the T-cell response. Although current studies show an induction of tolerance of gliadin peptides, it seems as if the vaccine may only be effective in patients with CD who are positive for the HLA DQ2 haplotype. There have been attempts to alter the immune response through infecting patients with CD with parasites. Unfortunately, further investigation was called into question because no benefit was observed in these clinical trials. Oral enzyme supplementation seems to be more promising, because researchers in Europe found that orally administered oligopeptidases allow the degradation of toxic gliadin peptides before they reach the small intestinal mucosa.[25]

Ideally, the optimal degradation of gluten should take place in the stomach, which limits the immune response in the proximal small intestine.[26] Probiotics are currently popular, because they have demonstrated to have a beneficial effect in those with small intestinal bacterial overgrowth, lactose intolerance, and irritable bowel syndrome (IBS). Unfortunately, studies have not demonstrated a significant effect in those with CD.[27] It is well known that glucocorticoids and biologic therapies modulate the inflammatory reaction and are often used in refractory CD.

In summary GFD is the only treatment available for CD.

REFRACTORY CELIAC DISEASE

Refractory CD must be considered if symptoms persist, despite being on a GFD, and histologic damage of the small intestinal mucosa continues. Refractory CD is classified as type 1 and 2, where type 1 is responsive to corticosteroids. Type 2 is considered a premalignant condition where almost 50% of patients develop enteropathy-associated T-cell lymphoma within 5 years of diagnosis. Type 2 refractory CD is diagnosed from biopsy specimens that show monoclonality and occurs when an individual loses antibodies to tTG and there is infiltration of lymphocytes in the intestinal epithelium that lack expression of CD8, CD4, and TCRs.[28]

MONITORING

Multiple guidelines call for routine monitoring of patients with CD, because this is a lifelong inflammatory condition. At time of diagnosis, all patients should have extensive nutrition counseling with an experienced dietician, because a GFD is the core management strategy. Patients should also be encouraged to join their local and/or national celiac support group.[5] Patients should be examined every 6 months in their first year of diagnosis to monitor symptoms, dietary adherence, nutrition, and serologic features.[29,30] It is recommended that tTG IgA should be measured after 6 months of adhering to a GFD. At this time, there should be a decline in the value, which provides an indirect indicator of dietary adherence and recovery. This marker should, again, be measured at 12 months after the diet to monitor adherence to the GFD. All patients should have annual hematologic and biochemical profiles. Because bone mineral density is one of the more common extraintestinal manifestations of CD, a dual-energy x-ray absorptiometry scan is recommended in the first year of diagnosis.[30] The most controversial aspect of monitoring patients with CD concerns the timing and role of repeat endoscopy with small bowel biopsies. Patients should understand that seroconversion with a GFD does not necessarily imply healing of the small intestine. The only accurate method available to verify intestinal healing is biopsy.[31]

NONCELIAC GLUTEN SENSITIVITY

According to the Oslo Definitions for CD, nonceliac gluten sensitivity (NCGS) is defined as being one or more of a variety of immunologic, morphologic, or symptomatic manifestations that is precipitated by the ingestion of gluten in individuals in whom CD has been excluded.[32] Whereas gluten-related disorders is an umbrella term to describe all conditions related to the dietary exposure to gluten, NCGS specifically references a clinical scenario in which a patient has symptoms with gluten exposure and has resolution with removal of gluten, without having a diagnosis of CD. This was first described in 1980 by Cooper and colleagues[33] and has recently been the subject of much research to help diagnose, evaluate, and manage individuals who describe symptoms that mimic other conditions, such as CD, wheat allergy, IBS, and lactose/fructose malabsorption.

Epidemiology

The incidence of NCGS is unknown. The condition is often self-diagnosed and managed with a GFD without the input of a physician. Cited rates of prevalence have ranged from less than 1% to 6% of the population.[34] This wide range is likely caused by different definitions and varying study designs. It is thought to be more common than CD, which is approximately 1% of the general population. There is a female predominance of 3:1, but no specific risk factors for the development of NCGS have been identified, nor have long-term consequences.[35]

Pathophysiology

The pathophysiology of NCGS is also unknown. It had been shown that in contrast to CD, there is normal intestinal permeability. The duodenal mucosa of patients with NCGS does not show inflammatory marker expression when incubated with gliadin in vitro and there is also no basophil activation, as compared with patients with CD.[36] Wheat amylase-tryptase inhibitors, which are a family of proteins in wheat that are highly resistant to proteolysis, may drive the innate immune system toward an inflammatory state in NCGS and these amylase-tryptase inhibitors are proteins that are resistant to proteolysis.[37]

Clinical Features

The prevalence of specific clinical features of NCGS is lacking, although there have been studies describing relative incidences of symptoms, both intestinal and extraintestinal in the study population. The manifestations can occur soon after ingestion of gluten and regress with gluten withdrawal. They then reappear when gluten is reintroduced in hours to days after re-exposure. NCGS, clinically, is similar to IBS with abdominal pain, bloating, and changes in bowel characteristics (diarrhea and/or constipation). There are also reported systemic features of "brain fog," headaches, joint pain, fatigue, depression, extremity numbness, dermatitis, and anemia. Other features include weight loss, gas, glossitis, and behavior changes.[38] In children with NCGS, gastrointestinal symptoms tend to dominate, but the most common extraintestinal manifestation is reported to be fatigue.[39]

Of note, as compared with the CD patient population, there is no increased prevalence of comorbid autoimmune diseases, such as type 1 diabetes mellitus and autoimmune thyroiditis, in patients with NCGS.[40] The psychiatric comorbid conditions of CD, such as anxiety and depression, are similar in patients with NCGS and CD. Whether there is a role of NCGS in neuropsychiatric illness is still being debated, because it has been implicated by some to be a cause of schizophrenia, autism spectrum disorders (ASD), and depression.[41]

ASD is the fastest growing group of developmental disorders in the United States that has long been associated with gluten sensitivity. Linking ASDs with CD has been unconvincing, because there has been no serologic evidence to support a relationship between the two disorders.[42] However, one treatment modality, the gluten-free casein-free diet, has been popular in the management of children with ASDs. The role of a leaky gut enabling gluten peptides to advance to the blood brain-barrier and then interfere in neurotransmission has been suggested and there has been research into the prevalence of a leaky gut in children with ASDs to support this hypothesis.[43] Despite the popularity of the gluten-free casein-free diet as a treatment of ASDs, convincing evidence to support its use is lacking.

IBS and NCGS have significant clinical overlap. Some patients labeled with IBS may have improvement in symptoms with withdrawal for gluten from their diet. This was particularly true for the patients with IBS-D with HLA DQ2 and/or DQ8 genotypes who showed more frequent bowel movements on a gluten-containing diet and which was also associated with an increase in small intestinal permeability while on that diet.[44] Other than gluten, wheat, and wheat derivatives, there are other components that may trigger symptoms in patients with IBS, such as fructans, and therefore it is not clear to what component these patients may be responding to when gluten is eliminated. Patients with IBS also improve with the use of a FODMAP (fermentable oligo-, di-, and monosaccharide and polyols) diet, which removes highly fermentable, poorly absorbed, osmotic, short-chain carbohydrates, which can also be found in wheat. Whether it is the gluten or the FODMAP removal that results in clinical improvement is debatable. The difficulty of a clinical diagnosis in this condition, given its overlap with other diseases, is what is driving the need for the identification of specific biomarkers to help estimate the prevalence of this condition, and to aid in its diagnosis.

Evaluation

The frequency of self-diagnosis of gluten sensitivity has led to a large number of patients either presenting to the physician for evaluation while on a GFD or having tried it in the past. Of the utmost importance is determining whether or not the patient has CD. **Fig. 2** describes an algorithm to help differentiate between the two conditions. The specific antibodies for the diagnosis of CD are negative in patients with NCGS. However, some recent studies have shown this population may, in fact, have a high rate of positivity for AGA IgG. Patients with NCGS were demonstrated to have an elevated AGA IgG at 56.4% compared with 81.2% in untreated CD. This is far higher than the rates for autoimmune liver disease (21.5%), connective tissue disorders (9%), and healthy blood donors (2%–8%).[45] There are also concerns about the possibility of a wheat allergy arising in patients for whom a GFD results in symptoms improvement. In this population, IgE-based assays should also be considered.

Genotyping remains a component of the diagnostic algorithm in several scenarios. It may be necessary to evaluate patients already on a GFD in whom serologic testing is not an option, and in patients with borderline serology to help determine whether obtaining histologic evidence is warranted. Patients with NCGS have a prevalence rate for HLA-DQ2 and DQ-8 of approximately 50% as compared with 95% in CD and 20% of the general population.[46]

In patients with NCGS there is biopsy evidence of mild inflammation of the mucosa (Marsh 0–1) as compared with partial or subtotal villous atrophy and crypt hyperplasia in patients with CD.[47] The level of CD3[+] intraepithelial lymphocytosis present in those with NCGS is somewhere between healthy control subjects and patients with CD. There are other possible histologic findings in patients with NCGS, such as activated circulating basophils and increased incidence of eosinophilic infiltration in the duodenum and/or the ileum.[38,48]

Diagnosis

For the clinician, it is important to keep the diagnosis of NCGS as a possibility for patients presenting with intestinal and extraintestinal complaints that improve on a GFD, but also not to mistake it for CD or a wheat allergy. These two conditions should always be excluded before diagnosing NCGS. A diagnostic algorithm shown in **Fig. 5** rests on excluding CD by obtaining celiac serologies while on a gluten-containing diet. If these serologies are negative and the patient is not IgA deficient, then the patient is unlikely to have CD and NCGS may be the more likely diagnosis. Other

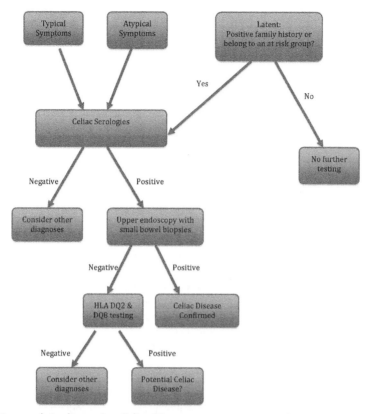

Fig. 5. Approach to diagnosing Celiac Disease.

supportive factors of this diagnosis include a lack of a personal history of autoimmune disease or family history of CD and absence of the features of malabsorption. If this is the case, further testing is not warranted. Those with equivocal serology would benefit from HLA typing to determine whether a biopsy is needed.[49] Once CD and wheat allergy are excluded, the patient should be placed on a GFD for at least 4 to 6 weeks. This typically results in significant improvement in several days and a subsequent gluten challenge should then be done to confirm the diagnosis.

Management

It is preferable to institute a gluten-limited diet in patients diagnosed with NCGS only after CD has been excluded. The need for a complete GFD versus a gluten-diminished diet depends on the patient's clinical response. Patients who remain on a GFD require nutritional support to ensure that macronutrient and micronutrient requirements are being met. In addition, because it is unknown whether this is a permanent or transitory condition, it is important to reassess the patient periodically (eg, every 6–12 months). This is particularly true of the pediatric population in whom dietary restrictions are onerous and may lead to other nutritional deficiencies. If the symptoms persist despite a gluten-restricted/GFD, other diagnoses should be entertained, such as lactose intolerance, IBS, fructose malabsorption, and small intestinal bacterial overgrowth.

REFERENCES

1. Marietta EV, David CS, Murray JA. Important lessons derived from animal models of celiac disease. Int Rev Immunol 2011;30:197–206.
2. Branski D, Fasano A, Troncone R. Latest developments in the pathogenesis and treatment of celiac disease. J Pediatr 2006;149:295–300.
3. Hill ID, Dirks MH, Liptak GS, et al. Guideline for the diagnosis and treatment of celiac disease in children: recommendations of the North American Society for Pediatric Gastroenterology, Hepatology and Nutrition. J Pediatr Gastroenterol Nutr 2005;40:1–19.
4. Barton SH, Murray JA. Celiac Disease and autoimmunity in the gut and elsewhere. Gastroenterol Clin North Am 2008;37(2):411–28.
5. Mocan O, Dumitrascu DL. The broad spectrum of celiac disease and gluten sensitivity enteropathy. Clujul Med 2016;89(3):335–42.
6. Rewers M. Epidemiology of celiac disease: what are the prevalence, incidence and progression of celiac disease? Gastroenterology 2005;128:S47–51.
7. Branski D. New insights in celiac disease. Rambam Maimonides Med J 2012; 3(1):e0006.
8. Kagnoff MF, Austin RK, Hubert JJ, et al. Possible role for a human adenovirus in the pathogenesis of celiac disease. J Exp Med 1984;160:1544–57.
9. Kelly CP, Bai JC, Liu E, et al. Advances in diagnosis and management of celiac disease. Gastroenterology 2015;148:1175–86.
10. Leffler DA, Schuppan D. Update on serologic testing in celiac disease. Am J Gastroenterol 2010;105:2250–4.
11. Dieterich W, Ehnis T, Bauer M, et al. Identification of tissue transglutaminase as the autoantigen of celiac disease. Nat Med 1997;3:797–801.
12. Holding S, Abuzakouk M, Doré PC. Antigliadin antibody testing for coeliac disease in children under 3 years of age is unhelpful. J Clin Pathol 2009;62:766–7.
13. Green PH, Jabri B. Coeliac disease. Lancet 2003;362(9381):383–91.
14. Oberhuber G, Granditsch G, Vogelsang H. The histopathology of celiac disease: time for a standardized report scheme for pathologist. Eur J Gastroenterol Hepatol 1999;11(10):1185–94.
15. Marsh MN. Gluten, major histocompatibility complex, and the small intestine. A molecular and immunobiologic approach to the spectrum of gluten sensitivity ('celiac sprue'). Gastroenterology 1992;102(1):330–54.
16. Rubio-Tapia A, Hill ID, Kelly CP, et al. Diagnosis and management of celiac disease. Am J Gastroenterol 2013;108:656–76.
17. Husby S, Koletzko S, Korponay-Szabó IR, et al. European Society for Pediatric Gastroenterology, Hepatology, and Nutrition guidelines for the diagnosis of coeliac disease. J Pediatr Gastroenterol Nutr 2012;54:136–60.
18. Szaflarska-Poplawska A. Non-dietary methods in the treatment of celiac disease. Prz Gastoenterol 2015;10(1):12–7.
19. Lee AR, Ng DL, Diamond B, et al. Living with celiac disease: survey results from the USA. J Hum Nutr Diet 2012;25:233–8.
20. Stace CA. Triticale: a case of nomenclatural mistreatment. Taxon 1987;36(2): 445–52.
21. Faulkner-Hogg KB, Selby WS, Loblay RH. Dietary analysis in symptomatic patients with celiac disease on a gluten-free diet: the role of trace amounts of gluten and non-gluten food intolerances. Scand J Gastroenterol 1999;34(8):784–9.

22. Baskshi A, Stephen S, Borum ML, et al. Emerging therapeutic options for celiac disease: potential alternatives to a gluten-free diet. Gastroenterol Hepatol 2012;8: 582–8.
23. Khaleghi S, Ju JM, Lamba A, et al. The potential utility of tight junction regulation in celiac disease: focus on larazotide acetate. Therap Adv Gastroenterol 2016; 9(1):37–49.
24. Paterson BM, Lammers KM, Arrieta MC, et al. The safety, tolerance, pharmacokinetic and pharmacodynamic effects of single doses of AT-1001 in celiac disease subjects: a proof of concept study. Aliment Pharmacol Ther 2007;26:757–66.
25. Watson P, Ding A, McMillan SA, et al. Implications of enzymatic detoxifications of gluten in celiac disease. Gastroenterology 2008;134:A213.
26. Ehren J, Govindarajan S, Morón B, et al. Protein engineering of improved propyl endopeptidases for therapy. Protein Eng Des Sel 2008;21:699–707.
27. Harnett K, Myers SP, Rolfe M. Probiotics and the microbiome in celiac disease: a randomized controlled trial. Evid Based Complement Alternat Med 2016; 2016:904.
28. Schuppan D, Junker Y, Barisani D. Celiac disease: from pathogenesis to novel therapies. Gastroenterology 2009;137:1912–33.
29. Bai JC, Fried M, Corazza GR, et al. World Gastroenterology Organisation global guidelines on celiac disease. J Clin Gastroenterol 2013;47:121–6.
30. Rubio-Tapia ID, Hill ID, Kelly CP, et al. ACG clinical guidelines: diagnosis and management of celiac disease. Am J Gastroenterol 2013;108:656.
31. Rubio-Tapia A, Rahim MW, See JA, et al. Mucosal recovery and mortality in adults with celiac disease after treatment with celiac disease after treatment with a gluten-free diet. Am J Gastroenterol 2010;105:1412–20.
32. Ludvigsson JF, Leffler DA, Bai JC, et al. The Oslo definitions for celiac disease and related terms. Gut 2013;62(1):43–52.
33. Cooper BT, Holmes GK, Ferguson R, et al. Gluten-sensitive diarrhea without evidence of celiac disease. Gastroenterology 1980;79:801–6.
34. Leonard MM, Vasagar B. US perspective on gluten-related disease. Clin Exp Gastroenterol 2014;7:25–37.
35. Catassi C, Bai JC, Bonaz B, et al. Non-celiac gluten sensitivity: the new frontier of gluten related disorders. Nutrients 2013;5(10):3839–53.
36. Bucci C, Zingone F, Russo I, et al. Gliadin does not induce mucosal inflammation or basophil activation in patients with non-celiac gluten sensitivity. Clin Gastroenterol Hepatol 2013;11:1294–9.
37. Sapone A, Leffler DA, Mukherjee R, et al. Non-celiac gluten sensitivity where are we now in 2015? Pract Gastroenterol 2015;142:40–8.
38. Mastrototaro L, Castellaneta S, Gentile A, et al. Gluten sensitivity in children: clinical, serological, genetic and histological description of the first paediatric series. Dig Liver Dis 2012;44:S254–5.
39. Volta U, Tovoli F, Cicola R, et al. Serological tests in gluten sensitivity nonceliac gluten intolerance. J Clin Gastroenterol 2012;46(8):680–5.
40. Lionetti E, Leonardi S, Franzonello C, et al. Gluten psychosis: confirmation of a new medical entity. Nutrients 2015;7(7):5532–9.
41. Batista I, Gandolfi L, Nobrega YK, et al. Autism spectrum disorder and celiac disease: no evidence for a link. Arq Neuropsiquiatr 2012;70:28–33.
42. De Magistris L, Familiari V, Pascotto A, et al. Alterations of the intestinal barrier in patients with autism spectrum disorders and in their first-degree relatives. J Pediatr Gastroenterol Nutr 2010;51:418–24.

43. Vazquez-Roque MI, Camilleri M, Smyrk T, et al. A controlled trial of gluten-free diet in patients with irritable bowel syndrome-diarrhea: effects on bowel frequency and intestinal function. Gastroenterology 2013;144(5):903–11.
44. Sapone A, Bai JC, Ciacci C, et al. Spectrum of gluten-related disorders: consensus on new nomenclature and classification. BMC Med 2012;7:10–3.
45. Sapone A, Lammers KM, Mazzarella G, et al. Differential mucosa IL-17 expression in two gliadin-induced disorders: gluten sensitivity and the autoimmune enteropathy celiac disease. Int Arch Allergy Immunol 2010;152(1):75–80.
46. Carroccio A, Mansueto P, Iacono G, et al. Non-celiac wheat sensitivity diagnosed by double-blind placebo-controlled challenge: exploring a new clinical entity. Gastroenterol 2012;107(12):1898–906.
47. Holmes G. Non celiac gluten sensitivity. Gastroenterol Hepatol Bed Bench 2013; 6(3):115–9.
48. Mansueto P, Seidita A, D'Alcamo A, et al. Non-celiac gluten sensitivity: literature review. J Am Coll Nutr 2014;33(1):39–54.
49. Kabbani TA, Vanga RR, Leffler DA, et al. Celiac disease or non-celiac gluten sensitivity? An approach to clinical differential diagnosis. Am J Gastroenterol 2014;109(5):741–6.

Pediatric Inflammatory Bowel Disease

Máire A. Conrad, MD, MS[a], Joel R. Rosh, MD[b],*

KEYWORDS

• Pediatrics • Adolescents • Inflammatory bowel disease • Crohn • Ulcerative colitis

KEY POINTS

• Inflammatory bowel disease (IBD) is a chronic immune-mediated condition of the gastro-intestinal (GI) tract in which the goal of treatment is to induce and maintain durable remission.
• There is a wide spectrum of presenting symptoms in pediatric IBD, but esophagogastro-duodenoscopy and colonoscopy are imperative to confirm the diagnosis.
• Treatment goals include achieving mucosal healing of the GI tract, reaching growth potential, limiting medication toxicities, and optimizing quality of life for all patients and families.

INTRODUCTION

IBD is a chronic immune-mediated condition of the GI tract in which the goal of treatment is to induce and maintain durable remission. Although classically divided into Crohn disease (CD) and ulcerative colitis (UC), IBD actually has a wide range of phenotypes with varied responses to therapy, which makes the natural history of this chronic disease difficult to predict. Pediatric IBD has several unique considerations in comparison to adult IBD, namely related to growth, development, pubertal maturation, bone health, and the psychological impact on the patient and family. Additionally, the longevity of disease burden and its consequent morbidity is significantly more in children than in adults diagnosed with IBD. The growing incidence and prevalence of IBD further highlight the importance of pediatric primary care providers being knowledgeable about and closely involved in the care of these patients.

Disclosure Statement: J.R. Rosh: Advisor/Consultant: Abbvie, Janssen; Grant/Research Support: Abbvie, Janssen.
[a] Division of Gastroenterology, Hepatology and Nutrition, The Children's Hospital of Philadelphia, Perelman School of Medicine, University of Pennsylvania, 3401 Civic Center Boulevard, Philadelphia, PA 19104, USA; [b] Pediatric Gastroenterology, Clinical Development and Research Affairs, Goryeb Children's Hospital/Atlantic Health, Icahn School of Medicine at Mount Sinai, 100 Madison Avenue, Morristown, NJ 07962, USA
* Corresponding author.
E-mail address: joel.rosh@atlantichealth.org

IBD can be categorized into CD, UC, and IBD-unspecified. CD may involve any portion of the GI tract, typically with serpiginous and aphthous ulcers often in patchy distribution, known as skip lesions. The pathognomonic feature of CD is noncaseating epithelioid granulomas, but the presence of granulomas is not essential for a diagnosis of CD. Most commonly, children have ileocolonic involvement and approximately one-third have upper tract involvement as well.[1,2] The inflammation in CD is typically trans-mural, which can lead to disease complications, including fistulae and subsequent intra-abdominal or perianal abscess formation. Perianal disease, including anal skin tags, fissures, fistulae, and abscesses, are associated only with Crohn disease. A sub-set of pediatric CD patients presents with stricturing disease at diagnosis, but the nat-ural history of the disease shows that many patients progress from an inflammatory phenotype to stricturing disease over their lifetime.

UC is characterized by continuous mucosal inflammation of the colon starting from the rectum and extending proximally. UC is unique from CD because it does not have small bowel involvement other than the possibility of backwash ileitis (typically nonspecific inflammation in the terminal ileum in UC patients with pancolitis and no ileocecal valve changes) and does not have granulomas on histopathology.[3] Addition-ally, the depth of inflammation is much more superficial and largely limited to the mu-cosa in UC.

IBD-unspecified describes those patients with colonic disease but who otherwise have features that are not specific for CD or UC. The full range of clinical phenotypes and the complexity of IBD suggest a multifactorial pathophysiology. The etiology is not completely understood, but it is hypothesized to be the result of a dysregulated im-mune response to commensal and/or pathogenic organisms in genetically susceptible hosts.

Genome-wide association studies in adults and older children have identified approximately 200 IBD risk-associated loci. This highlights the polygenic nature of the disease, and many of the identified gene polymorphisms associated with CD and UC influence immune-mediated pathways, leading to dysregulation in autophagy, cell-mediated immune responses, or innate immune responses. This dysregulation al-lows for an altered intestinal microbial composition resulting in dysbiosis, which may induce intestinal inflammation.[4,5]

EPIDEMIOLOGY

The incidence of IBD in the general population is rising.[6,7] High suspicion and recog-nition by general practitioners are imperative because IBD is not uncommon in chil-dren, with up to 25% of patients with IBD diagnosed before age 20.[8] Environmental factors have been implicated in the rapid rise in IBD especially with the recognition that children who emigrate from underdeveloped countries where the incidence of IBD is low take on an increased risk of IBD when they are established in Western so-cieties.[9,10] Additionally, the prevalence in children younger than age 20 with CD and UC is higher in the northeast United States than in Western US states.[11]

Although the average age of diagnosis of pediatric IBD is 10 years to 12 years, a growing subcohort of pediatric IBD includes very-early-onset IBD (VEO-IBD). VEO-IBD is diagnosed in children who present with symptoms by age 5 years and accounts for up to 15% of pediatric IBD cases. VEO-IBD may have a distinct phenotype that favors a colonic disease distribution, does not respond to conventional therapies, and can include primary immunodeficiencies with GI manifestations. Monogenic causes of VEO-IBD have been described and whole-exome sequencing has been innovative in identifying these rare novel variants.[12]

PRESENTATION

IBD can initially present with a heterogeneous constellation of symptoms, including but not limited to abdominal pain, diarrhea, rectal bleeding, weight loss or growth failure, constipation, fever, mouth sores, pallor, dizziness, and dehydration. In some rare cases, patients present with peritonitis, small bowel obstruction, appendicitis, or other surgical emergencies. IBD should be considered in previously healthy children who present with an acute intestinal surgical emergency, giving close attention to growth and chronic symptoms that may have been subtle prior to the acute onset of severe symptoms. In pediatrics, growth is one of the most critical factors and a slowed height velocity may precede apparent signs or symptoms of IBD, especially in cases of Crohn disease. Extraintestinal symptoms can involve dermatologic, musculoskeletal, hepatic, ophthalmologic, renal, pancreatic, or hematologic systems, as outlined in **Table 1**.

One of the main distinctions between pediatric IBD and adult IBD is the impact of the disease on growth and development. Growth retardation and pubertal delay are common at the time of diagnosis of CD and less commonly associated with UC.[13] Growth failure may be attributed to poor caloric intake as well as the direct effects of inflammation causing growth hormone resistance.[13] Diagnosing and intervening with appropriate medical or surgical therapy before a child has completed puberty are integral for optimizing a patient's final adult height. Delayed puberty, including absence of breast development, testicular enlargement, or delayed menarche, can lead to growth retardation in itself as well as decreased bone mineralization. It can also lead to psychological sequelae as a child recognizes differences in his/her own sexual maturation compared with other children of similar age.

DIFFERENTIAL DIAGNOSIS

The differential diagnosis of IBD can vary widely based on the presenting symptoms and disease location in both adults and children (**Table 2**). The most common

Table 1	
Extraintestinal manifestations of inflammatory bowel disease	
Dermatologic	Pyoderma gangrenosum
	Erythema nodosum
	Alopecia
	Bowel-associated dermatosis-arthritis syndrome
Rheumatologic	Arthritis
	Enthesitis
	Sacroiliitis
	Ankylosing spondylitis
Ophthalmologic	Uveitis
	Episcleritis
	Iritis
Hepatic/pancreas/biliary	Primary sclerosing cholangitis
	Autoimmune hepatitis
	Pancreatitis
	Cholelithiasis
Musculoskeletal	Osteopenia
	Osteoporosis
Hematologic	Anemia — iron deficiency or chronic disease
	Venous thrombosis
Urologic	Nephrolithiasis

Table 2
Differential diagnosis of inflammatory bowel disease

Infectious	C difficile
	Salmonella
	Shigella
	Campylobacter
	Yersinia
	Giardia
	Cryptosporidium
	Enteroviruses
	Other bacterial, viral, or parasitic infections
Inflammatory	Appendicitis
	Celiac disease
	Microscopic colitis
Malabsorptive	Lactose intolerance
	Fructose intolerance
	Small intestinal bacterial overgrowth
Allergy/immunology	Eosinophilic GI diseases
	Food protein–induced enterocolitis
	Primary immunodeficiency
	Acquired immunodeficiency
	Autoimmune enteropathy
Rheumatology	Henoch-Schönlein purpura
	Behçet syndrome
	Sarcoidosis
	Systemic lupus erythematosus
Oncologic	Lymphoma
	Neuroblastoma
	Sarcoma
Other	Irritable bowel syndrome
	Eating disorders
	Laxative abuse
	Lymphoma
	Radiation enteritis
	Ischemia

symptoms include diarrhea with or without blood, abdominal pain, and poor growth. An acute onset of symptoms, such as abdominal pain, diarrhea, and low-grade fever, suggests infectious gastroenteritis or colitis or acute appendicitis in the differential diagnosis. Celiac disease can present with diarrhea, abdominal pain, weight loss, poor growth, and low bone mineral density but is not associated with bloody diarrhea. Eosinophilic GI disorders are less common but can present similarly and typically are only delineated from other diagnoses by endoscopy. Lactose intolerance with chronic abdominal pain and frequent diarrhea should also be considered but should resolve with dietary changes and not affect growth. Eating disorders, including anorexia nervosa, should be considered in children with weight loss, abdominal pain, and vomiting as well as laxative abuse in children with diarrhea. Additional rare considerations include oncologic etiologies, sarcoidosis, and ischemic colitis. Finally, functional disorders, including irritable bowel syndrome, are likely the most common cause of chronic and recurrent abdominal pain, diarrhea, and/or constipation in children.

Primary immunodeficiencies should be considered in children with a significant infectious history prior to diagnosis as well as in all children who are presenting with symptoms before age 5. The intestinal mucosa is in close proximity to gut-associated lymphoid tissue and is the site of host-microbe interactions, which are critical to the appropriate development of the immune system. Primary immunodeficiencies, including chronic granulomatous disease, common variable immunodeficiency, Wiskott-Aldrich syndrome, Hermansky-Pudlak syndrome, B-cell defects and T-cell defects, phagocyte defects, and antibody-mediated defects, can initially present with an IBD phenotype.[14]

DIAGNOSTIC EVALUATION

The diagnostic evaluation in a patient suspected of having IBD begins with a thorough history to characterize abdominal pain and diarrhea as well as identify red flags, including blood in stool, nocturnal awakenings to defecate, tenesmus, defecation urgency, fevers, weight loss, mouth ulcers, joint swelling, redness, warmth, and pain (**Table 3**).

First and foremost, a detailed review of the World Health Organization growth chart to determine if there is a decreased height velocity or change in growth percentiles for age must be performed in every patient in whom there is suspicion for IBD. The physical examination should assess the abdomen for focal tenderness, peritoneal signs, and palpable masses that could be related to stricturing or penetrating disease. A perianal examination and rectal examination should not be overlooked due to the frequency of perianal abscesses and fistulae that are present at the time of diagnosis.[15] Some patients have no discomfort associated with perianal lesions and others are reticent to disclose these details to a physician. Rectal strictures may form if there has been long-standing local inflammation. Additional physical examination findings may be shallow, whitish ulcers in the oropharynx, a flow murmur due to anemia, hepatomegaly, joint swelling, redness or effusions, or limited lumbar spine range of motion. Rashes associated with IBD are typically on the lower extremities, including erythema nodosum, depicted as deep erythematous painful nodules, and pyoderma gangrenosum, characterized by ulceration, necrosis, and vasculitis. Clubbing of digits can be seen in CD as well.

The laboratory evaluation for a patient suspected of having IBD is outlined in **Table 4**. Normal laboratory results do not exclude the possibility for IBD. IBD serologies, including anti–*Saccharomyces cerevisiae* and perinuclear antinuclear cytoplasmic antibody, have been identified as immunologic markers found in some individuals with IBD. The diagnostic role of serology has undergone much study and debate in pediatrics and has been found considerably less sensitive than C-reactive protein (CRP) and erythrocyte sedimentation rate (ESR) for the presence of IBD.[16–19] The high cost and poor overall predictive value make this a less useful addition to the diagnostic work-up for IBD.

Table 3	
Red flags in history and physical examination of patients suspected of having inflammatory bowel disease	
History	**Physical Examination**
Blood in stool	Fevers
Nocturnal awakenings to defecate	Weight loss, decreased height velocity
Tenesmus	Abdominal tenderness, peritoneal signs, palpable mass
Defecation urgency	Perianal fistulae, abscesses, rectal stricture
Fevers	Mouth ulcers
	Cardiac flow murmur
	Hepatomegaly
	Joint swelling, erythema, warmth, or effusion
	Skin rashes, including nodules and ulcerations

Table 4
Laboratory evaluation in patients suspected of having inflammatory bowel disease

Initial Laboratory Considerations	Abnormalities Seen with Inflammatory Bowel Disease
Complete blood cell count with differential	Leukocytosis, microcytic anemia, thrombocytosis
Electrolytes	Acidosis and elevated BUN:Cr due to GI losses
Liver function tests	Hypoalbuminemia, elevated AST, ALT, GGT
CRP	Elevated marker of inflammation
ESR	Elevated marker of inflammation
Stool tests	
Stool culture	Rule out infectious enteritis causes, including salmonella, shigella, yersinia, and campylobacter
Rapid giardia and cryptosporidium antigen	Rule out parasitic infections
Stool C *difficile* toxin	Rule out C *difficile*
Stool calprotectin	Elevated marker of inflammation

Abbreviations: ALT, alanine aminotransferase; AST, aspartate aminotransferase; BUN, blood urea nitrogen; Cr, creatinine; GGT, gamma-glutamyl transferase.

Infectious stool studies must be performed to rule out other causes of chronic diarrhea or bloody diarrhea before proceeding with endoscopy, which is the diagnostic gold standard. *Clostridium difficile* testing; stool culture for *Salmonella*, *Shigella*, and *Campylobacter*; and ova and parasite testing, including *Giardia* and *Cryptosporidia* antigens, are particularly important. If one of these are detected, the patient should be treated or observed appropriately and further evaluation considered if symptoms persist.

In addition to ruling out infection by stool studies, fecal calprotectin has been used to screen for active inflammation. Calprotectin is a calcium-binding and zinc-binding neutrophilic cytosolic protein that can be detected in stool as an indicator of gut inflammation. Testing for fecal calprotectin has been established as a useful screening tool prior to considering endoscopy.[20,21] Additionally, it correlates closely with endoscopic activity of IBD, and there is growing evidence for serial monitoring as a marker of disease activity and treatment response.[22] Importantly, although fecal calprotectin has a high sensitivity, it is not specific to IBD, especially in children. Other causes of gut inflammation can lead to elevated calprotectin, including nonsteroidal anti-inflammatory drug use, infectious enterocolitis, inflammatory polyps including juvenile polyps, and oncologic processes. Therefore, calprotectin cannot take the place of endoscopic evaluation.

Children and adolescents with suspicion for IBD should be referred for evaluation by a pediatric gastroenterologist. On review of this evaluation, esophagogastroduodenoscopy and colonoscopy should both be performed for appropriate and complete evaluation. In pediatrics, biopsies during these procedures are essential to ensure the diagnosis and that histology is consistent with the chronic inflammation that is characteristic of IBD.

Diagnosis of IBD in very young children who developed symptoms before the age of 5 or those with a suspicious history, including recurrent infections, should have an immunologic evaluation to rule out primary immunodeficiencies, including chronic granulomatous disease and common variable immunodeficiency, among others. This may include dihydrorhodamine flow cytometry assay; measuring immunoglobulin (Ig) A, IgG, IgE, and IgM; and vaccine titers to diphtheria, tetanus, and pneumococcus to assess appropriate specific antibody response in children who have been vaccinated.[23]

A complete evaluation for IBD includes small bowel imaging to assess the intestine that is not evaluable by conventional endoscopy.[24] Upper GI study with small bowel follow-through has been a common method of evaluation for many years but does provide significant exposure to ionizing radiation and has low sensitivity and specificity. More recently, magnetic resonance enterography of the abdomen/pelvis has been growing in popularity because it prevents this radiation exposure. It requires a child to drink contrast and lie still for a prolonged period of time, which may be difficult for certain ages.[25]

MANAGEMENT

Once a diagnosis has been confirmed, the goal of treatment of pediatric IBD is to induce and maintain clinical remission, achieve normal growth, provide the best quality of life, promote psychological health, and minimize toxicity as much as possible. Additionally, the gold standard of optimal therapy is to achieve mucosal healing endoscopically to change the natural history and prevent complications of progressive bowel destruction, including hospitalization, surgery, and increased risk for colorectal cancer.[26] There are not yet tools to predict which therapy can meet this goal in individual patients, but there is ongoing research to identify genetic, serologic, and microbiome markers for this purpose. In observational adult studies of predicting outcomes in IBD, young age at onset of disease is repeatedly considered high risk for poor prognosis, which reinforces the need for a highly effective treatment approach in children. Treatment of IBD should be handled by a child and family focused multidisciplinary team of practitioners, including a pediatric gastroenterologist, pediatric surgeon, nurse, dietician, psychologist, and social worker to provide holistic care.

There are a few approaches to initiating and optimizing treatment of IBD. In Crohn disease, the oldest treatment paradigm includes step-up therapy. This non–evidence-based approach traditionally started with locally active agents, including 5-aminosalicylate (5-ASA) preparations or antibiotics, followed by prednisone or budesonide to control symptoms due to ongoing inflammation, and then escalated to immunomodulators, biologics, and, finally, after failing all medical therapies, surgery. This approach has been shown to potentially provide symptomatic management without necessarily achieving mucosal healing and changing the natural history of Crohn disease. The top-down approach to therapy, which initiates treatment with immune-modifying therapy, has demonstrated a definitively positive impact on clinical outcomes in children and adolescents, in particular those who have moderate to severe disease, likely due to the true and rapid induction of mucosal healing.[27] Future and ongoing studies intended to identify clinical markers useful in risk stratification will help provide the most personalized therapeutic plans for patients.

In UC, the mucosal confinement of the inflammatory process leads to a somewhat different treatment paradigm. 5-ASA medications, including mesalamine, balsalazide, and sulfasalazine, are locally acting anti-inflammatory agents, which topically treat the intestinal mucosa. They are well established, effective, and safe medications for adults with mild to moderate UC and can provide long-term steroid-free remission in up to 40% of pediatric UC patients.[28–31] These agents can be administered orally or rectally and overall are well tolerated with few dose-related adverse effects. Although these have a clear role in the maintenance of remission in pediatric UC, a majority of patients require an initial course of corticosteroids to induce that remission.

Intestinal dysbiosis is a major tenet of the pathophysiology of IBD, and, as a result, antibiotics have been a longstanding therapeutic approach.[32] Adult studies have shown metronidazole and rifaximin lead to clinical improvement in Crohn disease.[33–35]

Metronidazole and ciprofloxacin are typically first-line medical treatment of perianal fistulae but had the best efficacy in combination with anti–tumor necrosis factor (TNF)-α agents.[36] More recent studies have looked at combinations of antibiotics, including an 8-week trial of azithromycin and metronidazole in pediatric CD with improvement in clinical activity index and CRP.[37] Recent evidence has also emerged for using triple antibiotics (amoxicillin, doxycycline, and metronidazole) as salvage therapy for acute severe UC.[38] Alternatively, there have been several studies linking antibiotic exposure with developing IBD and there is clear dysbiosis shown with the use of antibiotics in intestinal microbiome studies.[39–42] The risks and benefits of prolonged antibiotic exposure must be weighed depending on individual cases.

Along with pharmacologic treatment approaches, dietary therapies for IBD continue to be explored. Enteral nutrition (EN) therapy, in which 100% of total calories are delivered by commercial formula and whole table foods are excluded from the diet, is the only nutritional therapy to date proved to induce remission and decrease steroid exposure in children and adolescents. There is evidence to support that 80% to 90% of calories from EN may be as effective.[43] EN provides additional support for the role of diet and the gut microbiota in the pathogenesis of IBD.

The appeal of EN compared with pharmacologic agents is that there are no serious associated side effects. Although proved an effective therapy in CD, the mechanism of action of nutritional therapy has not been fully characterized. A recent study of pediatric CD patients on exclusive EN (EEN) (90% of total caloric intake by dietary formula) compared with partial EN (53% by formula) showed EEN was superior at improving symptoms and quality of life as well as inducing mucosal healing, suggesting that the thorough elimination of solid table foods may be the key to why EN is therapeutic.[44] In addition, the alteration of the gut microbiota may be another possible mechanism of action. In the same study of pediatric CD patients, effective EEN therapy changed the microbiota within 1 week and reduced the dysbiosis seen initially.[40] Additionally, EN to induce remission has been shown to have an increased benefit to improving growth velocity over corticosteroids over 6 months.

Immunomodulators, including thiopurine analogs (azathioprine and 6-mercaptopurine), were one of the first classes of medications shown to effectively maintain remission in refractory, steroid-dependent Crohn disease.[45] Despite the efficacy of these medications, the long-term safety profile has come into question with the observation of a slightly increased risk of non-Hodgkin lymphoma as well as the observation of a small cohort of predominately male patients who develop an almost uniformly fatal form of hepatosplenic T-cell lymphoma. Alternatively, methotrexate has also been shown an effective immunomodulator in this setting.[46] Methotrexate has not been as extensively studied in IBD, but there are no reports of associated hepatosplenic T-cell lymphoma to date.[47]

Corticosteroids have been considered effective first-line therapy to induce remission in IBD among all age groups for more than 50 years. Unfortunately, the side effects of systemic steroids, including growth failure, bone demineralization, secondary adrenal insufficiency, acne, and increased infectious complications and emotional labiality make them an unfavorable therapeutic option. Avoiding ongoing use of systemic corticosteroids is now emphasized in adult and pediatric IBD. Nonsystemic corticosteroids, such as budesonide, have offered targeted therapy for IBD with high first-pass hepatic metabolism, resulting in less systemic glucocorticoid exposure than prednisone. In a pediatric randomized controlled trial, budesonide was just as effective as prednisone at inducing remission in CD by 12 weeks with less severe cosmetic side effects.[48] Neither budesonide nor prednisone is particularly effective at maintaining remission, although this has largely been studied in adults.[49,50]

Biologic agents, including anti-TNF antibodies and antiintegrin antibodies, have greatly improved the ability to treat moderate to severe CD and UC. The safety and efficacy of anti–TNF-α antibodies are well established, even demonstrating a significant response to a single infusion.[51] In children, infliximab is efficacious in inducing and maintaining remission in pediatric CD and UC.[52,53] Adalimumab has had similar success in pediatric Crohn disease, but studies of adalimumab for pediatric UC are ongoing.[54,55] Furthermore, studies have shown that early use of anti-TNF therapy is more effective in children than immunomodulators in inducing remission.[27,56] One of the profound outcomes from infliximab and adalimumab therapy in pediatrics has been the increase in height particularly in children diagnosed with CD early in puberty or before puberty.[56]

Vedolizumab is a humanized anti-$\alpha4\beta7$ integrin, IgG1 monoclonal antibody, which down-regulates intestinal inflammation by inhibiting T-cell migration in the GI tract. Vedolizumab has been shown to have modest improvement in clinical response and remission in both adult UC and CD patients. In children, observational studies of vedolizumab have demonstrated similar efficacy and safety.[57,58]

Therapeutic drug monitoring available for infliximab and adalimumab has helped optimize medication dosing for individual patients, which can help achieve improved clinical, biochemical, and endoscopic outcomes, increase the rate of remission, and decrease the incidence of antibody formation resulting in loss of response to these drugs.[59–61] Low or undetectable serum trough concentrations of infliximab are associated with worse clinical outcomes and worse disease activity as measured by CRP and antibodies to infliximab increase the clearance of the drug, which can lead to low trough levels.[62]

Despite medical advances, surgical intervention is still sometimes warranted in refractory pediatric IBD. In UC, total colectomy with end ileostomy can be curative for failure of medical management, resulting in transfusion dependent anemia and other sequelae of inadequate disease control. In 1 or 2 subsequent surgeries, takedown of the ileostomy and ileal pouch anal anastomosis can be performed.[63] For severe colitis in patients with CD or indeterminate colitis, diverting ileostomy has become a preferable option to resection or colectomy due to the high risk of complications long term in this subpopulation. This diverts the fecal stream away from the inflamed colonic mucosa, allowing for potential healing. Finally, CD patients may require intestinal resections, most commonly ileocecectomy. Surgical resection in childhood and adolescence is an increased risk for postoperative recurrence during adulthood and requires continued medical therapy and careful endoscopic surveillance postoperatively.

HEALTH MAINTENANCE

Health maintenance is critically important in the developing and growing child or adolescent with IBD. Monitoring growth is crucial to detecting subtle changes that may be indicative of ongoing disease activity. Detecting poor linear growth early is crucial to adequate therapy and disease control to ensure that patients with IBD meet their growth potential. Patients are at risk of malnutrition as well as obesity, which should be addressed during regular nutrition assessments.[64,65] Small intestinal disease or history of small intestinal resection increases risk for malabsorption and resulting malnutrition.

On diagnosis, the immunization status of each patient should be reviewed and kept up to date.[66,67] Vaccines should not be delayed in IBD patients, except that live vaccines should be avoided in patients treated with immune-modifying agents, including corticosteroids, thiopurines, methotrexate, and biologics. Patients with IBD on aminosalicylate monotherapy are not immunosuppressed. Ideally, vaccines should be administered when off of immune-modifying agents; therefore, catch-up immunizations should be administered at the time of diagnosis prior to initiating these therapies. Four weeks after varicella vaccine is given and 6 weeks after measles-mumps-rubella live vaccines are given are the acceptable time periods before starting immunosuppression.[68,69] The risks and benefits of holding immunizations versus postponing therapy for IBD should be discussed between pediatrician and gastroenterologist to determine the appropriate timing.

In addition to reviewing immunization status, tuberculosis exposure and hepatitis B status should be assessed. Purified protein derivative tuberculin or interferon assay testing should be completed prior to starting biologics. Hepatitis B surface antigen and antibody should be checked to ensure no active disease and appropriate immunization status. If hepatitis B surface antibody is negative, repeat hepatitis B vaccine series should be given, especially in those receiving anti-TNF therapy.

Due to their immunosuppressed status, IBD patients' treating pediatric gastroenterologists should be contacted during an infectious illness, especially if a patient is receiving biologics, immunomodulators, or high-dose corticosteroids. In particular, active or recent Epstein-Barr virus (EBV) should be discussed due to the possible complications, including lymphoma and hemophagocytic lymphohistiocytosis (HLH), especially in those on thiopurines. IBD patients with EBV should be monitored closely for evidence of laboratory test abnormalities, including cytopenia, hyperferritinemia, hypertriglyceridemia, and hypofibrinogenemia, which require emergent evaluation for HLH.[70] In uncomplicated EBV, a gastroenterologist may consider discontinuing immunosuppression until EBV serology is consistent with past infection (viral capsid antigen–IgG positive).[67]

A nutritional assessment should be obtained at each routine pediatric visit to ensure patients are meeting caloric requirements appropriate for age. Extra consideration is recommended for children with active inflammatory disease because they likely have higher caloric needs. Nutritional deficiencies, including iron, vitamin D, and zinc, may be apparent. Vitamin B_{12} deficiency should also be considered in children who have had surgical resections, particularly of the terminal ileum. A pediatric dietician with experience in IBD can provide additional recommendations for children with ongoing malnutrition or poor growth. Supplemental oral and, if needed, enteral nasogastric tube feeds may be required to provide adequate caloric intake for the malnourished patient.

Bone health can be adversely affected in patients with IBD due to inflammation, malnutrition, corticosteroid use, and low physical activity. Up to 40% of children newly diagnosed with IBD have been reported to have deficit in bone mass, which can have an impact long term on risk of fractures and overall linear growth. Bone mineral density is measured by dual energy x-ray absorptiometry scan, whose result is expressed as a z score, which measures the difference in bone mineral density from the normal mean for gender and age. Vitamin D deficiency (mild–moderate 25-hydroxy vitamin D level, 10–24 ng/mL, and severe level, <10 ng/mL) is prevalent among children with IBD, especially in those with severe disease and upper GI tract involvement.[71,72] Aside from the benefits for bone health, vitamin D and its receptors may inhibit colitis by protecting the mucosal epithelial barrier.[73–75] The 25-hydroxyvitamin D level should be monitored every 6 months to 12 months, depending on if a patient is deficient or not. Supplementation with cholecalciferol to maintain a 25-hydroxyvitamin D level greater than 30 ng/mL is suggested.[66]

The toll of a chronic disease on both physical and mental health can be extensive and lead to depression, anxiety, social isolation, and altered self-image.[76,77] In pediatrics, this burden extends to the entire family of a patient with a chronic disease. For patients with IBD, the relapsing and remitting nature of the disease can have a great impact on quality of life and the ability to fully participate in school. Regular assessment of major psychosocial stressors, school performance, and attendance as well as depression and suicide screening should be performed at all office visits. Up to 25% of adolescent patients with IBD may have symptoms of depression that often are undetected.[76] Psychological support is highly encouraged for families affected by pediatric IBD, especially for the patients, to provide strategies for coping with a chronic disease long term, and cognitive behavioral therapy is a useful tool in treating depression and anxiety. Pediatric IBD support groups are also effective venues for helping patients discover other children coping with similar scenarios and stressors.

This article outlines the unique features and considerations necessary for the appropriate care of pediatric IBD. Many medical advances in the past 10 years to 20 years have optimized the ability to care for these patients. Heightened awareness on the part of primary care providers as to the presentation of pediatric IBD allows for early diagnosis and the best prognosis. Each child and family requires the collaborative care of the primary care provider team as well as the pediatric gastroenterology team to ensure the best long-term outcomes and quality of life for the patient.

REFERENCES

1. Lemberg DA, Day AS. Crohn disease and ulcerative colitis in children: an update for 2014. J Paediatr Child Health 2015;51(3):266–70.
2. Castellaneta SP, Afzal NA, Greenberg M, et al. Diagnostic role of upper gastrointestinal endoscopy in pediatric inflammatory bowel disease. J Pediatr Gastroenterol Nutr 2004;39(3):257–61.
3. North American Society for Pediatric Gastroenterology Hepatology, Nutrition, Colitis Foundation of America, Bousvaros A, et al. Differentiating ulcerative colitis from Crohn disease in children and young adults: report of a working group of the North American Society for Pediatric Gastroenterology, Hepatology, and Nutrition and the Crohn's and Colitis Foundation of America. J Pediatr Gastroenterol Nutr 2007;44(5):653–74.
4. Haberman Y, Tickle TL, Dexheimer PJ, et al. Pediatric Crohn disease patients exhibit specific ileal transcriptome and microbiome signature. J Clin Invest 2014; 124(8):3617–33.
5. Sartor RB. Therapeutic manipulation of the enteric microflora in inflammatory bowel diseases: antibiotics, probiotics, and prebiotics. Gastroenterology 2004; 126(6):1620–33.
6. Molodecky NA, Soon IS, Rabi DM, et al. Increasing incidence and prevalence of the inflammatory bowel diseases with time, based on systematic review. Gastroenterology 2012;142(1):46–54.e42 [quiz: e30].
7. Eszter Muller K, Laszlo Lakatos P, Papp M, et al. Incidence and Paris classification of pediatric inflammatory bowel disease. Gastroenterol Res Pract 2014;2014: 904307.
8. Turunen P, Kolho KL, Auvinen A, et al. Incidence of inflammatory bowel disease in Finnish children, 1987-2003. Inflamm Bowel Dis 2006;12(8):677–83.
9. Barreiro-de Acosta M, Alvarez Castro A, Souto R, et al. Emigration to western industrialized countries: a risk factor for developing inflammatory bowel disease. J Crohns Colitis 2011;5(6):566–9.
10. Benchimol EI, Mack DR, Guttmann A, et al. Inflammatory bowel disease in immigrants to Canada and their children: a population-based cohort study. Am J Gastroenterol 2015;110(4):553–63.

11. Kappelman MD, Moore KR, Allen JK, et al. Recent trends in the prevalence of Crohn's disease and ulcerative colitis in a commercially insured US population. Dig Dis Sci 2013;58(2):519–25.

12. Kelsen JR, Dawany N, Moran CJ, et al. Exome sequencing analysis reveals variants in primary immunodeficiency genes in patients with very early onset inflammatory bowel disease. Gastroenterology 2015;149(6):1415–24.

13. Sanderson IR. Growth problems in children with IBD. Nat Rev Gastroenterol Hepatol 2014;11(10):601–10.

14. Snapper SB. Very-early-onset inflammatory bowel disease. Gastroenterol Hepatol (N Y) 2015;11(8):554–6.

15. Keljo DJ, Markowitz J, Langton C, et al. Course and treatment of perianal disease in children newly diagnosed with Crohn's disease. Inflamm Bowel Dis 2009;15(3): 383–7.

16. Benor S, Russell GH, Silver M, et al. Shortcomings of the inflammatory bowel disease Serology 7 panel. Pediatrics 2010;125(6):1230–6.

17. Olives JP, Breton A, Hugot JP, et al. Antineutrophil cytoplasmic antibodies in children with inflammatory bowel disease: prevalence and diagnostic value. J Pediatr Gastroenterol Nutr 1997;25(2):142–8.

18. Ruemmele FM, Targan SR, Levy G, et al. Diagnostic accuracy of serological assays in pediatric inflammatory bowel disease. Gastroenterology 1998;115(4): 822–9.

19. Khan K, Schwarzenberg SJ, Sharp H, et al. Role of serology and routine laboratory tests in childhood inflammatory bowel disease. Inflamm Bowel Dis 2002;8(5): 325–9.

20. van Rheenen PF, Van de Vijver E, Fidler V. Faecal calprotectin for screening of patients with suspected inflammatory bowel disease: diagnostic meta-analysis. BMJ 2010;341:c3369.

21. Henderson P, Anderson NH, Wilson DC. The diagnostic accuracy of fecal calprotectin during the investigation of suspected pediatric inflammatory bowel disease: a systematic review and meta-analysis. Am J Gastroenterol 2014;109(5): 637–45.

22. Sipponen T, Kolho KL. Fecal calprotectin in diagnosis and clinical assessment of inflammatory bowel disease. Scand J Gastroenterol 2015;50(1):74–80.

23. Uhlig HH, Schwerd T, Koletzko S, et al. The diagnostic approach to monogenic very early onset inflammatory bowel disease. Gastroenterology 2014;147(5): 990–1007.e3.

24. Levine A, Koletzko S, Turner D, et al. ESPGHAN revised porto criteria for the diagnosis of inflammatory bowel disease in children and adolescents. J Pediatr Gastroenterol Nutr 2014;58(6):795–806.

25. Anupindi SA, Grossman AB, Nimkin K, et al. Imaging in the evaluation of the young patient with inflammatory bowel disease: what the gastroenterologist needs to know. J Pediatr Gastroenterol Nutr 2014;59(4):429–39.

26. Schnitzler F, Fidder H, Ferrante M, et al. Mucosal healing predicts long-term outcome of maintenance therapy with infliximab in Crohn's disease. Inflamm Bowel Dis 2009;15(9):1295–301.

27. Walters TD, Kim MO, Denson LA, et al. Increased effectiveness of early therapy with anti-tumor necrosis factor-alpha vs an immunomodulator in children with Crohn's disease. Gastroenterology 2014;146(2):383–91.

28. Sutherland L, Macdonald JK. Oral 5-aminosalicylic acid for induction of remission in ulcerative colitis. Cochrane Database Syst Rev 2006;(2):CD000543.

29. Sutherland L, Macdonald JK. Oral 5-aminosalicylic acid for maintenance of remission in ulcerative colitis. Cochrane Database Syst Rev 2006;(2):CD000544.

30. Sandborn WJ. Oral 5-ASA therapy in ulcerative colitis: what are the implications of the new formulations? J Clin Gastroenterol 2008;42(4):338–44.

31. Zeisler B, Lerer T, Markowitz J, et al. Outcome following aminosalicylate therapy in children newly diagnosed as having ulcerative colitis. J Pediatr Gastroenterol Nutr 2013;56(1):12–8.

32. Wang SL, Wang ZR, Yang CQ. Meta-analysis of broad-spectrum antibiotic therapy in patients with active inflammatory bowel disease. Exp Ther Med 2012; 4(6):1051–6.

33. Scott FI, Osterman MT. Medical management of crohn disease. Clin Colon Rectal Surg 2013;26(2):67–74.

34. Prantera C, Lochs H, Grimaldi M, et al. Rifaximin-extended intestinal release induces remission in patients with moderately active Crohn's disease. Gastroenterology 2012;142(3):473–81.e4.

35. Su JW, Ma JJ, Zhang HJ. Use of antibiotics in patients with Crohn's disease: a systematic review and meta-analysis. J Dig Dis 2015;16(2):58–66.

36. Schwartz DA, Ghazi LJ, Regueiro M. Guidelines for medical treatment of Crohn's perianal fistulas: critical evaluation of therapeutic trials. Inflamm Bowel Dis 2015; 21(4):737–52.

37. Levine A, Turner D. Combined azithromycin and metronidazole therapy is effective in inducing remission in pediatric Crohn's disease. J Crohns Colitis 2011;5(3): 222–6.

38. Turner D, Levine A, Kolho KL, et al. Combination of oral antibiotics may be effective in severe pediatric ulcerative colitis: a preliminary report. J Crohns Colitis 2014;8(11):1464–70.

39. Margolis DJ, Fanelli M, Hoffstad O, et al. Potential association between the oral tetracycline class of antimicrobials used to treat acne and inflammatory bowel disease. Am J Gastroenterol 2010;105(12):2610–6.

40. Lewis JD, Chen EZ, Baldassano RN, et al. Inflammation, antibiotics, and diet as environmental stressors of the gut microbiome in pediatric Crohn's disease. Cell Host Microbe 2015;18(4):489–500.

41. Card T, Logan RF, Rodrigues LC, et al. Antibiotic use and the development of Crohn's disease. Gut 2004;53(2):246–50.

42. Shaw SY, Blanchard JF, Bernstein CN. Association between early childhood otitis media and pediatric inflammatory bowel disease: an exploratory population-based analysis. J Pediatr 2013;162(3):510–4.

43. Gupta K, Noble A, Kachelries KE, et al. A novel enteral nutrition protocol for the treatment of pediatric Crohn's disease. Inflamm Bowel Dis 2013;19(7):1374–8.

44. Lee D, Baldassano RN, Otley AR, et al. Comparative effectiveness of nutritional and biological therapy in North American children with active Crohn's disease. Inflamm Bowel Dis 2015;21(8):1786–93.

45. Markowitz J, Grancher K, Kohn N, et al. A multicenter trial of 6-mercaptopurine and prednisone in children with newly diagnosed Crohn's disease. Gastroenterology 2000;119(4):895–902.

46. Turner D, Grossman AB, Rosh J, et al. Methotrexate following unsuccessful thiopurine therapy in pediatric Crohn's disease. Am J Gastroenterol 2007;102(12): 2804–12 [quiz: 2803–13].

47. Sunseri W, Hyams JS, Lerer T, et al. Retrospective cohort study of methotrexate use in the treatment of pediatric Crohn's disease. Inflamm Bowel Dis 2014;20(8): 1341–5.

48. Levine A, Weizman Z, Broide E, et al. A comparison of budesonide and prednisone for the treatment of active pediatric Crohn disease. J Pediatr Gastroenterol Nutr 2003;36(2):248–52.
49. Ford AC, Bernstein CN, Khan KJ, et al. Glucocorticosteroid therapy in inflammatory bowel disease: systematic review and meta-analysis. Am J Gastroenterol 2011;106(4):590–9 [quiz: 600].
50. Simms L, Steinhart AH. Budesonide for maintenance of remission in Crohn's disease. Cochrane Database Syst Rev 2001;(1):CD002913.
51. Targan SR, Hanauer SB, van Deventer SJ, et al. A short-term study of chimeric monoclonal antibody cA2 to tumor necrosis factor alpha for Crohn's disease. Crohn's disease cA2 study group. N Engl J Med 1997;337(15):1029–35.
52. Hyams J, Damaraju L, Blank M, et al. Induction and maintenance therapy with infliximab for children with moderate to severe ulcerative colitis. Clin Gastroenterol Hepatol 2012;10(4):391–9.e1.
53. Hyams J, Walters TD, Crandall W, et al. Safety and efficacy of maintenance infliximab therapy for moderate-to-severe Crohn's disease in children: REACH open-label extension. Curr Med Res Opin 2011;27(3):651–62.
54. Rosh JR, Lerer T, Markowitz J, et al. Retrospective evaluation of the safety and effect of adalimumab therapy (RESEAT) in pediatric Crohn's disease. Am J Gastroenterol 2009;104(12):3042–9.
55. Hyams JS, Griffiths A, Markowitz J, et al. Safety and efficacy of adalimumab for moderate to severe Crohn's disease in children. Gastroenterology 2012;143(2): 365–74.e2.
56. Walters TD, Gilman AR, Griffiths AM. Linear growth improves during infliximab therapy in children with chronically active severe Crohn's disease. Inflamm Bowel Dis 2007;13(4):424–30.
57. Singh N, Rabizadeh S, Jossen J, et al. Multi-center experience of vedolizumab effectiveness in pediatric inflammatory bowel disease. Inflamm Bowel Dis 2016; 22(9):2121–6.
58. Conrad MA, Stein RE, Maxwell EC, et al. vedolizumab therapy in severe pediatric inflammatory bowel disease. Inflamm Bowel Dis 2016;22(10):2425–31.
59. Maser EA, Villela R, Silverberg MS, et al. Association of trough serum infliximab to clinical outcome after scheduled maintenance treatment for Crohn's disease. Clin Gastroenterol Hepatol 2006;4(10):1248–54.
60. Seow CH, Newman A, Irwin SP, et al. Trough serum infliximab: a predictive factor of clinical outcome for infliximab treatment in acute ulcerative colitis. Gut 2010; 59(1):49–54.
61. Adedokun OJ, Sandborn WJ, Feagan BG, et al. Association between serum concentration of infliximab and efficacy in adult patients with ulcerative colitis. Gastroenterology 2014;147(6):1296–307.e5.
62. Vande Casteele N, Khanna R, Levesque BG, et al. The relationship between infliximab concentrations, antibodies to infliximab and disease activity in Crohn's disease. Gut 2015;64(10):1539–45.
63. Baillie CT, Smith JA. Surgical strategies in paediatric inflammatory bowel disease. World J Gastroenterol 2015;21(20):6101–16.
64. Long MD, Crandall WV, Leibowitz IH, et al. Prevalence and epidemiology of overweight and obesity in children with inflammatory bowel disease. Inflamm Bowel Dis 2011;17(10):2162–8.
65. Kugathasan S, Nebel J, Skelton JA, et al. Body mass index in children with newly diagnosed inflammatory bowel disease: observations from two multicenter North American inception cohorts. J Pediatr 2007;151(5):523–7.

66. Breglio KJ, Rosh JR. Health maintenance and vaccination strategies in pediatric inflammatory bowel disease. Inflamm Bowel Dis 2013;19(8):1740–4.
67. Rufo PA, Denson LA, Sylvester FA, et al. Health supervision in the management of children and adolescents with IBD: NASPGHAN recommendations. J Pediatr Gastroenterol Nutr 2012;55(1):93–108.
68. Wasan SK, Baker SE, Skolnik PR, et al. A practical guide to vaccinating the inflammatory bowel disease patient. Am J Gastroenterol 2010;105(6):1231–8.
69. Lu Y, Bousvaros A. Immunizations in children with inflammatory bowel disease treated with immunosuppressive therapy. Gastroenterol Hepatol (N Y) 2014; 10(6):355–63.
70. Imashuku S. Systemic type Epstein-Barr virus-related lymphoproliferative diseases in children and young adults: challenges for pediatric hemato-oncologists and infectious disease specialists. Pediatr Hematol Oncol 2007;24(8):563–8.
71. Pappa HM, Gordon CM, Saslowsky TM, et al. Vitamin D status in children and young adults with inflammatory bowel disease. Pediatrics 2006;118(5):1950–61.
72. Kabbani TA, Koutroubakis IE, Schoen RE, et al. Association of vitamin D level with clinical status in inflammatory bowel disease: a 5-year longitudinal study. Am J Gastroenterol 2016;111(5):712–9.
73. Liu W, Chen Y, Golan MA, et al. Intestinal epithelial vitamin D receptor signaling inhibits experimental colitis. J Clin Invest 2013;123(9):3983–96.
74. Meckel K, Li YC, Lim J, et al. Serum 25-hydroxy vitamin D concentration is inversely associated with mucosal inflammation in patients with ulcerative colitis. Am J Clin Nutr 2016;104(1):113–20.
75. Stio M, Retico L, Annese V, et al. Vitamin D regulates the tight-junction protein expression in active ulcerative colitis. Scand J Gastroenterol 2016;51(10):1193–9.
76. Szigethy E, Levy-Warren A, Whitton S, et al. Depressive symptoms and inflammatory bowel disease in children and adolescents: a cross-sectional study. J Pediatr Gastroenterol Nutr 2004;39(4):395–403.
77. Szigethy E, McLafferty L, Goyal A. Inflammatory bowel disease. Child Adolesc Psychiatr Clin N Am 2010;19(2):301–18, ix.

Motility Disorders in Children

Samuel Nurko, MD, MPH

KEYWORDS

- High-resolution manometry • Motility studies • Children
- Motor disorders of esophagus

KEY POINTS

- Motility disorders in children represent an important problem.
- Anatomic, mucosal, and systemic diseases need to be excluded before a motility disorder is considered.
- New advances, like high-resolution manometry (HRM), are providing new insights into the pathophysiology of motor disorders.
- New approaches to treatment have evolved based on the pathophysiology of motor disorders.

INTRODUCTION

One of the main functions of the gastrointestinal (GI) tract is to allow for the ingestion of nutrients, their transport through different specialized areas of the GI tract to allow digestion and absorption, and the expulsion of unused portions at times when it is socially acceptable.[1,2] Each area of the GI tract has a specific motility pattern that allows it to perform its necessary function and is the result of a complex interaction between the muscles, the myenteric plexus, the peripheral nervous system, and the brain.[1,3] Diseases that affect this movement through the GI tract are known as motility disorders,[3] which are the main focus of this article. The general approach to a child with a suspected motility disorder and clinical presentation, evaluation, and treatment of primary motility disorders in children are addressed.

EVALUATION OF THE PEDIATRIC PATIENT WITH A SUSPECTED MOTILITY DISORDER

Pediatric gastrointestinal (GI) motility disorders are common.[1,3] **Box 1** shows the main motility disorders. As seen, motility disorders can be a result of diseases that affect primarily the muscles and innervation of the GI tract (achalasia, gastroparesis [GP],

Nothing to disclose.
Center for Motility and Functional Gastrointestinal Disorders, Boston Children's Hospital, 300 Longwood Avenue, Boston, MA 02155, USA
E-mail address: samuel.nurko@childrens.harvard.edu

Box 1
Motility disorders

Primary

Affect the intrinsic/extrinsic innervation of the GI tract
  Achalasia
  GP
  Pseudo-obstruction

Common disorders in which there is underlying motility dysfunction
  Gastroesophageal reflux
  Constipation

Malformations that affect the motility of the GI tract
  Tracheoesophageal fistula
  Anorectal malformations
  Congenital malformations (diaphragmatic hernia, omphalocele, gastroschisis)
  Other

Secondary

Systemic diseases
  Neuromuscular diseases
    Scleroderma, neurologic problems
  Metabolic/endocrine diseases
    Thyroid problems, mitochondrial disease

Medications

Iatrogenic
  Surgery

---

pseudo-obstruction, and Hirschsprung disease [HD]), congenital malformations that are accompanied by alterations in motility function (tracheoesophageal fistula, gastroschisis, and so forth), common pediatric diseases that have motility disturbances as part of their pathophysiology (gastroesophageal reflux disease and constipation) or non-GI processes that affect the GI motility secondarily (systemic diseases, iatrogenic problems, drugs, and so forth).

Given that motility disorders can affect so many different areas, their presentations vary according to the area of the GI tract that is affected (**Box 2**). Therefore, the signs

---

Box 2
Presenting symptoms of motility disorders according to the affected organs

- Esophagus
  - Dysphagia, odynophagia, oropharyngeal dysphagia, regurgitation/vomiting, chest pain, aspiration, respiratory problems, retching, gagging, weight loss

- Stomach
  - Early satiety, abdominal distention, vomiting, pain, dyspepsia, nausea, inability to tolerate food, retching, weight loss

- Small bowel
  - Abdominal distention/bloating, pain, vomiting, inability to tolerate food, diarrhea, nausea, bacterial overgrowth, weight loss

- Colon/anorectum
  - Abdominal distention, constipation, incontinence, pain

---

and symptoms are characteristic to the area that is affected but are not specific and can result from nonmotility problems. Therefore, when symptoms suggest that there may be a GI motility disorder, careful exclusion of anatomic, mucosal, or metabolic disorders should be undertaken before a motility disorder is diagnosed or specific motility studies are initiated (**Box 3**).[1–4]

Exclude Anatomic Problems

Excluding an anatomic cause is the most important first step after a careful history and physical examination (see **Box 3**). For areas that cannot be examined with a physical

---

Box 3
Approach to the patient with a suspected motility disorder

- Exclude anatomic obstruction
  - Physical examination
  - Imaging studies
    - Plain radiographs
    - Contrast studies. Detection of most upper or lower GI malformations, complications of disease processes or after surgery
    - CT/MRI. In patients with known pseudo-obstruction who have had previous surgery, who present with obstructive symptoms, particularly if the symptoms differ from the usual presentation of the patient, CT is indicated to look for the presence of transition points, or other complications.
  - Endoscopy

- Look for an etiology
  - Extraintestinal
    - Gallbladder, pancreas
    - Renal
    - Central nervous system
  - Mucosal
    - Celiac disease, eosinophilic esophagitis
  - Metabolic/endocrine
    - Electrolyte problems
    - Thyroid dysfunction
  - Systemic diseases
    - Connective tissue
    - Musculoskeletal problems
    - Mitochondrial disease
    - Cystic fibrosis
  - Drugs
    - Anticholinergic effects
    - Opiates
  - Psychological problems

- Evaluate transit
  - Radiograph with radiopaque markers. Defecation problems
  - Nuclear medicine. Mostly used for GE, where a 4-hour test is now the gold standard. Also used for esophageal transit and can be used for colonic transit.
  - Impedance
    - Esophagus
  - Breath testing. Use to evaluate GE: ^{13}C octanoic acid ^{13}C-Spirulina
  - Wireless motility capsule. Gastric, intestinal, and colonic transit

- Motility testing
  - Manometry testing. Esophageal manometry, antroduodenal manometry, colonic manometry, and ARM
  - Wireless motility capsule, not validated yet

examination, the most effective way to exclude anatomic problems is with the use of radiographic and/or endoscopic studies. Often the opacification of the GI tract with the use of contrast is necessary and can suggest the presence of a motility disorder (bird's beak in achalasia or transition zone in HD), an obstructive lesion, or a complication from the disease (strictures or necrotizing enterocolitis) or surgery. More advanced imaging like CT scan or MRI is often used to detect other processes, malformations, or, in particular, the presence of adhesions or postoperative complications.[1]

Look for an Underlying Disease Process

A thorough work-up needs to be completed to exclude processes that may have an indirect impact on the motor function[1] (see **Box 3**). Before embarking on an extensive motility evaluation, attempts to correct the underlying problem should be done first, because the treatment of the underlying condition may result in normalization of the motility problem (eg, hypothyroidism).

Transit Studies

Transit studies provide objective data that show how movement may be altered throughout the different segments of the GI tract and may indicate fast, slow, or normal transit measurements that have clinical implications as the treatment varies accordingly.[2,5,6]

Box 3 shows the different available techniques that include radiopaque markers, scintigraphic evaluation,[6,7] breath testing, impedance, or the wireless motility capsule that allows the determination of total body transit, gastric, small bowel, and colonic transit.[8] Witeless motility capsule use for the evaluation of motility patterns has not been validated (**Fig. 1**).

Manometry Studies

Manometric studies are used to directly evaluate the contractile patterns of the different segments of the GI tract and allow the definition of the underlying pathophysiology by

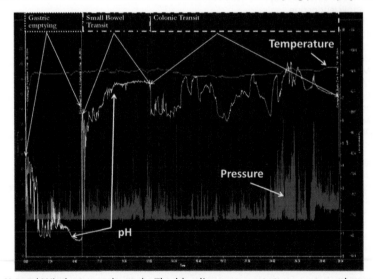

Fig. 1. Normal Wireless capsule study. The blue line represents temperature, the green line pH and the red waves pressure measurements. The different segments of the upper GI tract are identified by their respective pH, and the transit through each segment can then be calculated. The temperature is necessary to establish ingestion and excretion of the capsule.

demonstrating if the alteration is in the muscle strength or the nerve regulation.[1,2,5,6,9] GI manometry provides direct evidence about the contractile events of the organ that is studied. Each digestive organ has a characteristic motility pattern that has evolved to provide the most efficient motor function (**Figs. 2–7**).[1,2,5,6,9]

The role of manometric evaluation in children has been more clearly defined for anorectal manometry (ARM),[1,4,5,7,9,10] esophageal manometry,[1,4,5,7,9,10] antroduodenal manometry,[1,4,5,7,9,10] and colonic manometry[1,4,5,7,9,10] (**Box 4**). GI manometry has evolved during the past years and has changed from a research technique to a useful diagnostic tool.[1,4,5,7,9] The performance of motility studies in the pediatric population has certain important characteristics that make this more challenging, including technical aspects related to catheter size as well as developmental abnormalities and cooperation.[1,4,11]

Given that monomeric studies cannot be performed in asymptomatic controls, the normal patterns have been established after studied patients are deemed normal and by comparison with adult patterns. Given these limitations, it is therefore important to recognize that the manometric evaluation may detect aberrations that may be clinically insignificant,[12] and care needs to be exerted to avoid overinterpretation.[1,12,13]

A major technical advance that has occurred in recent years has been the development HRM[9,10,14] (see **Figs. 2–7**). HRM is achieved first by increasing the number of recording sites and decreasing the spacing between them and then by using specialized software that transforms the data into contour plots. This allows a better definition of the intraluminal pressure environment without spatial gaps and with minimal movement-related artifacts.[15,16] In children, the main impact of the technology has been in the simplification of the intubation, tolerability and performance of the test.[16]

The major impact of HRM has been in the study of esophageal motor function (see **Figs. 2** and **3**). New parameters of motility have been defined (**Table 1**)[10,11] and have been incorporated in a new classification (Chicago Classification) of esophageal

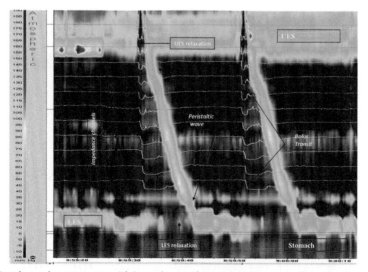

Fig. 2. Esophageal manometry with impedance. This represents a normal esophageal manometry using High resolution manometry. Normal relaxation of the upper esophageal and lower esophageal sphincter can be seen, as can the peristaltic wave. The tracing also has impedance waves, that allow the measurement of bolus transit.

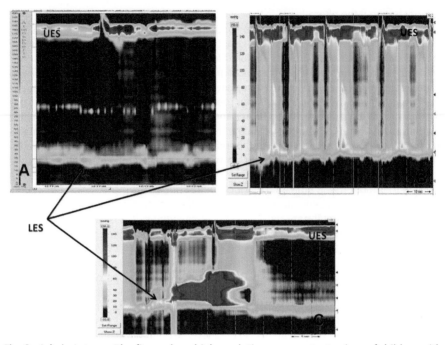

Fig. 3. Achalasia types. The figure show high resolution manometry tracings of children with the different achalasia subtypes. (*A*) Type 1 (characterized by lack of esophageal body contraction. (*B*) Type II (characterized by pressurization waves), and (*C*) Type III (characterized for having spastic contractions). See table for exact definitions of the subtypes.

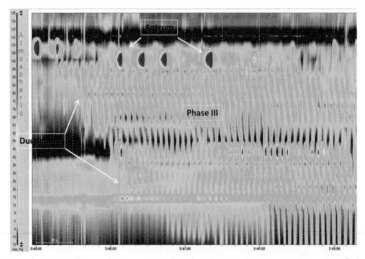

Fig. 4. Normal AD. High resolution antroduodenal manometry. A phase III of the motor migrating complex can be appreciated starting in the antrum (3 cycles per minute, and migrating distally into the small bowel (12 cycles per minute).

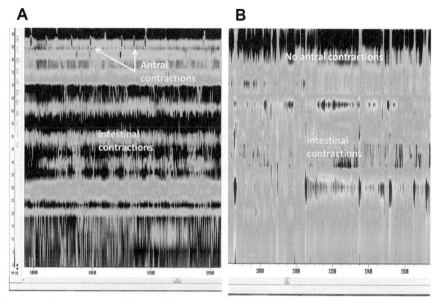

Fig. 5. Fed response and Gastroparesis. (*A*) shows a normal fed response with presence of antral and small bowel contractions, and (*B*) shows a patient with gastroparesis in which there are no antral contractions.

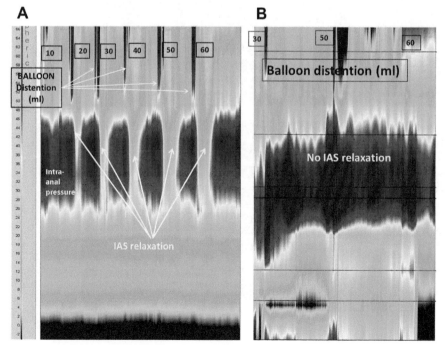

Fig. 6. Anorectal manometry tracing. (*A*) shows normal relaxation of the internal anal sphincter (IAS) after balloon distention. A normal dose response curve can be seen. In (*B*) the tracing represents a patient with Hirschsprung's disease. There is npo relaxation of the internal anal sphincter after balloon distention.

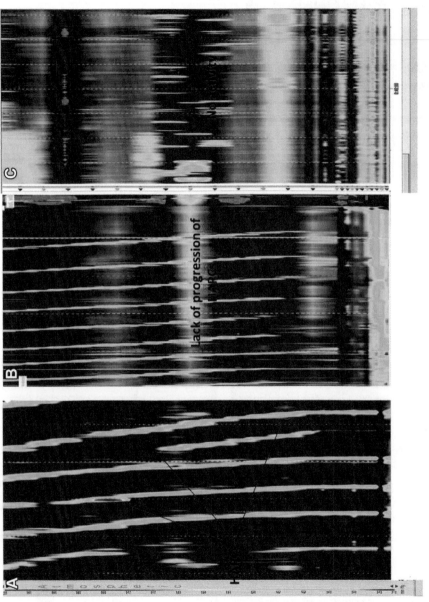

Fig. 7. High resolution colonic manometry. The figure shows the different patterns of colonic motility that can be seen in patients with constipation. (*A*) shows a normal study with the presence of high amplitude propagating contractions (HAPCs) migrating from the cecum all the way down to the rectosigmoid. (*B*) shows abnormal propagation of the HAPCs, and (*C*) shows no activity.

Box 4
Indications for manometry studies

Esophageal manometry

Esophageal dysfunction that is not explained by anatomic or well-defined problems

Dysphagia, odynophagia

Diagnosis of achalasia and other primary esophageal motor disorders

Support the diagnosis of connective tissue diseases, or other systemic illness.

Evaluation of patients with achalasia post-treatment and recurrent symptoms

Noncardiac chest pain

Patients with gastroesophageal reflux, where the diagnosis is not clear (to exclude primary motility disorders)

Before a fundoplication when a severe motility disorder is suspected

Localize lower esophageal sphincter before pH probe placement in patients with abnormal anatomy (like hiatal hernia).

Anorectal manometry

Diagnose a nonrelaxing internal anal sphincter.

Diagnose pelvic floor dyssynergia.

Evaluate postoperative patients with HD who have obstructive symptoms and for the effect of botulinum toxin.

Evaluate patients with fecal incontinence.

Evaluate postoperative patients after imperforate anus repair.

Decide if patient is a candidate for biofeedback therapy.

Antroduodenal manometry

Establish the presence of pseudo-obstruction. It has been shown extremely useful when the study demonstrates normal motility in patients unable to tolerate enteral feedings.

Classify pseudo-obstruction into myopathic or neuropathic forms.

Exclude a motility problem as the basis of a patient's symptoms. Showing normal findings in children with apparent intestinal failure

Evaluation of unexplained nausea and vomiting

Distinguish between rumination and vomiting

Exclude generalized motility dysfunction in patients with dysmotility elsewhere, for example, before colectomy.

It is indicated in patients with pseudo-obstruction considered for intestinal transplantation.

May be useful to predict outcome after feeding or after drug use in patients with pseudo-obstruction

May suggest unexpected obstruction

Colonic motility

Evaluation of selected patients with intractable constipation, because it can be helpful to differentiate functional fecal retention from colonic pseudo-obstruction.

Evaluation of children with pseudo-obstruction to establish presence of colonic involvement and to characterize the relationship between motor activity and persistent symptoms.

Establish the pathophysiology of persistent symptoms in selected children with HD, imperforate anus, and other colorectal problems.

Assess colonic motor activity prior to intestinal transplant.

Data from Di Lorenzo C, Hillemeier C, Hyman P, et al. Manometry studies in children: minimum standards for procedures. Neurogastroenterol Motil 2002;14(4):411–20; and Rodriguez L, Sood M, Di Lorenzo C, et al. An ANMS-NASPGHAN consensus document on anorectal and colonic manometry in children. Neurogastroenterol Motil 2017;29(1).

motility disorders proposed initially for adults but used widely in children (see **Table 1**).[14,17] Future studies are needed to establish if the same cutoff values used in adults also apply to children. Preliminary studies have shown that adjustments for size and age may be needed in children.[11,17] The addition of impedance measurements to HRM has provided the opportunity of studying the relationship between motility events and esophageal bolus flow (see **Fig. 2**). New objective parameters have been proposed and are providing new impact in the assessment of esophageal function. An automated impedance manometry method for the objective, reliable, and reproducible assessment of pharyngeal function in relation to ineffective pharyngeal swallowing and deglutitive aspiration has been described and shown predictive of aspiration.[18] The same analysis has been applied to study esophageal function and its relationship to dysphagia as well as resistance to flow through the esophagus gastric junction.[10]

Table 1 Chicago Classification	
Achalasia and esophagogastric gastric outflow obstruction	
Achalasia type I	Classic achalasia: mean IRP > upper limit of normal (usually 15 mm Hg), 100% failed peristalsis
Achalasia type II	Achalasia with esophageal compression: mean IRP > upper limit of normal, no normal peristalsis, panesophageal pressurization ≥20% of swallows
Achalasia type III	Mean IRP > upper limit of normal, no normal peristalsis, preserved fragments of distal peristalsis or premature (spastic) contractions (DCI 450 mm Hg.s.com ≥20% of swallows
Esophagus gastric junction outflow obstruction	Mean IRP > upper limit of normal, some instances of intact peristalsis, such that the criteria for achalasia are not met
Major disorders of peristalsis	
Distal esophageal spasm	Normal mean IRP ≥20% premature contractions (DCI >450 mm Hg.s.cm
Hypercontractile esophagus	At least 2 swallows with DCI >8000 mm Hg.s.cm
Absent contractility	Normal mean IRP, 100% of swallows with failed peristalsis
Minor disorders of peristalsis	
Ineffective esophageal motility	≥50% ineffective swallow
Fragmented peristalsis	≥50% fragmented contractions with DCI >450 mm Hg.s.cm

Abbreviations: DCI, distal contractile integral; IRP, integrated relaxation pressure.
Adapted from Kahrilas PJ, Bredenoord AJ, Fox M, et al. The Chicago Classification of esophageal motility disorders, v3.0. Neurogastroenterol Motil 2015;27(2):160–74.

HRM has also become the standard for ARM (see **Fig. 6**) and recently for antroduodenal (see **Figs. 4** and **5**) and colonic studies (see **Fig. 7**).[9]

PRIMARY MOTILITY DISORDERS IN CHILDREN

This discussion focuses on the most common primary motility disorders in children.

Esophageal Primary Motor Disorders

Achalasia

Clinical presentation Esophageal achalasia is a primary esophageal motor disorder that presents with obstructive symptoms at the gastroesophageal junction. It is uncommon, with a prevalence of 1 in 100,000 people.[19–21] It is estimated that less than 5% of patients with achalasia develop symptoms before 15 years of age.[20] A majority of cases are of unknown etiology, although in certain parts of the world, Chagas disease may have similar clinical presentation.[3,19,22] The median age for the diagnosis in children is approximately 8 years, and infant cases have been reported.[21] Genetic disorders associated with achalasia include Allgrove (or Triple A) syndrome (achalasia, adrenal insufficiency, and alacrima), Alport syndrome, and Down syndrome.[3,22] The pathogenesis of esophageal achalasia is unknown, and proposed causes include decreased nitric oxide synthase–containing nerve fibers and interstitial cells of Cajal in the distal esophagus.[3,19]

The presentation varies according to age.[22] In a review of 475 pediatric achalasia cases, 80% presented with vomiting, dysphagia in 76%, weight loss in 61%, respiratory symptoms in 44%, thoracic pain in 38%, growth failure in 31%, and nocturnal regurgitation in 21%.[22] In general, the youngest children have more respiratory symptoms. The dysphagia is often gradual and progressive, initially involving solids and progressing toward intermittent liquid involvement, regurgitation, and vomiting of undigested food.[3]

Diagnosis Achalasia can be suspected by upper Gastrointestinal series, in which a bird's beak appearance of the GEJ is usually seen. The diagnosis, however, requires esophageal manometry.[19,23] Achalasia is characterized by a lack of esophageal peristalsis and lower esophageal sphincter dysfunction.[19,23,24] With the advent of HRM, 3 subtypes of achalasia have been described[14,19,23,24]: type 1, classic achalasia with 100% failed peristalsis; type 2, no normal peristalsis and panesophageal pressurization with ≥20% of swallows; and type 3, no normal peristalsis with preserved fragments of distal peristalsis or premature [spastic] contractions with ≥20% of swallows (see **Fig. 3**).

Therapy Therapy is directed toward decreasing resistance to flow at the GEJ.[19,23,24] Choices include pharmacotherapy,[19,22–24] *Clostridium botulinum* toxin injection,[19,22–24] pneumatic balloon dilatation,[19,22–24] or esophagomyotomy performed by minimally invasive methods.[19,21–24] Botulinum toxin is now used only in equivocal cases, and pharmacologic therapy only for short periods of time, as a temporizing bridge until a more definitive therapy is offered. The best long-term treatment has not been established, but large prospective randomized studies performed in adults suggest that myotomy and pneumatic balloon dilation are equivalent.[19,23,24] There are no studies in pediatrics, and both have been shown effective, although those undergoing pneumatic balloon dilation usually require repeated treatments.[21] The preference of which modality to use rests more on the providers and the existing expertise. It has been suggested for the first time that the type of underlying manometric pattern may predict response to therapy in adults.[19,24] Recently a new approach using endoscopic techniques to perform a myotomy (peroral endoscopic myotomy [POEM]) has been shown effective in adults and children, and it is possible that it will become the gold standard therapy in the future.[25,26]

Stomach Motor Disorders

Gastroparesis

Clinical presentation GP, or delayed gastric emptying (GE) without obstruction, occurs in children, but the exact incidence and prevalence are not known.[27–29] The most common symptoms of GP in children include vomiting (42%–68%), abdominal pain (35%–51%), and nausea (28%–29%).[27,28] Children commonly present with vomiting, whereas adolescents primarily report nausea and abdominal pain.[27,28] Concurrent nausea, bloating, and other dyspeptic symptoms may also be associated. Vomiting classically occurs late postprandially and commonly contains foods eaten many hours previously.[27,28] Some patients with GP complain of regurgitation secondary to reflux. There is a significant overlap between the symptoms of GP and those of other disorders, in particular functional dyspepsia (FD). FD is characterized by pain or burning in the epigastrium, early satiety, and/or fullness—symptoms similar to those of GP and the differentiation can be difficult.[30,31]

The prevalence and etiology of GP in children have not been extensively examined. It has been suggested that only 20% of children have identifiable contributing factors. Idiopathic GP occurs in the absence of a systemic disease or other identifiable etiology.[28] Postviral GP is often suggested by a history of fevers, myalgias, nausea, or diarrhea occurring prior to presentation and may be confirmed in the laboratory.[3,28] Other causes in children include diabetes mellitus, vagotomy, medications, endocrinologic abnormalities (eg, hypothyroidism), foregut developmental abnormalities (eg, gastroschisis), neurologic disorders, and genetic/metabollic disorders.[3,28]

Diagnosis The diagnosis in children is often made through nuclear medicine scintigraphy, in particular the 4-hour GE test,[3,6,8] although standardization of this evaluation in children is lacking. As discussed previously, noninvasive techniques using breath testing can also be used.[3,6,8] The smart pill has also been shown to be a reliable noninvasive test to measure GE in adults, but there is limited information in children.[8] Finally there are other more invasive techniques to assess antral function, like antroduodenal manometry, which may demonstrate antral contractile abnormalities, in particular hypomotility. Although this test is believed to be sensitive and specific, it is more invasive[4,32] (see **Fig. 5**).

Therapy Therapy includes addressing any secondary causes, discontinuing medications known to slow GE, modifying a child's diet to decrease gastric distention, and appropriate nutritional support.[4,28,32,33] Given that liquids empty more quickly than solids, high residual undigestible solid food should be avoided. At times, nasogastric feedings or jejunal feedings may be needed to provide enteral nutrition. Pain needs to be treated aggressively.[4,28,32,33]

Pharmacotherapy may include conventional antiemetics (eg, Ondasentron) to decrease nausea and vomiting. Cyproheptidine has shown effective in the treatment of nausea.[34] Prokinetic drugs designed to improve GE have improved treatment of GP in children, with response rates close to 50% reported,[28,34] although the evidence is sparse. These drugs include erythromycin, metoclopramide, domperidone, and cisapride. Erythromycin is used as a first-line agent. Other macrolides, such as azithromycin, have been shown to improve GE and antral motility patterns in adults. An investigational new drug application and institutional review board approval is required for domperidone usage. Cisapride has been removed from the market in the United States due to its association with cardiac fatalities and is available through limited access protocols. Baclofen has been shown to improve GE in 1 pediatric study.[35] Endoscopic pyloric botulinum toxin injection has been reported to have an overall 67% response rate in children, with a median duration of 3 months with no significant adverse effects,[33] although 2 placebo-controlled trials in adults did not find sufficient evidence to support its use.[33] The use of botulinum toxin injection should be limited to those patients who fail medical therapy before invasive surgical interventions are considered. Recently it has been suggested that gastric electrical stimulation is a treatment option. Even though studies show no effect on GE, there is an improvement in symptoms, quality of life, length of hospital stay, and medication use.[36,37]

Small Intestinal and Colonic Motor Disorders

The motor disorders that affect the small intestine and colon in children include conditions, such as HD, chronic intestinal pseudo-obstruction (CIPO), and intractable constipation.

Chronic intestinal pseudo-obstruction

Clinical presentation CIPO is a rare disorder that occurs in approximately 1 in every 270,000 live births.[38] CIPO is not a single clinical entity, rather an umbrella term for a range of different diseases leading to severe, end-stage gut motor failure.[38] It is defined as "a severe disabling disease characterized by repetitive episodes or continuous symptoms and signs of intestinal obstruction, including radiographic documentation of dilated intestines and air-fluid levels, in the absence of fixed lesion which is occluding the lumen of the intestine."[3] The motor alterations lead to the inability to normally transit nourishment and secretions along the GI tract. Pediatric symptoms in one review included abdominal distention (98%), vomiting (91%), constipation (77%), failure to thrive (62%), abdominal pain (58%), sepsis (34%), and diarrhea (31%).[39,40] Any segment of the intestinal tract may be affected, and symptoms represent this heterogeneity. Intestinal dilation and slow transit predispose the patient to bacterial overgrowth, which may lead to malabsoprtion, diarrhea, and malnutrition.[38–40] In 1 review of 105 CIPO pediatric cases, approximately 75% presented within the first year of life, with 67% presenting within the first month.[40]

CIPO may be primary or secondary due to different processes and may be part of syndromes, such as megacystis, microcolon, and intestinal hypoperistalsis syndrome,[38,40] where new genetic mutations like in ACTG2 have been identified.[41] A majority of infantile forms are primary and spontaneous, with a small minority hereditary familial processes. Primary and secondary forms or often classified into primarily myopathic processes or neuropathic processes. Secondary forms are due to a viral infection,[38] muscular disorders (eg, muscular dystrophy), autoimmune disorders (eg, dermatomyositis), endocrinologic disorders (eg, hypothyroidism), mitochondrial disorders, related to medications, or inflammatory processes (eg, Crohn disease).[38] Associated intestinal abnormalities, such as malrotation, gastroschisis, and atresias, are seen in more than 25% of pediatric CIPO cases.[39] Urinary abnormalities, such as megacystis and urinary tract infections, are seen in a majority of congenital myopathic processes and in a minority of neuropathic processes[38–40,42] and need to be taken in account for long-term management.

Diagnosis Diagnosis is made clinically, and radiographic studies are used to exclude mechanical obstruction.[39] Many children have more than 1 laparatomy before pseudo-obstruction is formally diagnosed. Unfortunately, abdominal surgeries make it challenging to differentiate pseudo-obstructive crises from obstruction caused by adhesions.

Antroduodenal and colonic manometry have been used to characterize the intestinal involvement in children with CIPO and may also predict successful enteral nutrition support[1,38,39] (see **Fig. 4**). When myopathy is present, there are low amplitude but normally organized contractions found. With advanced disease, there is an absence of contractions. In neuropathy, contractions are of normal amplitude but are poorly organized, with groups of nonperistaltic contractions, prolonged tonic contractions, and persistence of a fasting motor pattern despite alimentation.[1] Care must be taken in interpreting manometric studies when severe intestinal dilation is present. At times, manometric studies are most useful when normal motility is demonstrated in children with suspected intestinal failure that are able unable to tolerate enteral feedings.[1,13] Often persistent pain is the main symptom, and somatoform disorders need to be considered in those patients.

Therapy A specific therapy is not available and supportive measures are given. Special attention must be placed to avoid complications like malnutrition or bacterial overgrowth.[38–40,42] When possible, it is recommended that enteral nutrition be given. Liquid diets low in fat are more easily emptied by the stomach, and, when not possible, total parental nutrition may be needed.[39,40,42] Metabolic and electrolyte abnormalities need to be prevented. Medications that decrease GI motility should not be used, and bacterial overgrowth should be treated aggressively. Surgical decompression through gastrostomies and ileostomies is frequently necessary.[38] Prokinetics have occasionally been effective.[38–40,42]

Treatment of abdominal pain is important. Opioids worsen GI motility and cause dependence. Tricyclic antidepressants, clonidine, and short periods of epidural anesthesia may be benefical.[38–40,42] Psychiatric support for the patient and family is helpful and provides important benefits.

CIPO is a disease that has high mortality and morbidity.[38–40,42] Quality-of-life outcomes in children with CIPO and their families are significantly diminished.[38,39,42] Although parenteral nutrition has saved the lives of children who cannot be given sufficient enteral nutrition, it is associated with the complications of sepsis, thromboembolic events, and liver disease with progressive failure.[38–40,42] These complications lead to the majority of deaths seen in children with CIPO.[38–40,42] Small bowel transplantation may provide the only hope of cure in patients with the most severe disease.[38]

Colonic Motor Abnormalities

Defecation problems in children are common.[43,44] After the neonatal period, the most frequent cause of constipation in childhood is functional constipation. Discrete abnormalities in colonic motility are rarely an important pathogenic factor in these children. The differential diagnosis, however, includes primary motor disorders that should not be missed.[44]

Hirschsprung disease

The most common of these conditions is HD, with an incidence that varies from 1 in 5000 to 1 in 10,000 live births.[43–45] This is a congenital disease with varying degrees of aganglionosis starting distally from the internal anal sphincter and moving proximally. The aganglionic segment is in a constant contractile state, whereas segment of intestine proximal to this with ganglion cells becomes dilated due to the functional obstruction distal to it.[32] The length of the aganglionic segment varies. It is limited to the rectum and sigmoid in 75%, affects the entire colon in 7%, and rarely extends into the small intestine.[46] The median age at time of diagnosis has been decreasing over time. It is established in 15% in the first month, 40% to 50% in first 3 months, 60% at the end of the first year, and 85% by 4 years of age.[43–45] Recent advances have shown that in some cases, identifiable genetic mutations (eg, proto-oncogene RET mutations) are associated with it.[45,47,48] Symptoms vary with age and the length of aganglionosis. In newborns, HD may present with acute obstruction, bilious emesis, abdominal distention, and lack of meconium passage. If a diagnosis is not made, the infant presents with constipation, which may later be followed by abdominal obstruction, frequent episodes of impaction, or the development of enterocolitis. Enterocolitis may be involved in 15% to 50% of cases and may be the first sign of presentation in 12%. It continues to be the principal cause of death, with a mortality rate that can reach up to 20% to 50%.[32,49] From infancy though adulthood, constipation may be the only symptom, which should be differentiated from functional constipation. Using clinical characteristics alone does not always distinguish the 2, and therefore HD should be considered in all patients with intractable constipation.[44,50]

Diagnosis Diagnosis is established through biopsy. Given that obtaining biopsies carries risks, other less invasive techniques, such as barium enema and ARM, may aid in excluding HD, because it shows a nonrelaxing internal anal sphincter in cases of aganglionosis (see **Fig. 6**). ARM is superior to barium enema for the diagnosis of HD, and studies suggest ARM may be as sensitive as rectal biopsy,[44,51] although false-negative results may occur, particularly within the neonatal period. Diagnosis should be confirmed via biopsy in all patients with an abnormal barium enema or suggestive ARM.[44,51] Rectal biopsy is the method of choice to reach the diagnosis in the neonate.[44,51] Rectal suction biopsies may be used to make the diagnosis. If ganglion cells are present, the diagnosis is excluded. If ganglion cells are not present, surgical full-thickness biopsies are undertaken. The usage of specialized stains, such as the acetylcholinesterase stain, and lately calretinin, are important, particularly in superficial biopsies, because they may obviate further surgical biopsies.[52,53]

Therapy Definitive therapy is surgical, although initial medical management is important to stabilize the patient. This includes correction of electrolyte abnormalities and rectal decompression. In cases of enterocolitis, antibiotics should also be administered.[52,53] Surgery is aimed at resecting the aganglionic segment, followed by a pull-through of ganglionic segments to the rectum.[54] The most frequently performed operations include the Swenson, Duhamel, and Soave. Recent advances have allowed for use of transanal or laparoscopic techniques.[54,55] The choice of surgery is based on the training and experience of the pediatric surgeon. The complications and long-term outcomes after the different surgeries are similar.[52,53] Obstructive symptoms occur in a significant number of patients, and the treatment of these has included application of botulinum toxin directly to the sphincter.[32,49,56] Antegrade continence enemas may be placed in postsurgical HD patients with continued obstructive symptoms.[57]

Internal anal sphincter achalasia, formerly termed ultrashort HD, an entity in which rectal biopsies show ganglion cells but ARM demonstrates lack of internal anal sphincter relaxation, has been described. Children with this condition may have significant constipation, enterocolitis, and abdominal distention due to the lack of sphincter relaxation. Therapy includes first botulinum toxin injection[49] and may require eventually a posterior myectomy.[58]

Other Neuromuscular Diseases Involving the Colon

Neurologic lesions, such as spinal dysraphism, spinal cord lesions, and tethered cord have been reported in up to 9% of pediatric patients with intractable constipation.[44]

Progressive neuromuscular deficits, abnormal gait, back pain, and new onset of fecal and urinary incontinence may be among the presenting symptoms. ARM may show abnormal sphincter tone, prolonged internal anal sphincter relaxation, and/or abnormal recovery with sustained balloon inflation and anal spasms. The presence of anal spasms has been shown predictive of spinal abnormalities in 60% of children with IC.[44]

The evaluation of a child in which a colonic neuromuscular disease is suspected includes radiographic and manometric studies.[44,45,59,60] Transit with radiopaque markers, may differentiate generalized colonic diseases from defecatory obstructive processes. Recently the smart pill has been used as a noninvasive way to address colonic transit.[7] With generalized colonic dysmotility, the radiopaque markers are found throughout the colon for many days. A normal colonic transit with radiopaque markers has been shown to correlate with normal colonic motility. In recent years, in children with intractable constipation, studies with colonic manometry have been used to establish the severity of the affected intestine[9,44,45,59] and patterns of abnormal colonic motility have emerged.[9,44,45,59] These can include segmental abnormalities or more generalized dismotility[9] (see **Fig. 7**). Efforts to correlate motility patterns with underlying histologic abnormalities have yielded mixed results, although the most recent studies using high-resolution colonic motility have shown a correlation between certain patterns of dismotility and specific histopahtologic changes.[59] It is possible that in the future distinctive populations of colonic dysfunction will be able to be defined.[9]

Treatment is supportive. Laxatives and therapies directed at decreasing anal sphincter pressure are used. There are new laxatives that are beginning to be used in the treatment of constipation, like the secretagogues (like lubiprostone and linaclotide).[45,61] Rarely, surgical resections are required. Appendicostomies or cecostomies are also used to provide antegrade enemas.[44,45] These operations allow for access to the proximal colon through the creation of a conduit to the skin. The procedure may be done surgically, with interventional radiology, or with endoscopy.[44,45,62] The results have been positive, particularly in patients with fecal incontinence for neurologic problems and in patients with constipation.[63] Sacral nerve stimulation is another new promising technique that has been used in patients with intractable constipation, but large prospective studies are still needed.[45]

FUTURE ADVANCES

Genetic advances have allowed for the detection of genes responsible for intestinal development and function. As discussed previously, mutations that lead to HD have been found and are being extensively studied. The genetic basis of other intestinal motor disorders will likely be elucidated and greater insight into the pathophysiology of these disorders will continue to emerge.

Continued research on noninvasive diagnostic modalities may lead to less discomfort while maintaining a high degree of sensitivity and specificity for the diagnosis of these disorders. The utilization of new manometric techniques will allow for the better study of motility processes. The challenge with the increased pathophysiologic knowledge will be to develop new drugs for the treatment of GI motor disorders. With continued basic science advances into the function of the enteric nervous system, such as the identification new receptors, new compounds will surely emerge. Drugs addressing and allowing for modification of intestinal sensation are sorely needed. Further clinical studies within the pediatric population are anxiously awaited.

REFERENCES

1. Nurko SS. Gastrointestinal manometry. Methodology and indications. In: Walker WA, al. e, editors. Pediatric gastrointestinal disease. 5th edition. Philadelphia: B.C. Decker Inc; 2008. p. 1375–91.
2. Camilleri M, Hasler WL, Parkman HP, et al. Measurement of gastrointestinal motility in the GI laboratory. Gastroenterology 1998;115(3):747–62.
3. Chumpitazi B, Nurko S. Pediatric gastrointestinal motility disorders: challenges and a clinical update. Gastroenterol Hepatol 2008;4(2):140–8.
4. Di Lorenzo C, Hillemeier C, Hyman P, et al. Manometry studies in children: minimum standards for procedures. Neurogastroenterol Motil 2002;14(4):411–20.
5. Camilleri M, Bharucha AE, di Lorenzo C, et al. American Neurogastroenterology and Motility Society consensus statement on intraluminal measurement of gastrointestinal and colonic motility in clinical practice. Neurogastroenterol Motil 2008; 20(12):1269–82.
6. Chogle A, Saps M. Gastroparesis in children: the benefit of conducting 4-hour scintigraphic gastric-emptying studies. J Pediatr Gastroenterol Nutr 2013;56(4): 439–42.
7. Belkind-Gerson J, Tran K, Di Lorenzo C. Novel techniques to study colonic motor function in children. Curr Gastroenterol Rep 2013;15(8):335.
8. Green AD, Belkind-Gerson J, Surjanhata BC, et al. Wireless motility capsule test in children with upper gastrointestinal symptoms. J Pediatr 2013;162(6): 1181–7.
9. Rodriguez L, Sood M, Di Lorenzo C, et al. An ANMS-NASPGHAN consensus document on anorectal and colonic manometry in children. Neurogastroenterol Motil 2017. [Epub ahead of print].
10. Rommel N, Omari TI, Selleslagh M, et al. High-resolution manometry combined with impedance measurements discriminates the cause of dysphagia in children. Eur J Pediatr 2015;174(12):1629–37.
11. Goldani HA, Staiano A, Borrelli O, et al. Pediatric esophageal high-resolution manometry: utility of a standardized protocol and size-adjusted pressure topography parameters. Am J Gastroenterol 2010;105(2):460–7.
12. Baron HI, Beck DC, Vargas JH, et al. Overinterpretation of gastroduodenal motility studies: two cases involving Munchausen syndrome by proxy. J Pediatr 1995;126(3):397–400.
13. Hyman PE, Bursch B, Beck D, et al. Discriminating pediatric condition falsification from chronic intestinal pseudo-obstruction in toddlers. Child Maltreat 2002;7(2): 132–7.
14. Kahrilas PJ, Bredenoord AJ, Fox M, et al. The Chicago Classification of esophageal motility disorders, v3.0. Neurogastroenterol Motil 2015;27(2):160–74.
15. Bredenoord AJ, Fox M, Kahrilas PJ, et al. Chicago classification criteria of esophageal motility disorders defined in high resolution esophageal pressure topography. Neurogastroenterol Motil 2012;24(Suppl 1):57–65.
16. Staiano A, Boccia G, Miele E, et al. Segmental characteristics of oesophageal peristalsis in paediatric patients. Neurogastroenterol Motil 2008;20(1):19–26.
17. Singendonk MM, Kritas S, Cock C, et al. Applying the Chicago Classification criteria of esophageal motility to a pediatric cohort: effects of patient age and size. Neurogastroenterol Motil 2014;26(9):1333–41.
18. Ferris L, Rommel N, Doeltgen S, et al. Pressure-flow analysis for the assessment of pediatric oropharyngeal dysphagia. J Pediatr 2016;177:279–85.e1.

19. Krill JT, Naik RD, Vaezi MF. Clinical management of achalasia: current state of the art. Clin Exp Gastroenterol 2016;9:71–82.
20. Podas T, Eaden J, Mayberry M, et al. Achalasia: a critical review of epidemiological studies. Am J Gastroenterol 1998;93(12):2345–7.
21. Smits M, van Lennep M, Vrijlandt R, et al. Pediatric Achalasia in the Netherlands: incidence, clinical course, and quality of life. J Pediatr 2016;169:110–5.e3.
22. Nurko SS. The Esophagus: motor disorders. In: Walker WA, al. e, editors. Pediatric gastrointestinal disease. 3rd edition. Philadelphia: B.C. Decker Inc; 2000. p. 317–50.
23. Vaezi MF, Pandolfino JE, Vela MF. ACG clinical guideline: diagnosis and management of achalasia. Am J Gastroenterol 2013;108(8):1238–49 [quiz: 1250].
24. Vaezi MF, Felix VN, Penagini R, et al. Achalasia: from diagnosis to management. Ann N Y Acad Sci 2016;1381(1):34–44.
25. Zhang Y, Wang H, Chen X, et al. Per-oral endoscopic myotomy versus laparoscopic heller myotomy for achalasia: a meta-analysis of nonrandomized comparative studies. Medicine 2016;95(6):e2736.
26. Li C, Tan Y, Wang X, et al. Peroral endoscopic myotomy for treatment of achalasia in children and adolescents. J Pediatr Surg 2015;50(1):201–5.
27. Waseem S, Islam S, Kahn G, et al. Spectrum of gastroparesis in children. J Pediatr Gastroenterol Nutr 2012;55(2):166–72.
28. Rodriguez L, Irani K, Jiang H, et al. Clinical presentation, response to therapy, and outcome of gastroparesis in children. J Pediatr Gastroenterol Nutr 2012; 55(2):185–90.
29. Jung HK. The incidence, prevalence, and survival of gastroparesis in olmsted county, Minnesota, 1996-2006 (gastroenterology 2009;136:1225-1233). J Neurogastroenterol Motil 2010;16(1):99–100.
30. Hyams JS, Di Lorenzo C, Saps M, et al. Functional disorders: children and adolescents. Gastroenterology 2016;150:1456–68.
31. Ganesh M, Nurko S. Functional dyspepsia in children. Pediatr Ann 2014;43(4): e101–5.
32. Chumpitazi BP, Nurko S. Defecation disorders in children after surgery for Hirschsprung disease. J Pediatr Gastroenterol Nutr 2011;53(1):75–9.
33. Rodriguez L, Rosen R, Manfredi M, et al. Endoscopic intrapyloric injection of botulinum toxin A in the treatment of children with gastroparesis: a retrospective, open-label study. Gastrointest Endosc 2012;75(2):302–9.
34. Rodriguez L, Diaz J, Nurko S. Safety and efficacy of cyproheptadine for treating dyspeptic symptoms in children. J Pediatr 2013;163(1):261–7.
35. Omari TI, Benninga MA, Sansom L, et al. Effect of baclofen on esophagogastric motility and gastroesophageal reflux in children with gastroesophageal reflux disease: a randomized controlled trial. J Pediatr 2006;149(4):468–74.
36. Lu PL, Di Lorenzo C. Neurostimulation of the gastrointestinal tract in children: is it time to shock the gut? Curr Opin Pediatr 2016;28(5):631–7.
37. Teich S, Mousa HM, Punati J, et al. Efficacy of permanent gastric electrical stimulation for the treatment of gastroparesis and functional dyspepsia in children and adolescents. J Pediatr Surg 2013;48(1):178–83.
38. Di Nardo G, Di Lorenzo C, Lauro A, et al. Chronic intestinal pseudo-obstruction in children and adults: diagnosis and therapeutic options. Neurogastroenterol Motil 2017. [Epub ahead of print].
39. Connor FL, Di Lorenzo C. Chronic intestinal pseudo-obstruction: assessment and management. Gastroenterology 2006;130(2 Suppl 1):S29–36.

40. Faure C, Goulet O, Ategbo S, et al. Chronic intestinal pseudoobstruction syndrome: clinical analysis, outcome, and prognosis in 105 children. French-Speaking Group of Pediatric Gastroenterology. Dig Dis Sci 1999;44(5):953–9.
41. Matera I, Rusmini M, Guo Y, et al. Variants of the ACTG2 gene correlate with degree of severity and presence of megacystis in chronic intestinal pseudo-obstruction. Eur J Hum Genet 2016;24(8):1211–5.
42. Mousa H, Hyman PE, Cocjin J, et al. Long-term outcome of congenital intestinal pseudoobstruction. Dig Dis Sci 2002;47(10):2298–305.
43. Benninga MA, Faure C, Hyman PE, et al. Childhood functional gastrointestinal disorders: neonate/Toddler. Gastroenterology 2016;50:1443–55.
44. Tabbers MM, Dilorenzo C, Berger MY, et al. Evaluation and treatment of functional constipation in infants and children: evidence-based recommendations from ESPGHAN and NASPGHAN. J Pediatr Gastroenterol Nutr 2014;58(2):265–81.
45. Koppen IJ, Di Lorenzo C, Saps M, et al. Childhood constipation: finally something is moving! Expert Rev Gastroenterol Hepatol 2016;10(1):141–55.
46. Rudolph C, Benaroch L. Hirschsprung disease. Pediatr Rev 1995;16(1):5–11.
47. Knowles CH, Lindberg G, Panza E, et al. New perspectives in the diagnosis and management of enteric neuropathies. Nat Rev Gastroenterol Hepatol 2013;10(4):206–18.
48. Moore SW. Genetic impact on the treatment & management of Hirschsprung disease. J Pediatr Surg 2017;52(2):218–22.
49. Chumpitazi BP, Fishman SJ, Nurko S. Long-term clinical outcome after botulinum toxin injection in children with nonrelaxing internal anal sphincter. Am J Gastroenterol 2009;104(4):976–83.
50. Rudolph CD, Hyman PE, Altschuler SM, et al. Diagnosis and treatment of chronic intestinal pseudo-obstruction in children: report of consensus workshop. J Pediatr Gastroenterol Nutr 1997;24(1):102–12.
51. de Lorijn F, Kremer LC, Reitsma JB, et al. Diagnostic tests in Hirschsprung disease: a systematic review. J Pediatr Gastroenterol Nutr 2006;42(5):496–505.
52. Nurko SS. Treatment of Hirschsprung's disease. In: Wolfe MM, Cohen S, Davis G, editors. Therapy of digestive disease. New York: W.B. Saunders; 2000. p. 609–16.
53. Nurko SS. Complications after gastrointestinal surgery: a medical perspective. In: Walker WA, editor. Pediatric gastrointestinal disease. 3rd edition. Philadelphia: B.C. Decker Inc; 2000. p. 1843–76.
54. Thomson D, Allin B, Long AM, et al. Laparoscopic assistance for primary transanal pull-through in Hirschsprung's disease: a systematic review and meta-analysis. BMJ Open 2015;5(3):e006063.
55. Georgeson KE, Robertson DJ. Laparoscopic-assisted approaches for the definitive surgery for Hirschsprung's disease. Semin Pediatr Surg 2004;13(4):256–62.
56. Langer JC. Persistent obstructive symptoms after surgery for Hirschsprung's disease: development of a diagnostic and therapeutic algorithm. J Pediatr Surg 2004;39(10):1458–62.
57. Yagmurlu A, Harmon CM, Georgeson KE. Laparoscopic cecostomy button placement for the management of fecal incontinence in children with Hirschsprung's disease and anorectal anomalies. Surg Endosc 2006;20(4):624–7.
58. De Caluwe D, Yoneda A, Akl U, et al. Internal anal sphincter achalasia: outcome after internal sphincter myectomy. J Pediatr Surg 2001;36(5):736–8.
59. Giorgio V, Borrelli O, Smith VV, et al. High-resolution colonic manometry accurately predicts colonic neuromuscular pathological phenotype in pediatric slow transit constipation. Neurogastroenterol Motil 2013;25(1):70–8.e8-9.

60. Koletzko S, Jesch I, Faus-Kebetaler T, et al. Rectal biopsy for diagnosis of intestinal neuronal dysplasia in children: a prospective multicentre study on interobserver variation and clinical outcome. Gut 1999;44(6):853–61.
61. Hyman PE, Di Lorenzo C, Prestridge LL, et al. Lubiprostone for the treatment of functional constipation in children. J Pediatr Gastroenterol Nutr 2014;58(3): 283–91.
62. Chait PG, Shandling B, Richards HM, et al. Fecal incontinence in children: treatment with percutaneous cecostomy tube placement–a prospective study. Radiology 1997;203(3):621–4.
63. Siddiqui AA, Fishman SJ, Bauer SB, et al. Long-term follow-up of patients after antegrade continence enema procedure. J Pediatr Gastroenterol Nutr 2011; 52(5):574–80.

Intestinal Transplant in Children

Nidhi Rawal, MD[a], Nada Yazigi, MD[b],*

KEYWORDS

- Intestine • Short gut syndrome • Pediatric • Transplant

KEY POINTS

- Outcomes of intestinal transplantation have dramatically improved; pediatric recipient survival is up to 95% and 70% at 1 and 3 years, respectively.
- Aggressive and innovative intestinal rehabilitation efforts have improved outcomes of children suffering from short gut syndrome — intestinal transplantation is now an integrated treatment modality when rehabilitation efforts fail.
- Early referral to a transplant center is crucial to optimize transplantation option and outcomes.
- Long-term intestinal transplant outcomes depend on excellent compliance with follow-up and immunosuppressive regimen.
- Chronic rejection incidence is dramatically decreased with new immunosuppressive protocols but remains the Achilles heel of pediatric intestinal transplantation.

HISTORY

The first reported human intestinal transplant was performed by Lillihei and coworkers in 1968.[1] Many attempts followed over the next decades and were met with high failure rates due to graft rejection and infectious complications. The past decade has seen major advances in the field, ushering in a new era where intestinal transplantation is the treatment of choice for many with intestinal failure.

The international 1-year mortality from pediatric intestinal transplantation significantly declined over the past decade, from 30% to the current 10% to 15%. This has mainly been the fruit of a multidisciplinary approach adopted in transplant centers, spanning the spectrum of diagnosis and treatment of intestinal failure to short-term and long-term care of post-transplant patients. Pediatric age carries many additional special

Disclosure Statement: The authors have nothing to disclose.
[a] Division of Gastroenterology, Hepatology and Nutrition, Department of Pediatrics, University of Maryland Medical Center, 22 South Green Street, Baltimore, MD 21201, USA; [b] Pediatric Transplant Hepatology, Department of Transplantation, MedStar Georgetown University Hospital, MedStar Georgetown Transplant Institute, PHC#2, 3800 Reservoir Road, Northwest, Washington, DC 20007, USA
* Corresponding author.
E-mail address: nada.a.yazigi@gunet.georgetown.edu

Pediatr Clin N Am 64 (2017) 613–619
http://dx.doi.org/10.1016/j.pcl.2017.02.002
0031-3955/17/© 2017 Elsevier Inc. All rights reserved.

considerations along the spectrum of care that continue to cause challenges but also offers growth opportunities. In particular, pediatric intestinal transplantation indications and timing are changing as a result of new developments in diagnostic and treatment tools.

This article reviews updates on pediatric intestinal transplantation and highlights future directions.

INTESTINAL FAILURE AND REHABILITATION

Intestinal failure can be broadly defined as the inability of the intestines to function, which can either be secondary to anatomically short intestine or lack of adequate absorptive intestinal function.

Intestinal Failure Causes

- Anatomic loss
  - Intestinal resection (volvulus, NEC, gastroschisis, intestinal atresia, Crohn disease)
  - Intestinal bypass
- Congenital mucosal disorders
  - Microvillous inclusion disease
  - Tufting enteropathy
- Intestinal motility disorders
  - Hirschsprung disease
  - Intestinal pseudo-obstruction
  - Megacystis microcolon hypoperistaltic syndrome

Every effort should be made for intestinal rehabilitation in patients who have some preserved ileal length.[2,3] In addition to nutritional and fluid rehabilitation, surgical procedures are commonly used to increase the intestinal absorptive surface and control bacterial overgrowth resulting from intestinal stasis. Such procedures include but are not limited to bowel lengthening, such as serial transverse enteroplasty and longitudinal intestinal lengthening and tailoring.[4] Trials are ongoing with enteral growth hormones and glutamine to improve the mucosal health. In addition, control of bacterial overgrowth, avoiding infections, and minimizing lipids exposure have greatly decreased early liver failure, allowing more time for rehabilitation efforts.[5] For some patients, however, these efforts remain temporary bridges that only help to reduce morbidity and mortality while affected patients await transplantation.

Complications of Intestinal Failure

Intestinal failure is a debilitating condition that can result in life-threatening complications. Intestinal transplantation has been a life-saving treatment of such patients. The most serious encountered complications are parenteral nutrition (PN)–associated liver disease, sepsis and loss of intravenous access.[2,3]

PN liver disease or intestinal failure–associated liver disease has been reported in as many as 50% of patients with intestinal failure who received PN for more than 5 years. It is more frequently seen in infants and toddlers versus adolescents and adults. Progressive liver disease can be identified by persistent elevations in serum bilirubin for more than 3 months to 4 months. These patients are also at risk of developing other complications, such as portal hypertension, variceal bleeding, and liver failure. All efforts should be made to perform intestinal transplant in these children while the liver disease is still reversible. Once liver failure is established, survival on the transplantation wait list is greatly affected and remains at less than 50%. Recently, intravenous lipids minimization and the use of polyunsaturated lipids have helped improve the incidence of (and sometimes reverse) jaundice and halt the rapidity of liver disease progression. But once the liver fibrosis is established, patients also require liver transplantation.[2,5]

Sepsis is the most common complication of PN in children less than 2 years of age. Excellent central line care, controlling bacterial overgrowth, ethanol, and antibiotics central line locks have all been helpful in decreasing its incidence. Good sepsis control has also been shown to be liver protective. Infectious complications unfortunately remain a reality for all. They are more common in patients with motility disorders and ones with primary or secondary immune deficiencies. Sepsis indications for intestinal transplant include systemic and serious infections, such as endocarditis, brain abscess, and fungal or severe bacterial infections, resulting in multiorgan failure.

In patients who are fully dependent on an intravenous source of nutrition, loss of intravenous access is clearly a life-threatening complication. It is unfortunately frequently encountered in children with intestinal failure and can be the only manifestation of a thrombophilic state.[2]

INTESTINAL TRANSPLANTATION INDICATIONS AND EPIDEMIOLOGY

In children, anatomic short bowel syndrome (SBS) is the most common cause of intestinal failure, with an estimated incidence of 3 patients to 5 patients per 100,000 births per year. PN becomes the mainstay treatment and survival tool for these patients.

A retrospective review of the United Network for Organ Sharing database by Lao and colleagues[6] showed that the median age for transplant is 1 year, and median weight at the time of the intestinal transplant is 10.7 kg. Almost 70% of patients needed both intestinal and liver transplant. The most common diagnoses encountered in this database were gastroschisis (24%), necrotizing enterocolitis (NEC) (15%), volvulus (14%), other causes of short gut syndrome (19%), functional bowel syndrome (16%), and Hirschsprung disease (7%) (**Box 1**).

Box 1
Leading causes of intestinal transplant in children

End-stage intestinal failure due to permanent requirement for partial or complete intravenous alimentation that is no longer tolerated
1. Progressive liver disease with/without portal hypertension
2. Impending loss of adequate central venous access to deliver nutrition
3. Recurrent catheter-related sepsis

Anatomic SBS due to massive resection of intestine
1. In neonates
    Midgut volvulus
    NEC
    Jejunoileal atresia
    Gastroschisis
2. In older children
    Late-onset volvulus
    Massive abdominal trauma
    Crohn disease
    Desmoid tumors

Functional intestinal failure (despite adequate length) due to
1. Long-segment Hirschsprung disease
2. Idiopathic pseudo-obstruction
3. Congenital secretory diarrhea syndromes
    Microvillus inclusion disease
    Tufting enteropathy

Indications for Pediatric Intestinal Transplantation

Intestinal transplantation is currently the treatment of choice when intestinal failure is complicated by life-threatening complications, such as

- Cholestasis, PN-induced liver failure
- Recurrent severe central line sepsis
- Fungal sepsis
- Impending loss of venous access defined as loss of more than 2 central venous access
- Major and recurrent electrolytes and fluid changes
- Poor growth on maximized rehabilitation efforts

Some of the factors that additionally increase the risk for needing an intestinal transplant are initial postresection small bowel length less than 30 cm with no ileocecal valve and enterocolonic discontinuity.

Referral to an intestinal transplant center should be made in cases of any of these complications. It is also encouraged in any cases of extreme short gut regardless of a child's age.

Contraindications to Intestinal Transplantation

Just like any other solid organ transplant, there are a few absolute contraindications to small intestinal transplant. These are summarized in **Box 2**.

Box 2
Contraindications to intestinal transplantation in children

Active infection

Profound neurologic disorder

Life-threatening comorbidities (pulmonary, heart, and so forth)

Severe congenital and acquired immunologic deficiencies

Noncurable malignancies

Multisystemic autoimmune or metabolic disorders

Insufficient vascular patency

Significant psychosocial factors precluding ability of the caregivers to take care of the patient

---

Types of Intestinal Transplantation

There are 3 types of intestinal transplant: isolated intestinal transplant, composite liver and bowel transplant, and multivisceral transplant. In isolated intestinal transplant, only small intestine is transplanted. In composite transplant, small intestine along with liver, pancreas, and duodenum are transplanted. In multivisceral transplant, liver, small intestine, pancreas, duodenum, and the stomach are transplanted. Currently every effort is made to include a colon graft in all transplant based on proved improved outcomes with such a practice.

TRANSPLANT EVALUATION

Pretransplant evaluation of a patient includes a comprehensive multisystemic assessment of the patient intending not only to rule in absolute indications for transplantation but also to rule out any possibilities for intestinal rehabilitation and any absolute contraindication for transplantation. The evaluation includes a comprehensive assessment of intestinal and nutritional status and multiorgan health, including but not limited to cardiovascular, neurodevelopment, renal, immunologic, infectious, thrombotic risk, pulmonary, bone health, and psychosocial. The evaluation, therefore, includes in addition to blood testing and many imaging and organ-specific testing as well as specialized transplant-focused consultations.

At the conclusion of an evaluation, a patient's data are reviewed within the transplant selection multidisciplinary committee and listing decided on if it is believed that transplantation will offer a survival benefit with better quality of life.

WAITING FOR TRANSPLANTATION

Depending on the age and size of a patient, as well as the severity of liver disease, the wait for transplantation can be up to 6 months to 18 months. While waiting on a transplantation list, full support and ongoing efforts for intestinal rehabilitation should continue. Re-evaluation with any changes and at intervals is the rule. Close coordination between the rehabilitation and transplant teams is crucial to assure the patient is always optimized and ready for transplantation. This includes not only nutritional and growth issues but also updating immunizations, providing education about transplantation care, and maintaining support to all other organs. It is also worth mentioning the importance of preventing emergence of bacterial resistance, kidney disease, anti-HLA antibodies, and psychosocial strains in these patients, factors all known to negatively affect the outcomes of intestinal transplantation.[7]

POST-TRANSPLANT MANAGEMENT

The early post-transplantation course is dominated by surgical recovery.[8] Patients are expected to spend many days in the pediatric ICU and an average of 1 month to 2 months in the hospital. This is negatively affected by any comorbidities going into transplantation. Enteral elemental feedings are started after a week of transplant as long as there is no evidence of rejection/vascular problems/infection. Feedings are slowly advanced to full maintenance by 2 weeks to 3 weeks post-transplantation. Intensive graft and overall health monitoring continue during that period, including twice-a-week ileoscopies. Most patients achieve enteral sufficiency by 4 weeks to 6 weeks post-transplantation and PN is stopped. Eventually, patients are discharged to housing in the transplant center area that allows ongoing close follow-up, including biweekly ileoscopies, laboratory testing, and clinic visits. This early period remains notable for frequent needs for admissions most commonly to rule out infection or rejection and dehydration. Eventually, as long as there is no rejection or major infectious complications, the ileostomy is taken down by 3 months to 6 months post-transplantation. The patient returns to his/her home area as long as close follow-up and access to advanced pediatric care are available within an hour's driving distance.

Tacrolimus and prednisone are the mainstay immunosuppressive agents used in intestinal transplantation. They are lifelong medications although their target levels decrease with time as long as there is no rejection. Secondary agents like sirolimus are used to prevent chronic rejection. Antimicrobials, salts supplements, and specialized enteral formulas are mainstay medications in the first year post-transplantation. Often, hypertension, proteinuria, and insulin resistance are noted in the first year and require targeted treatment. Intensive psychosocial and neurodevelopmental support as well as occupational, physical, and speech therapies are needed to assure a timely progression to oral feeding and progressive weaning off the gastric tube feeds.

OUTCOMES OF INTESTINAL TRANSPLANT

The incidence of intestinal transplantation complications has decreased dramatically over the past decade but it remains high when compared with other solid organ transplantation.[8–10] Although acute rejection is currently down to less than 20%, complications overall happen in most patients and include but are not limited to

- Graft: ischemia and rejection
- Immune: infections, post-transplant lymphoproliferative disease, graft-versus-host disease, allergies, and hematologic anomalies
- Extraintestinal: insulin resistance, hypertension, chronic kidney disease, bone disease, neurodevelopmental problems, and psychosocial strain

Survival after intestinal transplant is strongly associated with the underlying disease resulting in intestinal failure. Patients with postnatal volvulus and those with uncomplicated NEC have the best long-term outcomes. Patients with intestinal atresia or motility disorders tend to have more complicated course likely related to innate immune disorders and high infectious risks as well as HLA sensitization. Death on the wait list has been greatly reduced with improved intestinal rehabilitation and liver-protective PN regimens. Compliance with treatment and close specialized follow-up in transplant centers correlate with best short-term and long-term outcomes in intestinal transplantation. New immunosuppressive medications and protocols as well as immune monitoring are moving the field to better long-term outcomes. The inclusion of a liver graft and the absence of HLA antibody were found the independent variables that best correlate with excellent long-term outcome. Recently reported outcome data reflect those major improvements.[10] The international Intestinal Transplantation Registry reported on the 2015 data, indicating actuarial patient survival rates of 76%, 56%, and 43% at 1, 5, and 10 years, respectively.[9] Unpublished center-specific data from the authors' center, MedStar Georgetown Transplant Institute, show in the same period patient and graft survival rates at 95% at 1 year and 65% at 5 years.

CURRENT CHALLENGES IN PEDIATRIC INTESTINAL TRANSPLANT

Despite significant progress made in the area of pediatric small intestinal transplantation, colossal challenges continue to be faced.[8,9] Early referral and optimized pre-transplant care are crucial and rely on excellent coordination between rehabilitation and transplant teams. More awareness is needed to encourage organ donation that improves the timeliness of intestinal transplantation. Novel immunosuppressive and anti-infectious therapies and regimen are likely to lead to improved morbidity and mortality rates post–intestinal transplantation. Protocols to foster tolerance and improved technology to diagnose early rejection and infection are dramatically changing the field. The Achilles heel of intestinal transplantation remains the arduous and meticulous ongoing intensive care it requires that challenges compliance, psychosocial, and financial support systems. All efforts are focused on identifying and palliating compliance hurdles along the spectrum of the transplant journey.

REFERENCES

1. Moore FD, Burch GE, Harken DE, et al. Cardiac and other organ transplantation. In the setting of transplant science as a national effort. JAM 1968;206(11):2489–500.
2. Cohran VC, Prozialeck JD, Cole CR. Redefining short bowel syndrome in the 21st century [review]. Pediatr Res 2017. [Epub ahead of print].

3. Dore M, Junco PT, Moreno AA, et al. Ultrashort bowel syndrome outcome in children treated in a multidisciplinary intestinal rehabilitation unit. Eur J Pediatr Surg 2017;27(1):116–20.
4. Höllwarth ME. Surgical strategies in short bowel syndrome [review]. Pediatr Surg Int 2016. [Epub ahead of print].
5. Wales PW, Allen N, Worthington P, et al, American Society for Parenteral and Enteral Nutrition. Teitelbaum D. A.S.P.E.N. clinical guidelines: support of pediatric patients with intestinal failure at risk of parenteral nutrition-associated liver disease [review]. JPEN J Parenter Enteral Nutr 2014;38(5):538–57.
6. Lao OB, Healey PJ, Perkins JD, et al. Outcomes in children after intestinal transplant. Pediatrics 2010;125(3):e550–8.
7. Lao OB, Healey PJ, Perkins JD, et al. Outcomes in children with intestinal failure following listing for intestinal transplant. J Pediatr Surg 2010;45(1):100–7 [discussion: 107].
8. Bharadwaj S, Tandon P, Gohel TD, et al. Current status of intestinal and multivisceral transplantation. Gastroenterol Rep (Oxf) 2017 [Epub ahead of print]. [review].
9. Grant D, Abu-Elmagd K, Mazariegos G, et al, Intestinal Transplant Association. Intestinal transplant registry report: global activity and trends. Am J Transplant 2015;15(1):210–9.
10. Smith JM, Skeans MA, Horslen SP, et al. OPTN/SRTR 2015 annual data report: intestine. Am J Transplant 2017;17(Suppl 1):252–85.

Neonatal Cholestasis

Erin Lane, MD, Karen F. Murray, MD*

KEYWORDS

- Neonatal cholestasis • Neonatal liver disease • Biliary atresia • Jaundice
- Cholestasis

KEY POINTS

- The initial evaluation of a jaundiced infant should always include measuring serum conjugated (or direct) and unconjugated (or indirect) bilirubin levels.
- Jaundice in an infant that is of very early onset (less than 24 hours of age), persistent beyond 14 days of life, or of new-onset is abnormal and should be investigated.
- Conjugated hyperbilirubinemia in an infant (direct bilirubin levels >1.0 mg/dL or >17 μmol/L, or >15% of total bilirubin) is never normal and indicates hepatobiliary abnormality.
- Infants with cholestasis should be evaluated promptly for potentially life-threatening and treatable causes whereby timing of intervention directly impacts clinical outcomes.

INTRODUCTION

Jaundice in the neonate is common, usually secondary to unconjugated or indirect hyperbilirubinemia, and is most typically not dangerous to the infant. However, even in the setting of the well-appearing neonate, jaundice should be investigated if it is of very early onset (less than 24 hours of life), prolonged beyond 14 days of life, of new-onset, or at high levels. In these settings, it is critical to evaluate for potentially life-threatening causes, such as infection or evolving hepatobiliary dysfunction, and determine if urgent therapeutic intervention is required. Conjugated hyperbilirubinemia warrants expedient evaluation as timing of invention in some cases directly impacts clinical outcomes.

Bile is primarily composed of bile acids, bilirubin, and fats, is formed in the liver, and is secreted into the canaliculus. From the canaliculus, bile flows into biliary ducts from where it is ultimately secreted into the intestine after transient storage within the gallbladder. Disruption of this process at any level results in cholestasis. Cholestasis is the end result of obstruction of the normal excretion of bile from the liver, resulting in the abnormal accumulation of bile salts, bilirubin, and lipids in liver and the blood. Although cholestasis is not synonymous with conjugated hyperbilirubinemia, the abnormal retention of bilirubin, elevated serum levels in cholestasis, low cost, and

Division of Gastroenterology, Seattle Children's Hospital, 4800 Sand Point Way Northeast, M/S OB 9.620, PO Box 50020, Seattle, WA 98115, USA
* Corresponding author.
E-mail address: Karen.murray@seattlechildrens.org

Pediatr Clin N Am 64 (2017) 621–639
http://dx.doi.org/10.1016/j.pcl.2017.01.006
0031-3955/17/© 2017 Elsevier Inc. All rights reserved.

wide availability of testing make serum-conjugated bilirubin the most clinically useful marker of cholestasis.

Clinically, cholestasis in the infant may present as jaundice, pruritus, fat-soluble vitamin deficiency, or may evolve during or following acute liver failure. Functional or anatomic biliary obstruction is often heralded by the presence of acholic stools. Although cholestasis is frequently the primary presenting symptom of neonatal hepatobiliary disease, it also commonly represents the final common pathway of any disease that affects the neonatal liver. As such, cholestasis is often classified by origin and is designated as either (1) biliary, referring to structural abnormalities and obstruction of extrahepatic or intrahepatic bile ducts; or (2) hepatocellular, resulting from impairment in bile transport, genetic or metabolic abnormalities, and infection.

This review presents an approach to the evaluation of the jaundiced infant. The authors discuss the most common causes, disease-specific evaluation, and clinical management of neonatal cholestasis. In addition, general concepts of supportive care for infants with cholestasis are reviewed.

EVALUATION OF THE JAUNDICED INFANT

Jaundice in the infant is usually clinically evident when the total serum bilirubin level exceeds 2.5 to 3.0 mg/dL (42–51 μmol/L) and is seen as scleral icterus or yellowing of the oral mucosa. However, visual estimates of serum bilirubin levels are inadequate and not precise,[1] and hence, levels should be determined when concern for elevation is raised. Although jaundice in neonates is common and can be physiologic, the continued presence of jaundice at 2 weeks of age should alert providers to the possibility of a pathologic process. A thorough examination and history evaluating for the possibility acute life-threatening conditions such as sepsis are paramount. In addition, clinical evaluation should survey for stigmata of hepatobiliary disease that may be heralded by the presence of dark urine or acholic stools or examination findings of hepatosplenomegaly and ascites. If the infant is exclusively breastfed and is well, the evaluation of serum bilirubin levels may be delayed up to 1 week (until 3 weeks of age) after repeat clinical evaluation.[2] However, if the infant is ill appearing, is formula fed, or carries any additional "red flags" such as poor growth or dysmorphic features, the provider should obtain total and fractionated (direct and indirect) serum bilirubin levels.[2] Conjugated hyperbilirubinemia in an infant (direct bilirubin levels >1.0 mg/dL or >17 μmol/L, or >15% of total bilirubin) is never normal and indicates hepatobiliary abnormality. The identification of elevated unconjugated hyperbilirubinemia warrants a different approach to management and is beyond the scope of this review.

If conjugated hyperbilirubinemia is identified, referral to a pediatric hepatologist is mandatory because timely identification of treatable causes of cholestasis can improve clinical outcomes. Secondary laboratory evaluations after cholestasis is identified may include serum alanine aminotransferase (ALT), aspartate aminotransferase (AST), gamma-glutamyl transpeptidase (GGT), alkaline phosphatase, prothrombin time and international normalized ratio (INR), and albumin levels. The initial diagnostic imagining should include an abdominal ultrasound (US), which can identify congenital anatomic or obstructive causes of cholestasis, including choledochal cysts and gallstones, and screen for vascular anomalies and evidence of portal hypertension such as splenomegaly. Liver biopsy often provides critical information to the diagnostic evaluation of neonates with cholestasis.

An algorithmic approach to the evaluation of the cholestatic infant is summarized in **Fig. 1**. Specific causes of neonatal cholestasis are reviewed in the text and tabulated in **Table 1**.

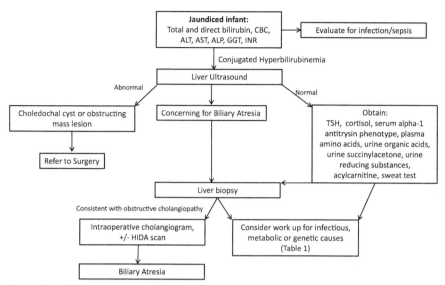

Fig. 1. Algorithmic approach to evaluation of neonatal cholestasis. ALP, alkaline phosphatase; CBC, complete blood count; TSH, thyroid stimulating hormone.

Structural (Biliary) Causes of Neonatal Cholestasis

Biliary atresia

Biliary atresia (BA) is the most common cause of infantile obstructive cholangiopathy and most frequent indication for liver transplantation in the pediatric population. The reported incidence of BA is 0.5 to 3.2 per 10,000 live births, but varies based on geography and ethnicity.[2–5] BA is characterized by progressive inflammation and fibrosis of the bile ducts, resulting in progressive obliteration of the extrahepatic and variably intrahepatic bile ducts.[6,7] The cause of BA is currently unknown. Hypotheses regarding pathogenesis range from abnormal genetic programming of bile duct formation, to viral infections, toxins, or autoimmune-mediated chronic biliary inflammation.[8–11]

BA is characterized anatomically, by the level of extrahepatic biliary obstruction.[12] Two clinical phenotypes exist: "classical" BA, which is not associated with extrahepatic congenital anomalies, and "biliary atresia with splenic malformation" that presents with other congenital anomalies, most frequently situs inversus, asplenia, or polysplenia, cardiac malformations, and intestinal malrotation.

BA presents most commonly with cholestasis between 2 and 5 weeks of life. Acholic stools may be present and indicate biliary obstruction; however, onset commonly follows the onset of jaundice. Unfortunately, if an affected infant has a preceding history of physiologic jaundice, the development of cholestasis may go unrecognized and delay appropriate evaluation and management. This clinical scenario highlights the importance of evaluating any prolonged or new jaundice in infants. Infants with delayed evaluation or presentation may demonstrate signs of chronic liver disease with portal hypertension such as hepatosplenomegaly or ascites. As chronic inflammation and cholestasis lead to malabsorption, many infants with BA present with inadequate weight gain and are characterized as failure to thrive.

Expedient differentiation of BA from other causes of neonatal cholestasis is critical, because surgical intervention before 2 months of age has been shown to improve surgical success and clinical outcome.[13–15] Without rapid intervention, the natural history

Table 1
Causes of neonatal cholestasis

Metabolic/genetic	Galactosemia
	Tyrosinemia type 1
	Dubin-Johnson syndrome
	Rotor syndrome
	Disorders of BAD
	A1AT deficiency
	CF
	Defects of bile transport (PFIC)
	Peroxisomal disorders
Syndromic	Trisomy 21
	Trisomy 13
	Trisomy 18
	Joubert syndrome
	Ivemark syndrome
	Beckwith-Weidemann syndrome
	Bardet-Biedl syndrome
Biliary	BA
	Choledochal cyst
	ALGS
	Choledocholithiasis
	Neonatal sclerosing cholangitis
	Caroli disease
	Obstruction from mass or stricture
Nutritional	Total parenteral nutrition
Cardiovascular	Heart failure
	Shock
	Hepatic ischemia
Infection	Herpes simplex virus
	Cytomegalovirus
	Adenovirus
	Hepatitis B
	Sepsis
	Urinary tract infection
	Cholecystitis
	Cholangitis
Endocrine	Hypothyroidism
	Panhypopituitarism
	Adrenal insufficiency

of BA is uniform fatality secondary to progressive end-stage liver disease by 2 years of age. Early in the course of disease, infants with BA typically demonstrate conjugated hyperbilirubinemia (direct bilirubin 2–7 mg/dL with total bilirubin levels between 5 and 12 mg/dL), with elevations in transaminases (ALT, AST) and GGT; the GGT elevation is usually more significant than that of ALT because the focus of the hepatocellular injury is in the bile ducts.[16]

Abdominal US is recommended early in the evaluation of a cholestatic infant. In the setting of BA, the US typically demonstrates absence, or nonfilling, of the gallbladder after adequate fasting, and an atretic extrahepatic bile duct; a normal gallbladder appearance, however, does not eliminate BA as the cause. The presence of an echogenic or fibrotic triangular cord at the porta hepatis representing the biliary remnant may be described as the "triangular cord sign" (**Fig. 2**) and has a diagnostic sensitivity

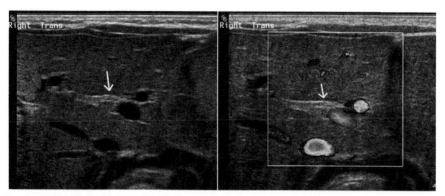

Fig. 2. Abdominal US in BA. Triangular-shaped homogenous echogenicity near the bifurcation of the portal vein consistent with triangular cord sign. *White arrows* indicate triangular cord of hyperechoic fibrous tissue seen at the porta hepatis. *Square* on figure at right indicates application of Doppler, highlighting vascular structures.

of 73%.[17] Functional abdominal imaging, including hepatobiliary scintigraphy with technetium-labeled iminodiacetic acid derivatives (HIDA scan), can assist in the differentiation between obstructive and nonobstructive causes of neonatal cholestasis. Pretreatment with phenobarbital (5 mg/kg/d) for 5 days before HIDA scan may increase the sensitivity of this test, but specificity is limited. On HIDA, the demonstration of rapid update of tracer but absence of excretion into the bowel at 24 hours is suggestive of BA (**Fig. 3**) or other obstructive process (eg, plugging in cystic fibrosis, CF); however, the low specificity (45%–72%) of the examination makes it better suited for exclusion rather than diagnosis of BA.[18,19] A normal HIDA does eliminate BA from the differential of possible diagnoses. A false "positive" nonexcreting HIDA scan finding may result from functional causes of cholestasis such as hypothyroidism.

In many cases, percutaneous liver biopsy is helpful in excluding alternate causes of neonatal cholestasis. Histopathological findings supportive of a diagnosis of BA include demonstration of bile ductular proliferation and bile duct plugging with relative preservation of normal hepatic lobular architecture (**Fig. 4**). Given the progressive nature of BA, however, the extent of liver fibrosis at the time of biopsy may vary, as can the extent of bile duct proliferation and destruction.

Failure to exclude BA, or a high suspicion for BA, necessitates surgical exploration with intraoperative cholangiogram. The diagnosis of BA is confirmed or excluded at the time of laparotomy, and intraoperative cholangiogram remains the gold standard for verifying a diagnosis of BA[16,20]; the identification of an atretic extrahepatic biliary tree confirms the diagnosis (**Fig. 5**). If BA is confirmed, surgical intervention at the time of initial laparotomy and intraoperative cholangiogram, with a Kasai hepatic portoenterostomy, is recommended. The Kasai aims to restore bile flow from the liver to bowel by excising the biliary obstruction and establishing biliary drainage through an anastomosis of the jejunal limb of a Roux-en-Y with the liver at the porta hepatis. The younger the age of diagnosis of BA and Kasai, the more likely the Kasai will be successful.[2,16] Although restoration of bile flow can significantly slow the progression of disease, most children progress to develop cirrhosis and portal hypertension despite effective bile drainage and ultimately require liver transplantation.

The importance of early diagnosis and surgical intervention implies a role for screening in the identification of BA. Screening for BA using stool color cards is currently used in Japan and Taiwan. Implementation of these programs, which use

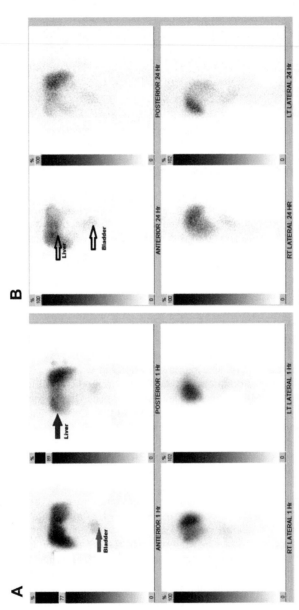

Fig. 3. HIDA scan in BA. Hepatobiliary scan at 1 hour (*A*) demonstrates rapid hepatic uptake (*red arrow*). Hepatobiliary scan at 24 hours (*B*) demonstrates lack of visualization of the biliary tree, gallbladder, and small bowel. Radiotracer is visualized in the kidneys and urinary bladder (*black arrow*). These findings are suggestive of, but not diagnostic for, BA.

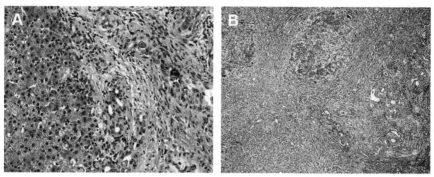

Fig. 4. BA histology. (*A*) Hematoxylin and eosin stain of a liver biopsy from a 3-month-old girl demonstrating a proliferation of bile ductules. Bile plugs are present (original magnification ×200). (*B*) Masson trichrome stain from the liver transplant specimen from the same girl at 8 months of age. Diffuse cirrhosis is identified with marked fibrous expansion of portal tracts. The portal triads lack bile ducts, but there is a marked bile ductule reaction, many containing bile plugs (original magnification ×40). (*Courtesy of* Dr Karen Chisholm, Seattle Children's Hospital, Seattle, WA.)

parents and caregivers to observe and report the infant's stool color at 1 month of age, has improved the timeliness of diagnosis and resulted in a significantly higher proportion of infants undergoing portoenterostomy before 60 days of age.[21–23] Stool color screening cards have not been widely adopted in North America or Europe, placing responsibility on primary care practitioners to have a high level of suspicion at the earliest routine well-child clinic visits.

Alagille syndrome
Alagille syndrome (ALGS) is a genetic disorder characterized by chronic, progressive cholestasis secondary to a paucity of intralobular bile ducts. The estimated prevalence

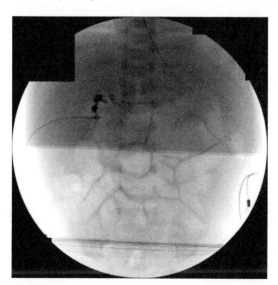

Fig. 5. Intraoperative cholangiogram. Catheter is demonstrated within a rudimentary gallbladder. Contrast injection does not show normal branching of extrahepatic or intrahepatic bile ducts concerning for BA.

is 1:30,000.[24] ALGS is inherited in an autosomal dominant fashion, but may occur sporadically due to de novo mutation. Most individuals with ALGS carry a mutation in *JAG1*, a gene located on chromosome 20, but a small number have mutations in *NOTCH2*.[25–29] The product of *JAG1* and *NOTCH2* is a ligand in the Notch signaling pathway, which plays a key role in embryogenesis.

Multiple organ systems are affected in infants with ALGS. Typically, ALGS is characterized by progressive cholestatic liver disease, stereotypical facial features, congenital heart disease, posterior embryotoxon, butterfly vertebrae, and renal disease. Most infants with ALGS present with cholestasis within the first 3 months of life. Those with severe congenital heart disease may present at birth or may initially come to attention after a cardiology evaluation. Although many forms of congenital heart disease have been associated with ALGS (eg, tetralogy of Fallot and transposition of the great arteries), the most common is peripheral pulmonary stenosis. The characteristic facial features are frequently difficult to appreciate in the neonatal period but include a prominent forehead and pointed chin, giving the face a triangular appearance, deep-set eyes with hypertelorism, and a saddle nose.

Care must be taken to discriminate ALGS from alternate causes of neonatal cholestasis, particularly BA. As in BA, standard neonatal cholestasis evaluation typically demonstrates conjugated hyperbilirubinemia associated with elevated serum aminotransferases and especially GGT, reflective of the biliary involvement. Recommended assessments for the extrahepatic manifestations include abdominal US, radiographs of the spine to identify hemivertebra or butterfly vertebra, echocardiogram, and ophthalmologic evaluation to identify the presence of posterior embryotoxon. Children with ALGS may also benefit from routine neuroimaging, because cerebrovascular anomalies, such as Moyamoya, resulting in increased risk of intracranial bleeding or stroke, have been described.[30]

Although a liver biopsy is not required for diagnosis when other stereotypical syndromic features are present, histologic evaluation may be needed when the diagnosis is in question or hepatic disease advancement is suspected of being advanced. The histopathology in ALGS is characterized by bile ductular paucity. The number of bile ducts is normally diminished in preterm infants, however, so care must be taken to not to make the diagnosis of pathologic paucity incorrectly[24] (**Fig. 6**). In term infants

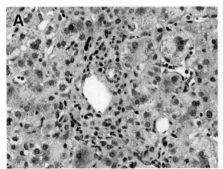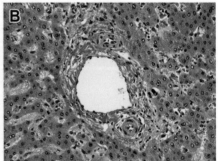

Fig. 6. ALGS histology. (*A*) Hematoxylin and eosin stain of a liver biopsy from a 3-month-old boy demonstrating loss of bile ducts in a portal triad. The adjacent hepatocytes are swollen and show hepatocanalicular cholestasis (original magnification ×400). (*B*) Hematoxylin and eosin stain of a different boy at 10 months of age who was transplanted for ALGS. His liver demonstrated paucity of bile ducts in the portal triads and mild hepatocanalicular cholestasis (original magnification ×200). (*Courtesy of* Dr Karen Chisholm, Seattle Children's Hospital, Seattle, WA.)

and older children, the normal bile duct to portal tract ratio ranges from 0.9 to 1.8, with ratios less than 0.9 suggestive of paucity. Without the other features of ALGS, infants with cholestatic jaundice and elevated GGT usually require a liver biopsy, hepatobiliary scintigraphy, and possibly an intraoperative cholangiogram to verify patency of the extrahepatic biliary system; care must be taken to interpret the intraoperative cholangiogram correctly, because the extrahepatic bile ducts in ALGS are typically very small due to few feeding intrahepatic ducts, but they are patent.

In addition to the syndromic features characteristic of ALGS, children with ALGS commonly suffer from severe metabolic bone disease, dyslipidemia, and refractory pruritis. Significantly elevated serum alkaline phosphatase typically reflects abnormal bone metabolism in addition to the biliary disease. Hypercholesterolemia and hypertriglyceridemia can lead to the development of xanthomas, which may appear most prominently on extensor surfaces and areas of minor trauma, such as the diaper area, plantar surfaces of the feet, abdomen, and neck. In addition, serum bile salt levels can be extremely elevated, even in the absence of jaundice, leading to intractable and refractory pruritis.

Treatment of ALGS is directed at maintaining adequate nutrition, treating the complications of cholestasis, and supporting cardiovascular health. Twenty-five percent to 50% of children with ALGS have debilitating and disfiguring pruritus despite medical therapy, or develop progressive liver disease, and ultimately require liver transplantation.[24]

Gallstones
Gallstones are uncommon in infants; however, sepsis, prematurity, and prolonged exposure to total parenteral nutrition may increase the risk of their development. Most infants identified to have gallstones have congenital biliary abnormalities or hemolytic disease (leading to development of black pigment stones).[31] For most infants, gallstones are incidental and asymptomatic. Screening studies have identified a prevalence of gallstones in approximately 2% of well children. In a cohort of children with incidentally identified gallstones followed over 15 years, there was only a 2% annual risk of biliary pain, and that risk decreased after 5 years.[31] Therefore, unless there is the development of obstruction (choledocholithiasis) or infection (cholecystitis or cholangitis), treatment is generally unnecessary. In select cases, ursodeoxycholic acid (ursodiol) may be considered an oral therapy for gallstone dissolution.[31]

Choledochal cysts
Choledochal cysts are congenital dilations or aneurysms of the biliary system. They may be single or multiple and may involve any part of the biliary system. The highest incidence is in Asia, occurring in approximately 1 in 1000 live births.[32] There are 5 types, classified by location of biliary dilation, with the most commonly seen (accounting for >85% of all choledochal cysts) variant being cystic or fusiform dilations of the common bile duct.[32] Most infants with choledochal cysts present with cholestasis; however, they may initially present with cholangitis or pancreatitis.

Diagnosis of choledochal cysts relies on imaging. Abdominal US is the diagnostic imaging modality of choice in evaluating intrahepatic and extrahepatic biliary anatomy. Secondary imaging may be required to delineate complicated biliary anatomy, including HIDA scans and magnetic resonance cholangiopancreatography. Serum laboratory testing may reveal elevated conjugated hyperbilirubinemia and GGT (reflecting biliary obstruction), and usually less dramatically elevated serum aminotransferases.

Definitive treatment is surgical resection, although treatment of pre-existing cholangitis or pancreatitis is necessary before surgical intervention. Surgical treatment is aimed at resolving biliary obstruction, restoring normal biliary drainage, and eliminating the long-term risk of cholangiocarcinoma or squamous cell carcinoma in any residual cyst.[32–35]

Genetic and Metabolic Causes of Neonatal Cholestasis

Alpha-1 antitrypsin deficiency

Alpha-1 antitrypsin (A1AT) deficiency is the most common genetic cause of liver disease and affects approximately 1 in 2000 live births.[36–38] The gene mutation leading to A1AT deficiency is inherited as an autosomal dominant disorder and results in a single amino acid substitution within the A1AT protein. This amino acid change causes abnormal molecular folding of the A1AT protein, and inability of the protein to be processed beyond and excreted from the endoplasmic reticulum. Inability of the abnormal protein to be excreted from hepatocytes leads to both low plasma levels of circulating A1AT and to hepatocellular injury from excessive accumulation. A1AT functions as a serine protease, which primarily acts to inhibit other proteases and elastases; without appropriate inhibition, the activities of proteases and elastases lead to cellular destruction.

The clinical phenotypes of A1AT deficiency include both liver and pulmonary manifestations, but penetrance is highly variable. Liver disease commonly presents in the neonatal period and is frequently characterized by transient cholestatic jaundice. Despite similar levels of circulating protein levels, advancement of the liver disease with stigmata of portal hypertension or the development of liver failure is uncommon, occurring in roughly 20% of homozygotically affected individuals. Pulmonary disease is a later development, manifesting in adulthood.

A1AT deficiency is diagnosed by protein phenotyping. Although widely available, the serum level of A1AT is less reliable for diagnosis because it can be misleadingly elevated into the normal range in times of systemic inflammation or infection (as an acute-phase reactant). A1AT phenotyping (Pi type) is the most specific and preferred diagnostic serum test. A1AT variants are named according to their electrophoretic migration pattern,[39] with normal A1AT protein designated M. The S and Z variants are the most common mutations leading to a reduction in serum A1AT, and disease when inherited homozygotically. The PiZZ variant, named for its slowest gel migration, causes the most severe clinical disease phenotype. Generally, liver disease manifests only in PiZZ, PiSZ, or rarely, PiSS variants.[40]

The classic, although not pathognomonic, histologic finding in A1AT deficiency is periodic acid Schiff-positive, diastase-resistant, eosinophilic globules within the hepatocytes. This finding represents the accumulated abnormal protein trapped within the endoplasmic reticulum. Liver histology may also demonstrate bile duct destruction, proliferation, and potentially bile duct paucity, making it important to distinguish from BA and ALGS.

Management of liver disease in A1AT is primarily supportive, because there are no specific or targeted therapies currently available. As cholestasis tends to be the primary clinical phenotype in neonates, fat malabsorption and fat-soluble vitamin deficiency are possible. Most infants will benefit from supplementation with medium-chain triglyceride (MCT) and fat-soluble vitamins as needed. Ursodeoxycholic acid may be used, but no study to date has demonstrated clear benefit. Although breastfeeding may be supported, there is no evidence that demonstrates clear benefit of breastfeeding over formula.[41,42]

Liver transplantation is indicated for infants and children with end-stage liver disease secondary to A1AT. Importantly, because A1AT is primarily manufactured in the liver, the recipient assumes the donor's Pi phenotype. Thus, after transplant, the recipient experiences normal serum levels of functional A1AT, a decreased risk of pulmonary disease, and no chance of recurrent disease in the transplanted organ.

To prevent the development of pulmonary manifestations, including early emphysema, avoidance of smoking and environmental pollution is critical. It should be noted that recombinant A1AT is available and approved for the treatment of pulmonary manifestations. However, recombinant A1AT has no role in the treatment or prevention of hepatic injury, because it has no effect on the direct hepatocellular injury caused by the presence of misfolded A1AT.

Cystic fibrosis liver disease
Although CF is common, affecting approximately 1:2500 live births in North America, CF-related liver disease affects less than 2% of infants.[43] Given the low incidence of CF-related liver disease in neonates, testing for CF in jaundiced infants should be reserved for infants affected with meconium ileus, inadequate weight gain despite theoretically adequate caloric intake, those with an obstructive cholangiopathy without other explanation, or those infants in whom alternate causes of cholestasis have been excluded. Diagnosis of CF-related liver disease relies on diagnosis of CF, commonly supported by newborn screening for immunoreactive trypsinogen. The gold standard remains sequencing of the CFTR gene or a positive sweat chloride test.

Disorders of bile acid synthesis
Cholic acid and chenodeoxycholic acid are the primary bile acids manufactured in humans; disruption in the normal synthetic pathways results in the accumulation of toxic intermediate metabolites. Liver injury is also mediated by abnormal accumulation of cholesterol, drugs, and other toxins within the liver from abnormal bile excretion. Although rare, disorders of bile acid synthesis (BAD) should be included in the differential for a neonate presenting with progressive cholestasis when alternate causes have been ruled out.

In the neonatal period, infants with disorders of BAD may present with persistent cholestasis, whereas others may present with acute hepatitis or liver failure. The most common clinical presentation of disorders of BAD includes neonatal jaundice, failure to thrive, hepatosplenomegaly, rickets, and bleeding. Some disorders of BAD are associated with neurologic disease, including seizures, developmental delay, deafness, blindness, and neuromuscular weakness.

Diagnosis of bile acid synthetic disorders should include serum and urine analyses of the bile acids. Serum tests may demonstrate low bile acid levels, elevated serum aminotransferases, normal GGT, and evidence of fat malabsorption. If serum bile acids are low, urinary bile acids should be measured to identify the particular synthetic defect; the subject must not be on ursodeoxycholic acid therapy at the time of the analysis. Hepatic histology is generally nondiagnostic and may demonstrate nonspecific canalicular bile plugging, inflammation without bile duct proliferation, or giant cell transformation.[44]

Treatment of inborn errors of BAD, when possible, focuses on suppressing production of toxic metabolites and supporting normal growth. For the most treatable forms of BAD, these objectives are best achieved by treatment with cholic acid. Ursodiol is not indicated because it does not suppress production of abnormal bile acid intermediates.

Progressive familial intrahepatic cholestasis
Progressive familial intrahepatic cholestasis (PFIC) is a group of disorders characterized by defective bile export and subsequent cholestasis. This group of autosomal

recessive disorders includes PFIC 1, PFIC 2, and PFIC 3 and is named based on the specific genetic mutation. In PFIC, liver disease results from the accumulation of bile salts within the hepatocytes, leading to profound cholestasis. Infants commonly present with profound pruritus, but may also present with jaundice or occasionally life-threatening hemorrhage secondary to vitamin K deficiency.

PFIC 1, also known as Byler disease, is caused by a mutation in the gene ATP8B1 on chromosome 18q21-22.[45] This gene codes for a protein flippase (FIC 1), which facilitates the flipping of aminophospholipids from the outer to inner canalicular membrane. Affected individuals typically present in infancy with recurrent episodes of jaundice within the first few months of life. Later, affected children may develop short stature, deafness, pancreatitis, and persistent diarrhea.

PFIC 2 results from a defect in the bile canalicular bile salt export pump (BSEP) caused by a mutation in the gene ABCB11 on chromosome 2q24.[45] BSEP is responsible for transporting bile acids from inside the hepatocyte to the canaliculus. Disruption of BSEP results in accumulation of bile acids within hepatocytes, resulting in severe cholestasis. PFIC 2 presents in infancy with rapidly progressive cholestasis that often progresses to liver failure within the first few years of life. Children with PFIC 2 have an increased risk of developing hepatocellular carcinoma and cholangiocarcinoma.[45]

PFIC 3 is caused by a mutation in the gene ABCB4 on chromosome 7q21, which encodes for multidrug resistance–associated protein 3 (MDR3). MDR3 is a "floppase," which mediates flopping of aminophospholipids from the inner to outer canalicular lipid bilayer, resulting in a deficiency in export of phospholipids. Bile in infants with PFIC3 has insufficient phospholipid concentration, making the micelles unstable and toxic to bile ducts, which ultimately leads to the development of progressive intrahepatic cholangiopathy. In contrast to PFIC 1 and 2, only a third of children with PFIC 3 present with cholestasis during infancy. When infants with PFIC 3 do present with liver disease, they commonly have concurrent cholesterol gallstones complicating their intrahepatic cholestasis.

Definitive diagnosis of PFIC is dependent on specific genetic testing. However, routine serum laboratory testing can suggest PFIC as a cause of neonatal cholestasis. Infants with PFIC generally have markedly elevated serum bile acid levels with only mildly elevated serum bilirubin. The characteristic biochemical marker of PFIC 1 and 2 is a normal or low GGT, normal serum cholesterol, and only mild transaminitis. PFIC 3 presents with an elevated GGT in the absence of extrahepatic biliary obstruction.

Treatment of PFIC initially focuses on nutritional support to optimize absorption of fat and fat-soluble vitamins and achieve weight gain, in the presence of profound cholestasis. Aggressive treatment of pruritus often requires multiple concurrent therapies, including ursodiol, cholestyramine, rifampin, and opioid antagonists. In medically refractory cases or in the presence of advanced liver disease, treatment may include partial biliary diversion, interruption of the enterohepatic circulation by surgical ileal exclusion, and liver transplantation.[16,45,46]

Disorder of amino acid metabolism: type 1 tyrosinemia

Type 1 tyrosinemia is a metabolic disorder of amino acid metabolism that results from deficiency of fumarylacetoacetate hydrolase, the enzyme responsible for the final step of tyrosine degradation.[47] Type 1 tyrosinemia is an autosomal recessive disorder with an incidence of 1:100,000. Tyrosinemia generally presents acutely in the neonatal period and should be included in the differential of acute neonatal liver failure. In addition to acute liver failure, neonates with tyrosinemia may present with failure to thrive, vomiting, ascites, coagulopathy, hypoglycemia, and hyperbilirubinemia. In older infants, a more chronic presentation characterized by growth failure, Fanconi syndrome, and neurologic manifestations may develop. Diagnosis of type 1 tyrosinemia is made by identifying elevated urinary succinylacetone.

Support of the infant diagnosed with tyrosinemia in the neonatal period consists of correcting any metabolic derangements, treating sepsis when present, and correcting coagulopathy as needed, followed by the restriction of dietary tyrosine. Usage of low-tyrosine formulas alone, however, results in less than 40% survival at 1 year of age.[48–50] More definitive treatment with NTBC (2-(2-nitro-4-trifluromethylbenzoyl)-1,3-cyclohexanedione, nitisinone) improves survival to greater than 85% at 1 year of age and is the standard of care.[51] NTBC works by inhibiting the formation of maleyl acetoacetic acid and fumaryl acetoacetic acid, the precursors to the hepatotoxic compound succinylacetone. Despite adequate treatment, children with tyrosinemia type 1 carry a long-term risk of developing hepatocellular carcinoma and therefore require close follow-up.

Galactosemia

Galactosemia results from an inability to metabolize galactose secondary to a deficiency in one of the following enzymes: galactokinase, galactose-1-phosphate uridyl transferase (Gal-1-PUT), or uridine diphosphate galactose-4-epimease. Gal-1-PUT deficiency is the most common cause of galactosemia and results in the inability to metabolize galactose into glucose-1-phosphate. It is an autosomal recessive disorder with an incidence of 1:60,000 live births.[47]

Abnormal galactose metabolism results in the accumulation of toxic metabolites in the liver, brain, kidney, and eye lens. Classically, galactosemia presents within the first few weeks of life after infants ingest breast milk or milk-based formulas that contain lactose. Presenting symptoms may include failure to thrive, jaundice, vomiting, and diarrhea. Infants with galactosemia are at increased risk for gram-negative sepsis and hence may present acutely with sepsis and associated severe acidosis, jaundice, and coagulopathy. Additional clinical findings may include hepatomegaly, ascites, bleeding, hypotonia, edema, and bulging fontanelle.

Many state-mandated newborn screening tests identify variants of Gal-1-PUT–deficient disease. Although diagnosis can be suggested by the presence of reducing substances in the urine, this is only sensitive when affected individuals are still ingesting galactose. Definitive diagnosis requires demonstration of a complete absence of Gal-1-PUT activity via a quantitative red blood cell (RBC) assay; analysis post-RBC transfusion will give unreliable results.

Treatment of galactosemia centers on the immediate stabilization of the critically ill infant and removal of dietary galactose. Stabilization with intravenous glucose, vitamin K, antibiotics, and initiation of a soy-based (non-galactose-containing) formula when well enough is usually effective. Continued avoidance of lactose and galactose-containing foods is required throughout life. Despite treatment, many children will have some degree of developmental delay residual from the presenting illness.

Other Causes of Neonatal Cholestasis

Infections

Congenital or perinatal infections and sepsis are common causes of neonatal liver cholestasis. For ill-appearing infants with cholestasis, a rapid evaluation for bacterial infection (such as sepsis or urinary tract infection) is mandatory. Judicial selection of antimicrobials must be considered, because several are known to exacerbate cholestasis by displacing bilirubin from albumin (eg, Ceftriaxone), or may be potentially hepatotoxic (eg, fluconazole and acyclovir).[52] In addition to common bacterial infections,

TORCH infections (toxoplasmosis, rubella, cytomegalovirus, herpes, and syphilis) as well as hepatitis B, parvovirus B19, adenovirus, and echoviruses can result in neonatal cholestasis and hepatitis.

Parenteral nutrition-associated liver disease

Parenteral nutrition-associated liver disease (PNALD) is an important and common cause of cholestasis, hepatitis, and liver-related morbidity in the neonatal period. Several clinical risk factors have been identified that contribute to the development of PNALD, and these include prematurity, low birth weight, lack of enteral feeding, sepsis, short gut syndrome, and necrotizing enterocolitis.[53,54] An estimated 33% to 85% of premature infants who receive parenteral nutrition for more than 7 days develop PNALD.[55,56] When TPN is used for less than 2 weeks, any associated liver inflammation generally completely resolves. However, prolonged use increases the risk for irreversible liver disease that may ultimately result in liver fibrosis and failure.[57,58] The diagnosis of PNALD is suggested by the presence of a serum conjugated bilirubin level greater than 2 mg/dL, ALT greater than 2 times the upper limit of normal, and elevated GGT.

Minimization of PNALD requires early initiation and continuation of enteral feeding as possible, use of intralipids at a dose not more than 1 g/kg/d, and prevention of infection. Ursodiol at a dose of 20 to 30 mg/kg/d in divided doses may be additionally used to improve bile flow.[59–61] Use of omega-6 fatty acid or fish oil–based, rather than soy-based, lipid formulations has been shown to be effective at resolving cholestasis.[62] Aggressive prevention of PNALD and bowel rehabilitation when appropriate is critical in preventing irreversible liver damage.

Idiopathic neonatal hepatitis

Idiopathic neonatal hepatitis is a term historically applied to infants presenting with neonatal cholestasis or hepatitis in whom a specific cause could not be identified. Typically, liver biopsies in these infants demonstrated nonspecific intrahepatic cholestasis and giant cell transformation of hepatocytes[63] (**Fig. 7**). However, now it is recognized that multinucleated giant cells represent a stereotypical response by

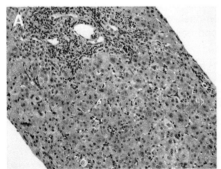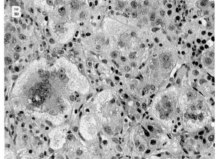

Fig. 7. Neonatal hepatitis histology. (*A*) Hematoxylin and eosin stain from a liver biopsy from a 6-week-old infant demonstrating hepatocyte ballooning and giant cell transformation. Extramedullary hematopoiesis is present, especially in the portal triad. Hepatocanalicular cholestasis is identified (original magnification ×200). (*B*) Higher power of a hematoxylin and eosin stain from a liver biopsy from a different 8-week-old infant highlights giant cell transformation of hepatocytes. Extramedullary hematopoiesis is present in the upper right (original magnification ×400). (*Courtesy of* Dr Karen Chisholm, Seattle Children's Hospital, Seattle, WA.)

the immature liver to many causes of hepatocyte injury, including infection, biliary obstruction, and metabolic disease. In addition, with advancements in next-generation DNA sequencing, the number of identifiable causes of neonatal cholestasis has increased, reducing the frequency of this nonspecific diagnosis.

Nutritional Support of the Cholestatic Infant

Nutritional support is critical and central to the medical management of infants with chronic cholestasis. Optimization of nutritional status can reverse, improve, and/or prevent complications of cholestasis, including fat-soluble vitamin (A, D, E, and K) deficiencies, bleeding secondary to progressive coagulopathy, and pathologic fractures (**Table 2**).[64] Growth failure in the cholestatic infant is common and occurs secondarily to malabsorption from inadequate bile flow and intestinal mucosal congestion from portal hypertension. In addition, infants with cholestasis often have increased caloric needs in the setting of chronic liver disease and may require a daily caloric intake exceeding 150% of those of healthy infants to achieve weight gain.

Enteral nutrition is the preferred modality, and when oral intake is inadequate, placement of a nasoenteric tube for supplemental feeding is recommended. Breast feeding is encouraged, but when growth is inadequate on breast milk alone, supplemental formula must be considered. The selection of formula should consider MCT content, because this fat source is directly absorbed into the portal venous system and does not require emulsification by bile acids or active transport, which is disrupted in cholestasis. Children with portal hypertension and ascites also benefit from sodium restriction; however, in the exclusively formula-fed infant, additional sodium restriction is unnecessary.

Table 2
Fat-soluble vitamin supplementation

Vitamin	Target Serum Level	Recommended Supplementation
Vitamin A (retinol)	19–77 μg/dL Retinol: RBP molar ratio >0.8	Dose in increments of 5000 IU (up to 25–50,000 IU/d) orally Or Monthly intramuscular administration of 50,000 IU Monitor serum levels very 1–2 mo
Vitamin D (25-hydroxy vitamin D)	>30 ng/mL	Serum 25(OH)D level 5–30 ng/mL: 1000–5000 IU daily for 3 mo Serum 25(OH)D level <5 ng/mL: 1000–8000 IU daily for 3 mo Or Calcitriol at 0.05–0.20 μg/kg daily Monitor serum levels every 1–3 mo
Vitamin E (α-tocopherol)	3.8–20.3 μg/mL Vitamin E: total serum lipids ratio >0.6 mg/g	Water-miscible vitamin E: 1 unit/kg daily Monitor serum levels every 1–2 mo
Vitamin K (phytonadione)	INR ≤1.2	Oral: 2.5–5 mg Or SQ, IM, IV: 1–10 mg/dose once INR may not correct with advanced liver failure

Abbreviations: IM, intramuscularly; IV, intravenously; RBP, retinol binding protein; SQ, subcutaneously.

Despite attempts at optimizing nutrition through enteral feeds, many infants with advanced liver disease may evolve to require parenteral nutrition in anticipation of liver transplantation.

Treatment of Pruritis in the Cholestatic Infant

Infants with chronic cholestasis often have significant discomfort from intractable pruritus secondary to abnormal retention and accumulation of bile salts in the skin. Treatment is largely aimed at symptomatic improvement, with resolution of symptoms only after definitive intervention of the underlying cause of the cholestasis. Pharmacologic treatments include antihistamines (diphenhydramine, hydroxyzine), ursodeoxycholic acid, cholestyramine, rifampin, and opioid antagonists.

SUMMARY

Although jaundice in the neonatal period is common and often physiologic, cholestasis is always pathologic and indicates hepatobiliary disease. A high level of suspicion and prompt investigation for all infants with early, persistent, or high levels of hyperbilirubinemia is required and warrants fractionating the bilirubin levels. If cholestasis is confirmed, urgent referral to a pediatric gastroenterologist or hepatologist is recommended to assist in diagnostic and therapeutic interventions to optimize clinical outcome.

REFERENCES

1. Moyer VA, Ahn C, Sneed S. Accuracy of clinical judgment in neonatal jaundice. Arch Pediatr Adolesc Med 2000;154:391–4.
2. Fawaz R, Baumann U, Ekong U, et al. Guideline for the Evaluation of Cholestatic Jaundice in Infants: Joint Recommendations of the North American Society for Pediatric Gastroenterology, Hepatology, and Nutrition (NASPGHAN) and the European Society for Pediatric Gastroenterology, Hepatology, and Nutrition (ESPGHAN). J Pediatr Gastroenterol Nutr 2016;64(1):154–68.
3. The NS, Honein MA, Caton AR, et al. Risk factors for isolated biliary atresia, National Birth Defects Prevention Study, 1997-2002. Am J Med Genet A 2007; 143A(19):2274–84.
4. Schreiber RA, Barker CC, Roberts EA, et al. Biliary atresia: the Canadian experience. J Pediatr 2007;151(6):659–65, 665.e1.
5. McKiernan PJ, Baker AJ, Kelly DA. The frequency and outcome of biliary atresia in the UK and Ireland. Lancet 2000;355(9197):25–9.
6. Hartley JL, Davenport M, Kelly DA. Biliary atresia. Lancet 2009;374:1704–13.
7. Balistreri WF, Grand R, Hoofnagle JH, et al. Biliary atresia: current concepts and research directions: summary of a symposium. Hepatology 1996;23:1682–92.
8. Sokol RJ, Mack C. Etiopathogenesis of biliary atresia. Semin Liver Dis 2001;21(4): 517–24.
9. Mack CL. The pathogenesis of biliary atresia: evidence for a virus-induced autoimmune disease. Semin Liver Dis 2007;27(3):233–42.
10. Schreiber RA, Kleinman RE. Genetics, immunology, and biliary atresia: an opening or a diversion? J Pediatr Gastroenterol Nutr 1993;16(2):111–3.
11. Bezerra JA. Potential etiologies of biliary atresia. Pediatr Transplant 2005;9(5): 646–51.
12. Karrer FM, Lilly JR, Stewart BA, et al. Biliary atresia registry, 1976-1989. J Pediatr Surg 1990;35:1076–81.
13. Ohi R. Surgery for biliary atresia. Liver 2001;21:175–82.

14. Shneider BL, Brown MB, Haber B, et al. A multicenter study of the outcome of biliary atresia in the United States, 1997-2000. J Pediatr 2006;148:467–74.

15. Murray KF, Horslen S, editors. Diseases of the liver in children. New York: Springer; 2014.

16. Hsu HY, Chang MH. Biliary atresia. In: Murray KF, Horslen S, editors. Diseases of the liver in children. 1st edition. New York: Springer; 2014. p. 257–67.

17. Lee HJ, Lee SM, Park WH, et al. Objective criteria of triangular cord sign in biliary atresia on US scan. Radiology 2003;229:395–400.

18. Kianifar HR, Tehranian S, Shojaei P, et al. Accuracy of hepatobiliary scintigraphy for differentiation of neonatal hepatitis from biliary atresia: systematic review and meta-analysis of the literature. Pediatr Radiol 2013;43(8):905–19.

19. Gilmour SM, Hershkop M, Reifen R, et al. Outcome of hepatobiliary scanning in neonatal hepatitis syndrome. J Nucl Med 1997;38(8):1279–82.

20. el-Youssef M, Whitington PF. Diagnostic approach to the child with hepatobiliary disease. Semin Liver Dis 1998;18(3):195–202.

21. Lien TH, Chang MH, Wu JF, et al. Effects of the infant stool color card screening program on 5-year outcome of biliary atresia in Taiwan. Hepatology 2011;53(1):202–8.

22. Chen SM, Chang MH, Du JC, et al. Screening for biliary atresia by infant stool color card in Taiwan. Pediatrics 2006;117(4):1147–54.

23. Schreiber RA, Masucci L, Kaczorowski J, et al. Home-based screening for biliary atresia using infant stool colour cards: a large-scale prospective cohort study and cost-effectiveness analysis. J Med Screen 2014;21(3):126–32.

24. Kamath BM, Piccoli DA. Alagille syndrome. In: Murray KF, Horslen S, editors. Diseases of the liver in children. 1st edition. New York: Springer; 2014. p. 227–46.

25. Li L, Kranz ID, Deng Y, et al. Alagille syndrome is caused by mutations in human Jagged 1, which encodes a ligand for Notch1. Nat Genet 1997;16:235–51.

26. Oda T, Elkahloun AG, Pike BL, et al. Mutations in the human Jagged1 gene are responsible for Alagille syndrome. Nat Genet 1997;16:235–42.

27. Warthen DM, Moore ED, Kamath BM, et al. Jagged1 (JAG1) mutations in Alagille syndrome: increasing the mutation detection rate. Hum Mutat 2006;27:436–43.

28. Kamath BM, Bauer RC, Loomes KM, et al. NOTCH2 mutations in Alagille syndrome. J Med Genet 2012;49:138–44.

29. McDaniell R, Warthen DM, Sanchez-Lara PA, et al. NOTCH 2 mutations cause Alagille syndrome, a heterogeneous disorder of the notch signaling pathway. Am J Hum Genet 2006;79:169–73.

30. Emerick KM, Rand EB, Goldmuntz E, et al. Features of Alagille syndrome in 92 patients: frequency and relation to prognosis. Hepatology 1999;29(3):822–9.

31. Giefer MJ, Kozarek RA. Gallstone disease in children. In: Murray KF, Horslen S, editors. Diseases of the liver in children. 1st edition. New York: Springer; 2014. p. 389–401.

32. Murray KF. Choledochal cysts and fibrocystic diseases of the liver. In: Murray KF, Horslen S, editors. Diseases of the liver in children. 1st edition. New York: Springer; 2014. p. 269–84.

33. Todani T, Watanabe Y, Toki A, et al. Carcinoma related to choledochal cysts with internal drainage operations. Surg Gynecol Obstet 1987;164(1):61–4.

34. Bismut H, Krissat J. Choledochal cysts malignancies. An Oncol 1999;10(Suppl 4):S94–8.

35. Voyles CR, Smadja C, Shands WC, et al. Carcinoma in choledochal cysts. Age-related incidence. Arch Surg 1983;118(8):986–8.

36. Perlmutter DH. Alpha-1-antitrypsin deficiency. Semin Liver Dis 1998;18(3): 217–25.

37. Perlmutter DH. Alpha-1-antitrypsin deficiency. Curr Treat Options Gastroenterol 2000;3(6):451–6.

38. Perlmutter DH. Alpha-1-antitrypsin deficiency. In: Suchy F, Sokol R, editors. Liver disease in children. 3rd edition. Cambridge (United Kingdom): Cambridge University Press; 2007. p. 545–71.

39. Pierce JA, Eradio BG. Improved identification of anti-trypsin phenotypes through isoelectric focusing with dithioerythritol. J Lab Clin Med 1979;94(6):826–31.

40. Ranes J, Stoller JK. A review of alpha-1-antitrypsin deficiency. Semin Respir Crit Care Med 2005;26(2):154–66.

41. Udall JN Jr, Dixon M, Newman AP, et al. Liver disease in alpha 1-antitrypsin deficiency. A retrospective analysis of the influence of early breast-vs bottle-feeding. JAMA 1985;253(18):2679–82.

42. Labrune P, Odievre M, Alagille D. Influence of sex and breastfeeding on liver disease in alpha-1-antitrypsin deficiency. Hepatology 1989;10(1):122.

43. Markewicz MR, Hurtado CW. Metabolic liver disease: part 2. In: Murray KF, Horslen S, editors. Diseases of the liver in children. 1st edition. New York: Springer; 2014. p. 185–214.

44. Setchell KD, Heubi JE. Defects in bile acid biosynthesis-diagnosis and treatment. J Pediatr Gastroenterol Nutr 2006;43(Suppl 1):S17–22.

45. Jacquemin E. Progressive familial intrahepatic cholestasis. Clin Res Hepatol Gastroenterol 2012;36:S26–35.

46. Englert C, Grabhorn D, Richter A, et al. Liver transplantation in children with progressive familial intrahepatic cholestasis. Transplantation 2007;84:1361–3.

47. Squires JE, Heubi JE. Metabolic liver disease: part 1. In: Murray KF, Horslen S, editors. Diseases of the liver in children. 1st edition. New York: Springer; 2014. p. 153–83.

48. McKiernan PJ. Nitisinone in the treatment of hereditary tyrosinaemia type 1. Drugs 2006;66:743–50.

49. Holme E, Lindstedt S. Tyrosinaemia type 1 and NTBC ((2-(2-nitro-4-trifluromethyl-benzoyl)-1,3-cyclohexanedione). J Inherit Metab Dis 1998;21:507–17.

50. Masurel-Paulet A, Poggi-Bach J, Rolland MO, et al. NTBC treatment in tyrosinaemia type 1: long-term outcome in French patients. J Inherit Metab Dis 2008;31: 81–7.

51. Mohan N, McKiernan P, Preece MA, et al. Indications and outcome of liver transplantation in tyrosinaemia type 1. Eur J Pediatr 1999;158(Suppl 2):S49–54.

52. Shah U. Infections of the liver. In: Murray KF, Horslen S, editors. Diseases of the liver in children. 1st edition. New York: Springer; 2014. p. 285–312.

53. Btaiche IF, Khalidi N. Parenteral nutrition-associated liver complications in children. Pharmacotherapy 2002;22(2):188–211.

54. Rangel SJ, Calkins CM, Cowles RA, et al. Parenteral nutrition-associated cholestasis: an American Pediatric Surgical Association Outcomes and Clinical Trials Committee systematic review. J Pediatr Surg 2012;47(1):225–40.

55. Koseesirikul P, Chotinaruemol S, Ukarapol N. Incidence and risk factors of PN-associated liver disease in newborn infants. Pediatr Int 2012;54:434–6.

56. Duro D, Mitchell PD, Kalish LA, et al. Risk factors for PN-associated liver disease following surgical therapy for necrotizing enterocolitis; a Glaser Pediatric Research Network Study. J Pediatr Gastroenterol Nutr 2011;52:595–600.

57. Nanji AA, Anderson FH. Sensitivity and specificity of liver function tests in the detection of parenteral nutrition associated cholestasis. JPEN J Parenter Enteral Nutr 1985;9(3):307–8.
58. Beath SV, Booth IW, Murphy MS, et al. Nutritional care and candidates for small bowel transplantation. Arch Dis Child 1995;73(4):348–50.
59. Kowdley KV. Ursodeoxycholic acid therapy in hepatobiliary disease. Am J Med 2000;108(6):481–6.
60. Chen CY, Tsao PN, Chen HL, et al. Ursodeoxycholic acid (UDCA) therapy in very-low-birth-weight infants with parenteral nutrition-associated cholestasis. J Pediatr 2004;145(3):317–21.
61. Al-Hathlol L, Al-Madani A, Al-Saif S, et al. Ursodeoxycholic acid therapy for intractable total parenteral nutrition-associated cholestasis in surgical very low birth weight infants. Singapore Med J 2006;47(2):147–51.
62. Blackmer AB, Btaiche IF, Arnold MA, et al. Parenteral nutrition-associated liver disease in pediatric patients: strategies for treatment and prevention. In: Murray KF, Horslen S, editors. Diseases of the liver in children. 1st edition. New York: Springer; 2014. p. 327–49.
63. Balistreri WF, Bezerra JA. Whatever happened to "neonatal hepatitis"? Clin Liver Dis 2006;10:27–53.
64. Shneider BL, Magee JC, Bezerra JA, et al, Childhood Liver Disease Research Education Network (ChiLDREN). Efficacy of fat-soluble vitamin supplementation in infants with biliary atresia. Pediatrics 2012;130(3):e607–14.

Hepatitis B and C

Wikrom Karnsakul, MD[a],*, Kathleen B. Schwarz, MD[b]

KEYWORDS

- Hepatitis B • Hepatitis C • Sustained virologic response • Pegylated interferon
- Direct-acting antiviral agents • Spontaneous viral clearance

KEY POINTS

- The disease burden for both hepatitis B virus (HBV) and hepatitis C virus (HCV) infection in the pediatric population is high because most infected children acquire the virus via maternal fetal transmission.
- Without spontaneous viral clearance or indications to treat, most HBV-infected and HCV-infected children will become adults with chronic viral hepatitis and liver disease.
- The treatment goal for HCV infection is to achieve a sustained virologic response (ie, sustained viral clearance). The treatment goal for HBV infection is to achieve a functional cure, meaning that circulating markers of viral infection are negative but there may be residual covalently closed circular (ccc) HBV DNA in the liver.
- Successful antiviral treatment in adults with HBV and HCV infection gives promise to guide therapy in children; however, there are differences between adults and children with these infections, including in natural history, pharmacokinetics, responses to therapy, and short-term and long-term adverse effects of antiviral agents.
- Apart from antiviral therapies, prevention of these diseases is important because transmission largely occurs during the perinatal period.

Disclosure Statement: W. Karnsakul has had a relationship with Gilead as a sponsor for an open-label, multicenter, multicohort, single-arm study to investigate the safety and efficacy of sofosbuvir plus ribavirin in adolescents and children with genotype 2 or 3 chronic HCV infection and a phase 2, open-label, multicenter, multicohort study to investigate the safety and efficacy of ledipasvir/sofosbuvir fixed-dose combination in adolescents and children with chronic HCV-infection and a long-term follow-up registry for adolescent and pediatric subjects who received a Gilead hepatitis C virus direct-acting antiviral in chronic hepatitis C infection trials. K.B. Schwarz: Research grants from NIDDK, Gilead, BMS, and Roche; consulting for Gilead, Roche/Genentech, and Up to Date.
[a] Pediatric Liver Center, Department of Pediatrics, Johns Hopkins University School of Medicine, 600 North Wolfe Street, CMSC 2-117, Baltimore, MD 21287, USA; [b] Pediatric Liver Center, Department of Pediatrics, Johns Hopkins University School of Medicine, 600 North Wolfe Street, CMSC 2-116, Baltimore, MD 21287, USA
* Corresponding author.
E-mail address: wkarnsa1@jhmi.edu

Viral hepatitis has been a global health concern and economic burden for the past century. Hepatitis B virus (HBV) and hepatitis C virus (HCV) are the most common causes of chronic viral hepatitis in the United States, as well as worldwide. However, the presentation depends on the type of virus and the age of the patients. Children with HBV rarely have acute severe hepatitis. Most children with HBV and HCV are asymptomatic during childhood but are at risk for developing cirrhosis and hepatocellular carcinoma (HCC) in adulthood. In this article, human immunodeficiency virus (HIV) coinfection is not discussed in depth.

HEPATITIS B VIRUS
Epidemiology and Natural History

The number of cases of chronic HBV (CHB) infection has been estimated at almost 400 million worldwide ($\sim$5% of world's population). HBV has 8 genotypes (A–H) which are associated with moderate differences in response to therapy.[1] Children with CHB (genotypes B and C) have a high frequency of hepatitis B envelope antigen (HBeAg) positivity and high HBV DNA levels compared with those with other genotypes. The timing of HBeAg seroconversion in genotype C is more delayed compared with genotype B. Genotype C results in more aggressive hepatitis and is associated with an increased risk of HCC.[2] However, the development of HCC was associated with genotype B in a Taiwanese pediatric study.[2] The prevalence of CHB infection in pregnant women in urban areas of the United States varies by race and ethnicity.[3] Although the highest rate was observed in Asian women (6%), the rates in black, white, and Hispanic women were 1, 0.6%, and 0.14%, respectively.

Maternal-fetal transmission is currently the most common route of HBV transmission because meticulous screening for HBV has been performed in individuals receiving transfusion of blood products. Perinatal transmission occurs at or close to the time of birth as a result of exposure to maternal blood and cervical secretions. Transplacental transmission is presumably responsible for perinatal infections, depending on risk factors, including maternal HBeAg positivity, hepatitis B surface antigen (HBsAg) titer, and HBV DNA level.[4] Infants born to mothers positive for HBeAg and mothers with very high serum DNA levels ($>= 10^9$ copies per mL) are at risk for acquiring HBV despite receiving active and passive immunization within 24 hours postpartum.[5–7] Transplacental transmission can occur due to leakage, such as during a threatened abortion. Amniocentesis in HBsAg-positive mothers can be another risk of HBV transmission.[8] Although HBsAg and HBV DNA can be detected in the colostrum and breast milk of HBV-infected mothers, several studies have shown that there is no additional risk of transmission of HBV to breast-fed infants of infected mothers, provided that completed active and passive immunoprophylaxis is received.[9,10]

Wang and colleagues[11] compared outcomes among 3 groups of infants of HBsAg-positive mothers: 144 born by spontaneous vaginal delivery, 40 by forceps or vacuum extraction, and 117 by cesarean section, all of whom received the HBV vaccine and the hepatitis B immunoglobulin (HBIG). Because the response rates to recommended passive and active immunoprophylaxis were similar in all groups, in the 1-year-old infants, hepatitis B surface antibody (anti-HBs) was detected in 78.9% of the infants born by normal vaginal delivery, 84.6% by forceps or vacuum extraction, and 86.4% by cesarean section, with CHB incidence of 7.3%, 7.7%, and 6.8%, respectively. The mode of delivery does not likely influence HBV transmission. A higher incidence of low birth weight and prematurity has been reported in infants born to mothers infected with HBV compared with those born to uninfected mothers.[12]

The spontaneous seroconversion rates of HBeAg (loss of HBeAg and development of the HBe antibody [anti-HBe]) for children infected via perinatal transmission are less than 2% per year for those under age 3 years, and 4% to 5% per year in those older than 3 years; whereas children infected after the perinatal period have higher rates of spontaneous HBeAg seroconversion, up to 70% to 80% over 20 years. The time to HBeAg clearance for individuals with HBV genotype C is longer than in patients with other genotypes.[13] Since the early 1990s, the incidence of acute HBV in the United States has declined.[14]

About one-third of older children and adolescents with acute HBV infection will develop classic symptoms of hepatitis. Cirrhosis and HCC, mostly in adulthood, may be anticipated in about 25% of those who acquire HBV infection during infancy or childhood. Approximately 90% of children infected as infants will develop CHB infection. The risk decreases to 25% to 50% for children who become infected after early infancy but before age 5 years and to only 5% to 10% for children who become infected in adolescence or adulthood. Most children with CHB are asymptomatic, growing and developing normally. Like adults, children and adolescents who are immune-active with persistent elevation of alanine aminotransferase (ALT) and histologic findings of liver inflammation and fibrosis have an increased risk of cirrhosis and HCC compared with those without evidence of hepatic inflammation.[15,16]

Diagnosis and Tests

The diagnosis of acute hepatitis B is based on the detection of HBsAg as an initial serologic marker and immunoglobulin (Ig)-M antibody to hepatitis B core antigen (anti-HBc). Early in the course of acute infection, HBeAg and HBV DNA are detected and are markers of active viral replication. As patients recover, serum HBV DNA significantly declines but may remain detectable by polymerase chain reaction (PCR) assay for up to several decades. Anti-HBc IgM is the initial antibody, which usually persists for several months. During the window period anti-HBc IgM may be present as the only marker of acute HBV infection (after HBsAg is cleared and before anti-HBs is detected). The development of anti-HBc IgG and anti-HBs indicates recovery from acute HBV infection. Seroconversion (HBeAg to anti-HBe) occurs and is followed by a decrease in serum HBV DNA levels and, eventually, HBsAg becomes undetectable. Persistence of HBsAg for longer than 6 months indicates an HBV carrier or progression to CHB. During the early phase of CHB, HBeAg and high serum HBV DNA levels are markers of HBV replication.

Different serologic patterns are observed at various phases of CHB (**Table 1**): immune tolerant phase, immune-active phase, inactive (HBeAg-negative), inactive (loss of HBsAg), and HBeAg-negative immune reactivation phase. The immune tolerant phase is characterized by normal or mildly elevated serum aminotransferases (ALT <1.5 times the upper limit of normal) and evidence of active HBV replication (HBV DNA >20,000 IU/mL or 10^5 copies/mL). HBsAg and HBeAg are positive. Children with maternal-fetal transmission may remain in this phase for up to several decades and are less likely to respond to antiviral therapies compared with immune-active children. Immune-active hepatitis is characterized by elevated serum aminotransferases (ALT>1.5–2 times the upper limit of normal) and active HBV replication (HBV DNA is typically >20,000 IU/mL or 10^5 copies/mL). HBsAg and HBeAg are positive. During this phase children are more likely to clear HBeAg spontaneously or to respond to antiviral therapies. Inactive CHB phase (HBeAg-negative), also known as the nonreplicative or latent phase, is characterized by normal levels of serum aminotransferases and low or undetectable levels of HBV replication. HBsAg is positive but HBeAg is negative. Up to 20% of children with the nonreplicative phase undergo reversions to the

Table 1
Different serologic patterns at various phases in patients with chronic hepatitis B

Phases	Other Terms	Serum Aminotransferases	HBV Replication	HBV DNA	HBsAg	HBeAg	Anti HBs	Covalently Closed Circular (ccc) DNA	Spontaneous Clearance	Response to Antiviral Therapy
Immune tolerant		Normal or mildly elevated (ALT <2 times the upper limit of normal)	Active	>20,000 IU/mL or 10^5 copies/mL	Positive	Positive	Negative	Positive	Less likely	Less likely
Immune-active		Elevated serum aminotransferases (ALT>1.5–2 times the upper limit of normal)	Active	>20,000 IU/mL or 105 copies/mL	Positive	Positive	Negative	Positive	Possible	Highly possible
Inactive	Nonreplicative or latent phase	Normal	Inactive	Low or undetectable levels	Positive	Negative	Negative	Positive	Possible (Up to 20% of children with the nonreplicative phase undergo reversions to the immune-active phase)	Possible (Up to 20% of children with the nonreplicative phase undergo reversions to the immune-active phase)
HBsAg or HBeAg-negative immune reactivation		Normal or elevated	Active	Increased	Becoming positive	Becoming positive	Negative	Positive	Less likely	Less likely
Inactive with loss of HBsAg	Functional cure	Normal	None	Undetected	Negative	Negative	Positive	Positive		
Inactive with loss of HBsAg	Clinical cure	Normal	None	Undetected	Negative	Negative	Positive	Negative		

immune-active phase, and 20% to 30% reactivate into HBeAg-negative HBV.[17] Inactive CHB (loss of HBsAg) occurs in a minority of children who clear HBeAg, as well as the HBV infection (clearance of HBsAg and appearance of anti-HBs). However, the state of negative serologic markers of active infection, including loss of HBsAg, is now referred to as a functional cure because such individuals probably have residual covalently closed circular (ccc) HBV DNA and, therefore, remain at risk for reactivation which receiving immunosuppressants such as chemotherapy for cancer. During the HBeAg-negative immune reactivation phase, children have increased HBV DNA levels with normal or elevated serum aminotransferases and have more virulent liver disease.[18]

Screening tests for HBV are recommended for children and adolescents with clinical signs of hepatitis or unexplained elevation of serum aminotransferases; for all internationally adopted children; for all pregnant adolescents; for adolescents who engage in high-risk behaviors, including the use of intravenous or intranasal drugs or unprotected sex with an infected partner or more than 1 partner; for men who have sex with men; and for those with a history of sexually transmitted disease, immigrants from high prevalence areas (HBsAg prevalence is >2%), including Africa and Asia, the Cape Verde islands, most of Eastern and Mediterranean Europe, the Caribbean, and parts of South America; for children living in communities where HBV is endemic; and for children born to immigrant parents from endemic areas. Because approximately 5% of infants born to HBsAg-positive mothers develop CHB even after optimal immunoprophylaxis, anti-HBs and HBsAg should be tested at 9 to 12 months of age, or 1 to 2 months after the last dose of hepatitis B vaccine given to an at-risk infant.[19,20]

Hepatitis delta (D) (HDV) infection can occur with CHB and an enzyme immunoassay for anti-HDV is commercially available. Negative anti-HBc IgM, positive HBsAg, and presence of anti-HDV suggest the diagnosis of HDV superinfection. Anti-HDV may take several weeks to develop. Acute and convalescent sera may be required. IgM anti-HDV is not useful because it can persist several months during chronic infection.

Prevention and Treatment

The combination vaccination strategy (HBIG and HBV vaccine series) for high-risk neonates significantly prevents vertical transmission to neonates born to HBV-infected mothers. Children and adolescents with CHB should be immunized against hepatitis A, if not already immune.

Not all children with CHB will benefit from antiviral therapy due to potential side effects and the development of antiviral resistance. Treatment should be considered for children with immune-active CHB regardless of HBe Ag status, or if liver biopsy shows moderate-to-severe inflammation or the presence of fibrosis.[21] The treatment goal for CHB is to suppress HBV replication, reduce liver inflammation, reverse hepatic fibrosis, and prevent the development of cirrhosis and HCC. There are currently several oral antivirals approved by the US Food and Drug Administration (FDA) for CHB in adults: 3 nucleoside drugs (lamivudine, entecavir, and telbivudine) and 2 nucleotides (adefovir dipivoxil and tenofovir disoproxil fumarate).

The first treatments for children with CHB to be FDA approved are thrice-weekly interferon (IFN)-alpha and daily lamivudine for 16 to 24 weeks for children between age 2 and 18 years.[22]

Although lamivudine is well-tolerated in young children, drug resistance is common in approximately 20% of patients per year; therefore, its use is currently rare. There have been promising results with pegylated-IFN (PEG-IFN) for adults with CHB and this treatment is currently being studied in children. Adefovir dipivoxil, a nucleotide analog, is approved for children 12-years-old and older but probably has a limited role because higher antiviral activity and lower rates of viral resistance compared with newer agents, such as PEG-IFN and entecavir.[23] Entecavir and tenofovir are FDA-approved for adults with CHB and tenofovir disoproxil is FDA-approved for children 12 years and older.[24] The pediatric approval for entecavir was based primarily on a phase 3 randomized trial (NCT01079806) in 180 children between 2 and 18 years of age who had not been previously treated with a nucleoside/nucleotide analog.

Side effects from nucleos(t)ide analogues usually are minimal during clinical trials but more have been reported after postmarketing surveillance. These analogues have activity against human mitochondrial DNA (mtDNA) polymerase gamma and can lead to mitochondrial dysfunction. All 5 approved agents carry an FDA black box warning of potential mitochondrial toxicity. Myopathy and neuropathy are commonly reported with lamivudine, nephrotoxicity is fairly common with adefovir and tenofovir, and pancreatitis may be associated with the use of lamivudine or adefovir. Antiviral therapy with nucleos(t)ide analogues for children in the immune-tolerant phase has not been associated with benefits but poses a theoretic risk for the development of antiviral drug resistance or adverse side effects.[25]

The best strategy to control HBV infection in children and adolescents is to implement a universal vaccination program. For newborn infants born to mother with CHB, the current recommendation is the administration of prophylaxis (HBIG and completion of hepatitis B vaccine series with the first dose of hepatitis B vaccine given within 12 hours of birth).[26] The efficacy of the combination of HBIG and HBV vaccine series is not yet 100% but somewhat higher (85%–95%) than that of HBV vaccine alone (65%–95%). The risk of maternal-fetal transmission exists despite double vaccination of infants born to mothers with positive HBeAg and/or a high HBV DNA level.[27] The American Association for the Study of Liver Diseases (AASLD) suggests antiviral therapy to reduce the risk of perinatal transmission of hepatitis B in HBsAg-positive pregnant women with a high viral load. Increasing evidence of the safety of exposing infants to antiviral therapy during pregnancy is available but long-term follow-up is required.[28] However, the exact viral load threshold and the timing of when to start therapy during the third trimester have not been clearly addressed. Mothers with CHB who have cracked nipples should avoid breastfeeding and should not donate their breast milk.

After a routine series of HBV vaccination, a circulating anti-HBs level of greater than 10 mIU/mL is considered to be seroprotective. In immune-competent children, seroprotective levels are achieved in at least 95% after 1 course of HBV vaccine. Peak vaccine-induced anti-HBs level is directly related to the waning of the antibody over time, which could increase the risk of HBV infection and of CHB carriage.[29]

Following an additional dose of a new HBV vaccine series (the fourth dose), 15% to 20% of patients who fail to respond to the first complete HBV vaccine series will develop a protective antibody response and 50% to 75% will develop such a response after 3 additional doses. Therefore, another complete 3-dose series of the HBV vaccine is recommended for nonresponders to routine HBV vaccination. Nonresponders after 3 additional doses are less likely to have any benefit after the sixth dose and should be tested for HBsAg to determine the possibility of CHB. Immunosuppression and certain genetic factors (both HLA and non-HLA genes) may explain such nonresponsiveness to routine and additional HBV vaccination.[29]

Special Considerations

The influence of age, mode of acquisition, ethnicity, and/or HBV genotype on the natural history of CHB in children is variable. Genotype testing is not routinely recommended in clinical practice. HBV genotyping may be considered for HBeAg-positive children who are being considered for IFN therapy. A response to IFN was more likely observed in genotype A and B than genotype C. HBV genotype may influence HCC development in children differently than in young adults.

The risk for HCC in children increases with age due to the duration of disease, the degree of histologic injury, and the replicative state of the virus (HBV DNA levels). HCC can occur even after viral replication ceases or early HBeAg seroconversion.[30] It is unclear how to monitor disease progression and the development of HCC in children. The monitoring protocol for HCC for adults with HBV that is recommended is the combined use of liver ultrasound and serum alpha-fetoprotein (AFP) every 12 months or more often in those with elevated AFP, cirrhosis, or a family history of HCC.[31]

The financial burden for children with CHB is undoubtedly high due to long-term exposure to the virus and risks of cirrhosis and HCC. To reduce the financial burden, an effective combination therapy using antiviral drugs is required to target the viral replication cycle rather than merely achieving prolonged suppression of viral replication.

Efforts have also focused on searching for natural products, such as alternative medicines with low cost and safety, for the antiviral therapy. In recent decades, a large number of clinical trials and preclinical studies using Chinese medicine have demonstrated potential benefit in several aspects of treatment of CHB. Many concerns include study design the quality of clinical trials and the inconsistent and unknown active ingredient components of Chinese medicines in the regimen.[32,33]

HEPATITIS C VIRUS
Epidemiology and Natural History

HCV infection is a global health burden affecting 170 million individuals worldwide. In the United States, there are approximately 7 million HCV-infected adults and 100,000 children.[34] In the third National Health and Nutrition Evaluation Survey, the HCV seroprevalence among children was estimated at 0.2% to 0.4% ($\sim$132,000 antibody-positive children).[35] US census results have estimated that 23,048 to 42,296 children are chronically infected with HCV and 7200 new cases occur annually.[36] Genotype 1, 1a and 1b, are the most common subtypes in the United States, followed by genotypes 2 and 3, and, less commonly, subtypes 4 to 6.[37]

Before 1992, HCV-infected children acquired the virus through transfusion of blood and blood-related products. Since 1992, blood units transfused have mostly been free of HCV, which is estimated to be 0.01% to 0.001% per transfusion.[38] Therefore, most new HCV-infected cases have occurred through maternal-fetal (vertical) transmission.[36] Vertical transmission accounts for greater than 60% of children with HCV and approximately 5% of infants are born to HCV-RNA–positive woman.[39] Mothers with high viral load (HCV-RNA >10^6 copies/ml) are more likely to transmit the virus to the fetus. HIV-coinfected mothers have a 4-fold to 5-fold increased risk of vertical transmission. Infants born to HCV-positive mothers are more likely to be of low birth weight, small for gestational age, and require neonatal intensive care unit admission and assisted ventilation compared with uninfected infants.[40]

Mok and colleagues[41] reported that one-third to one-half of infants with HCV had acquired HCV in utero from HCV-infected mothers. HCV was detected in breast milk and colostrum.[42,43] The HCV transmission rate was higher in infants exposed to HCV-RNA–positive breast milk.[44] Most studies, however, did not demonstrate an association between transmission and mode of infant feeding.[45,46] In contrast to HBV infection in children, children with HCV infection have a higher rate of spontaneous viral clearance. About 25% to 40% of infants who acquired HCV via vertical transmission have spontaneous clearance of HCV-RNA by 2 to 3 years, whereas

6% to 12% of children up to 7 years exhibit the spontaneous HCV clearance.[47–49] Spontaneous viral clearance more likely occurs with HCV genotype 3 infection.[50] Chen and colleagues[51] reported a study of 42 children chronically infected with HCV, with an RNA level below 4.5×10^4 IU/mL at enrollment, having a higher rate of spontaneous viral clearance.

On the other hand, children who acquire HCV via the parenteral transmission have highly variable viral clearance. In up to 3 decades of longitudinal cohorts, viral clearance ranged from 11% and 30% to 45% in studies of infants infected by an HCV-RNA–positive blood donor or contaminated blood products during surgery, respectively.[52–54] Children with elevated serum aminotransferases at onset of the illness have a greater chance of biochemical remission and loss of viremia compared with those with normal serum aminotransferases.[48,55]

Similar to HBV infection in children, most children ($\sim$80%) with chronic HCV (CHC) infection without spontaneous viral clearance have an asymptomatic clinical course with normal histology or mildly elevated serum aminotransferases and minimal changes in liver histopathology.[39,56] Up to 10% to 20% of HCV-infected children without viral clearance will have persistent elevation of serum aminotransferases and may have clinical manifestations of liver disease. An increase in the aspartate aminotransferase (AST)/ALT ratio (AST > ALT) may suggest the development of cirrhosis in individuals with CHC. Cirrhosis is reported in 1% to 2% of children, and progression to severe chronic liver disease and HCC occurs 20 to 40 years after infection.[57] Two HCV-infected adolescents developed HCC.[58] The first case was a 14-year-old African American girl with vertical transmission of HCV genotype 1a with end-stage liver disease requiring liver transplant. AFP concentration increased from 39.8 to 76.6 ng/mL (normal <8.9 ng/mL) within 5 months. The pathologic testing of her liver explant showed a single 1.5-cm nodule of well-differentiated HCC. The second case was a 13-year-old white girl with a T cell–depleted allogeneic stem cell transplant for recurrent acute myelogenous leukemia and elevated serum aminotransferases. HCV-PCR was positive and AFP concentration was elevated (2740 ng/mL–normal <10). Computerized axial tomography scan of the abdomen revealed 2 low-attenuation lesions in the right lobe of the liver. She underwent a right hepatectomy. Multinodular HCC with the margins of the sample free of tumor was noted in the excised liver. Six months after the HCV diagnosis, several low-attenuation lesions were noted in the left lobe of the liver, she had worsening of cholestasis and died after palliative biliary stent placement. The risk of HCC is significantly decreased among HCV-infected adult cases with a sustained viral response (SVR) compared with those without an SVR.[59,60]

Diagnosis and Tests

In general, the algorithm for testing and diagnosis of HCV infection begins with an antibody test in accordance with guidelines and recommendations provided by the AASLD in 2009[61] and the US Centers for Disease Control and Prevention in 2013.[62] Screening tests for HCV are recommended in children and adolescents with clinical settings of hepatitis or unexplained elevation of serum aminotransferases, with HIV infection, with a history of illicit injection drug use, sexual assault, multiple sexual partners, mothers who are known or suspected to be infected with HCV or have a history of intravenous drug use, and children who are international adoptees or refugees from countries with high prevalence rates, including Africa, China, Russia, Eastern Europe, and Southeast Asia.[63] In the setting of either a reactive or indeterminate HCV antibody result, HCV-RNA testing should be performed. The diagnosis of HCV infection is confirmed when HCV-RNA is detected.[61]

However, in young infants born to an HCV-positive mother, passive (transplacental) maternal antibodies can persist for up to 18 months. Therefore, the American Academy of Pediatrics recommends that infants born to HCV-infected mothers be screened by anti-HCV antibody at age 18 months postpartum.[64] In children in whom HCV-RNA is not detected, a reactive antibody could indicate either a past HCV infection with a viral clearance or the antibody test is false-positive. False-negative antibody testing could occur in immunocompromised patients, especially those with advanced HIV infection, hemodialysis, transplant recipients, or suspected cases with acute HCV infection. Because HCV-RNA can be detected within 10 to 14 days after infection, those with suspicion for acute HCV infection should have HCV-RNA testing performed concomitantly with the antibody testing.

As the initial assay for antibody testing for HCV, several different antibody tests are available, including laboratory-based immunoassays, rapid point-of-care tests, and home-based tests; and all can be used. The most common standard test to detect anti-HCV antibodies in serum and plasma is an immunoassay or enzyme-linked immunosorbent assay (EIA). The latest, third-generation EIA (EIA-3) generally detects antibodies to recombinant antigens from the core, NS3, NS4, and NS5 proteins of HCV.[65] These very high sensitivity and high-specificity EIA tests become positive as early as 8 weeks after exposure.[66] Most rapid tests for HCV antibodies have been developed for HCV testing outside of traditional clinical settings.[67]

Quantitative HCV-RNA assays are used to confirm the presence or absence of infection and to quantify the amount of HCV-RNA present, to determine SVR, and to guide decisions for a duration of antiviral therapy. False-positive HCV-RNA results can occur in the presence of carryover contamination. Fortunately, real-time PCR methods have largely eliminated this issue and replaced standard PCR methods in clinical laboratories for HCV level testing with greater sensitivity with lower detection limits of approximately 15 IU/mL.[68]

Prevention and Treatment

Children and adolescents should be immunized against hepatitis A and hepatitis B, if not already immune. Prevention of new HCV infections in older children and adolescents focuses mostly on counseling for high-risk behaviors, such as sex with multiple partners and the use of intravenous drugs and/or intranasal cocaine because of sharing of potentially contaminated equipment. Although commercial body piercing and tattooing are not definitely associated with the risk of acquiring HCV, self-tattooing and self-piercing with shared needles should be discouraged.[69]

The goal of treatment in HCV infection is achievement of an SVR. Currently, SVR is defined as undetectable HCV-RNA in peripheral blood 24 weeks after the end of the treatment. Late relapse is rare after SVR. The durability of undetectable serum HCV was observed in almost all cases (>99%) after SVR.[70] Treatment of HCV-infected children has been guided by clinical trials in adults. Several clinical trials in children were performed to address the efficacy and safety of these therapies. Historically, in small uncontrolled clinical trials of thrice-weekly IFN, reported SVR rates are better in children (30%–60%) than in adults (8%–35%).[71] In a small pilot study of long-acting IFN or weekly PEG-IFN-alfa-2a, HCV-infected children 2 to 8 years of age had an SVR of 43% (46% in genotype 1).[72] In an open-label, uncontrolled pilot study of the combination of PEG-IFN-alfa-2b plus oral ribavirin (RV) in HCV genotype 1, infected children 2 to 17 years of age achieved an SVR of 48%. This therapy was approved for use in children in the United States based on this single uncontrolled trial.[73] For CHC infection, the current FDA-approved standard of care for children ages 3 to 18 years is once-weekly PEG-IFN-alpha-2a or PEG-IFN-alpha-2b plus daily RV for 24 weeks in HCV genotypes 2 and 3, and for 48 weeks for HCV geno-types 1 and 4.[74]

The Pediatric Study of Hepatitis C (PEDS-C) was a prospective, randomized, controlled trial that demonstrated that early and sustained response rates are signifi-cantly increased when RV is added to PEG-IFN-alfa-2a versus PEG-IFN-alfa-2a plus placebo regardless of age, serum aminotransferases levels, and degree of histologic severity. The study indicates that children with CHC should not receive PEG monother-apy, except those with HCV-RNA levels less than 600,000 IU/mL who responded well.[56] A systematic review and meta-analysis included 8 trials in which 438 children ages 3 to 18 years were treated with PEG-IFN-alpha-2a or PEG-IFN-alpha-2b and RV.[75] In chil-dren with HCV genotype 2 or 3 infection, an SVR of 89% was reported; whereas, in chil-dren with HCV genotype 1 or 4 infection, the SVR at best occurred in up to 52%. Combined therapies with PEG-IFN and RV results in an SVR up to 100% in HCV geno-type 2 or 3 children but only 45% to 55% in those infected with genotype 1 or 4.

Adverse effects range from more common symptoms, including flu-like illness, myalgia, and neutropenia, to less commonly observed anemia and thrombocytopenia, thyroid-related symptoms, alopecia, neuropsychiatric manifestations from mood alter-ations, irritability, agitation, and aggressive behavior to depression, anxiety, and sui-cidal ideation.[39,56] Spastic diplegia was sporadically reported in young infants using IFNα.[76] Jonas and colleagues[77] previously reported that children had significant changes in body weight, linear growth, body mass index, and body composition during the treatment with PEG-IFN, which were reversible, although many had height Z scores that did not return to baseline by 2 years after cessation of treatment. Recently, long-term effects on growth were reported in children in children treated with PEG-IFN and RV for 48 weeks and then followed for 5 years; almost all returned to baseline rates of linear growth velocity.[78] Children who received PEG-IFN-alfa-2a and RV rarely devel-oped ophthalmologic complications, such as potential severity of ischemic retinopathy and uveitis; therefore, an ophthalmologic examination is recommended during and af-ter therapy.[79] RV may have effects on viral replication, error-prone mutagenesis, decreased intracellular inosine 5'-monophosphate dehydrogenase, and enhanced im-mune response.[80,81] The administration of RV requires extreme caution in childbearing-age adolescents with CHC given its teratogenic effects.[82]

Direct-acting antiviral agents (DAAs) have fundamentally changed the treatment of HCV infection. DAAs are uniquely designed to inhibit 3 viral proteins: NS3/4A prote-ase, NS5B RNA-dependent polymerase, and NS5A protein, so-called HCV protease inhibitors (PIs), nucleoside HCV polymerase inhibitors, and nonnucleoside HCV poly-merase inhibitors, respectively. When PIs (telaprevir and boceprevir) were added to baseline regimens of PEG alfa-2a and RV, SVR improved up to 75% in genotype 1 treatment-naïve patients.[83,84]

Both PIs entered pediatric trials in 2008.[85] Due to side effects of telaprevir, including severe rash and the black-box warning of Steven-Johnson syndrome and dysgeusia in boceprevir, both drugs were removed from the market.

Some children who are previous nonresponders with IFN-alpha therapy plus RV could potentially be retreated with PEG-IFN and RV. However, because the treat-ment using PEG-IFN-alpha-2a and RV is associated with several adverse effects, the efficacy and applicability can be limited in patients with CHC-induced liver dis-ease.[86] In addition, the treatment is relatively contraindicated in end-stage liver and renal disease. The improvement of existing therapies and development of new effective, safe, and tolerable drugs is, therefore, necessary. When risk-benefit ratio is considered, children with genotype 2 or 3, younger children with CHC genotype 1, and children with normal serum aminotransferases probably have milder hepatic disease, higher possibility of spontaneous viral clearance, lower risk of cirrhosis and HCC development, and could wait for more efficient antiviral therapy with fewer side effects. Excellent results from recent and ongoing trials with DAAs other than telaprevir and boceprevir in adults show shorter duration and high tolerance. The combination of newer NS3/4A PI (simeprevir) and NS5B RNA-dependent PI (sofosbuvir) can further improve response rates and reduce the length of antiviral treatment with or without IFN-alpha or RV regimen in both treatment-naive and previous non-responders with genotype 1 CHC.[87,88] Adverse effects of the regimen, such as fatigue, headache, and nausea, were reported to be mild.[89] Last but not least, 95% to 100% of patients with genotype 1 infection achieved an SVR at 12 weeks in a recent trial using a fixed-dose combination of sofosbuvir and the NS5A inhibitor ledipasvir alone or with RV administered for 8 to 12 weeks in both adults with a treatment history or the presence of compensated cirrhosis.[90] As of September 2016, 10 DAAs were approved for adults and combined into 6 regimens given for different durations, depending on HCV genotypes targeted. These therapeutic advances are currently leading to clinical trials in the pediatric population. Until DAAs are approved in children with HCV, an expectant approach is advocated and treatments that are FDA-approved for adults but not yet children should be considered only for those at high risk for more severe, progressive liver diseases.

Special Considerations and Controversies

Compared with adults with CHC, children have different modes of transmission, spontaneous and treatment rates of clearance, and slow progression of fibrosis.[91] The accumulative duration of HCV infection since birth theoretically makes children with vertical transmission of HCV at risk for cirrhosis and HCC by the time of the transition to adulthood. **Fig. 1** provides recommendations to pediatricians and pediatric gastroenterologists to monitoring and/or managing children with CHC. As hepatitis C therapy is rapidly progresses, DAAs have proven to be efficient therapy even in HCV-infected adults with compensated cirrhosis. Pretreatment liver histology does not necessarily predict the response. A new IFN-free, DAA-based combination: sofosbuvir (400 mg) plus ledipasvir (90 mg) in a single tablet was approved in 2014 in the United States for adults; clinical trials are ongoing to improve tolerability and compliance in children.[92]

A subgroup of high-risk children with end-stage or decompensated liver diseases may benefit from DAA trials before a consideration for liver transplantation because the outcome of liver transplantation in adults with CHC has been suboptimal with development of recurrent HCV infection in most recipients before the advent of DAA therapy.[93] Other factors to consider that may affect HCV and the treatment include obesity and vitamin D status.[94–96] Several pediatric studies indicate most children had mild or minimal hepatic fibrosis.[97] Therefore, the role of obtaining a liver biopsy before treatment of children with CHC is unclear. If liver fibrosis plays a pivotal role in the timing of an antiviral therapy or selecting appropriate therapies, noninvasive markers may guide treatment in children with CHC.[98] With the development of newer therapies in children, some factors, such as IL-28B receptor polymorphism or pretreatment HCV-RNA levels, may predict a higher SVR with shorter duration of therapy.[56,77,99] Currently, there is no definite consensus regarding longitudinal monitoring and timing of treatment of asymptomatic children with HCV infection. HCV-infected children with significant liver disease should have annual or biannual abdominal sonography and serum AFP.[74] This raises concerns to parents caring for children with CHC. Although global impairment in quality of life, cognitive, behavioral, or emotional functioning is not a concern in young children with HCV infection. Rodrigue and colleagues[100] reported that stress and strain on

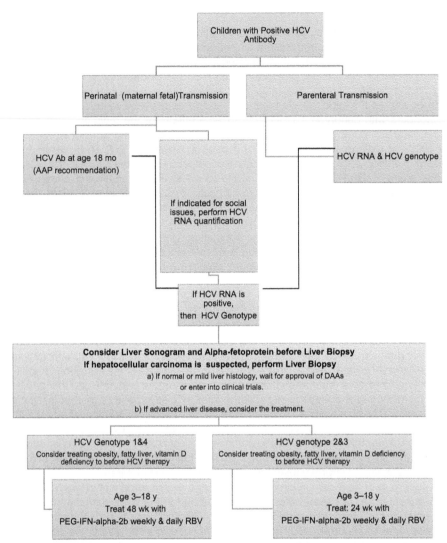

Fig. 1. Recommended approach to monitoring and/or managing children with CHC infection indicated as having HCV infection for greater than 6 months.

the family system in caregiver stress may be associated with some cognitive changes in children given a parental guilt because most cases were vertical transmission. After weighing the risk-benefit decisions toward treatment, there is always a fear of induction of drug resistance. Resistance-associated variants with reduced sensitivity to DAAs have been reported.[101] Considering treating children with CHC, the financial burden of HCV is high. Jhaveri and colleagues[36] estimated the direct medical costs for the care of children with CHC: US $26 million for screening, $117 to 206 million for monitoring, and $56 to 104 million for treatment costs. Because CHC is becoming a serious health issue in children transitioning to adulthood, increased efforts and resources to identify more effective prevention will certainly be cost-effective.

REFERENCES

1. Palumbo E. Hepatitis B genotypes and response to antiviral therapy: a review. Am J Ther 2007;14:306–9.
2. Chan HL, Hui AY, Wong ML, et al. Genotype C hepatitis B virus infection is associated with an increased risk of hepatocellular carcinoma. Gut 2004;53:1494–8.
3. Euler GL, Wooten KG, Baughman AL, et al. Hepatitis B surface antigen prevalence among pregnant women in urban areas: implications for testing, reporting, and preventing perinatal transmission. Pediatrics 2003;111:1192–7.
4. Xu DZ, Yan YP, Choi BC, et al. Risk factors and mechanism of transplacental transmission of hepatitis B virus: a case-control study. J Med Virol 2002;67:20–6.
5. Willner IR, Uhl MD, Howard SC, et al. Serious hepatitis A: an analysis of patients hospitalized during an urban epidemic in the United States. Ann Intern Med 1998;128:111–4.
6. Lin HH, Lee TY, Chen DS, et al. Transplacental leakage of HBeAg-positive maternal blood as the most likely route in causing intrauterine infection with hepatitis B virus. J Pediatr 1987;111:877.
7. Ohto H, Lin HH, Kawana T, et al. Intrauterine transmission of hepatitis B virus is closely related to placental leakage. J Med Virol 1987;21:1.
8. Alexander JM, Ramus R, Jackson G, et al. Risk of hepatitis B transmission after amniocentesis in chronic hepatitis B carriers. Infect Dis Obstet Gynecol 1999;7:283–6.
9. Beasley RP, Stevens CE, Shiao IS, et al. Evidence against breast-feeding as a mechanism for vertical transmission of hepatitis B. Lancet 1975;2:740.
10. Hill JB, Sheffield JS, Kim MJ, et al. Risk of hepatitis B transmission in breast-fed infants of chronic hepatitis B carriers. Obstet Gynecol 2002;99:1049.
11. Wang J, Zhu Q, Zhang X. Effect of delivery mode on maternal–infant transmission of hepatitis B virus by immunoprophylaxis. Chin Med J 2002;115:1510–2.
12. Shepard TH. Catalog of teratogenic agents. 9th edition. Baltimore (MD): Johns Hopkins University Press; 1998. p. p1309.
13. Livingston SE, Simonetti JP, Bulkow LR, et al. Clearance of hepatitis B e antigen in patients with chronic hepatitis B and genotypes A, B, C, D, and F. Gastroenterology 2007;133:1452–7.
14. Goldstein ST, Alter MJ, Williams IT, et al. Incidence and risk factors for acute hepatitis B in the United States, 1982–1998: implications for vaccination programs. J Infect Dis 2002;185:713–9.
15. Bortolotti F, Cadrobbi P, Crivellaro C, et al. Long-term outcome of chronic type B hepatitis in patients who acquire hepatitis B virus infection in childhood. Gastroenterology 1990;99:805–10.
16. Bortolotti F, Jara P, Crivellaro C, et al. Outcome of chronic hepatitis B in Caucasian children during a 20-year observation period. J Hepatol 1998;29:184–90.
17. Hsu YS, Chien RN, Yeh CT, et al. Long-term outcome after spontaneous HBeAg seroconversion in patients with chronic hepatitis B. Hepatology 2002;35:1522.
18. Haber BA, Block JM, Jonas MM, et al, Hepatitis B Foundation. Recommendations for screening, monitoring, and referral of pediatric chronic hepatitis B. Pediatrics 2009;124:e1007.
19. Workowski KA, Bolan GA, Centers for Disease Control and Prevention. Sexually transmitted diseases treatment guidelines, 2015. MMWR Recomm Rep 2015;64(RR-03):1.
20. American Academy of Pediatrics. Medical evaluation of internationally adopted children for infectious diseases. In: Pickering LK, Baker CJ, Kimberlin DW, et al,

editors. Red book: 2012 report of the committee on infectious diseases. 29th edition. Elk Grove Village (IL): American Academy of Pediatrics; 2012. p. 193.

21. Jonas MM, Block JM, Haber BA, et al. Treatment of children with chronic hepatitis B virus infection in the United States: patient selection and therapeutic options. Hepatology 2010;52:2192–205.

22. Sokal EM, Clonjeevaram HS, Roberts EA, et al. Interferon alfa therapy for chronic hepatitis B in children: a multinational randomized controlled trial. Gastroenterology 1998;114:988–95.

23. Jonas MM, Kelly D, pollack H, et al. Safety, efficacy, and pharmacokinetics of adefovir dipivoxil in children and adolescents (age 2 to <18 years) with chronic hepatitis B. Hepatology 2008;47:1863–71.

24. Murray KF, Szenborn L, Wysocki J, et al. Randomized, placebo-controlled trial of tenofovir disoproxil fumarate in adolescents with chronic hepatitis B. Hepatology 2012;56:2018–26.

25. Khungar V, Han S. A systematic review of side effects of nucleoside and nucleotide drugs used for treatment of chronic hepatitis B. Curr Hepat Rep 2010;9: 75–90.

26. Hepatitis B virus: a comprehensive strategy for eliminating transmission in the United States through universal childhood vaccination. Recommendations of the Immunization Practices Advisory Committee (ACIP). MMWR Recomm Rep 1991;40(RR-13):1–25.

27. Wong VC, Ip HM, Reesink HW, et al. Prevention of the HBsAg carrier state in newborn infants of mothers who are chronic carriers of HBsAg and HBeAg by administration of hepatitis-B vaccine and hepatitis-B immunoglobulin. Double-blind randomised placebo-controlled study. Lancet 1984;1:1–6.

28. Zeng H, Cai H, Wang Y, et al. Growth and development of children prenatally exposed to telbivudine administered for the treatment of chronic hepatitis B in their mothers. Int J Infect Dis 2015;33:97–103.

29. Hennig BJ, Fielding K, Broxholme J, et al. Host genetic factors and vaccine-induced immunity to hepatitis B virus infection. PLoS One 2008;3:e1898.

30. Wen WH, Chang MH, Hsu HY, et al. The development of hepatocellular carcinoma among prospectively followed children with chronic hepatitis B virus infection. J Pediatr 2004;144(3):397.

31. European Association for Study of Liver, European Organisation for Research and Treatment of Cancer. EASL-EORTC clinical practice guidelines: management of hepatocellular carcinoma. Eur J Cancer 2012;48:599–641.

32. Wang G, Zhang L, Bonkovsky HL. Chinese medicine for treatment of chronic hepatitis B. Chin J Integr Med 2012;18:253–5.

33. Zhang L, Wang G, Hou W, et al. Contemporary clinical research of traditional Chinese medicines for chronic hepatitis B in China: an analytical review. Hepatology 2010;51(2):690–8.

34. Jonas M. Children with hepatitis C. Hepatology 2003;36:S173–8.

35. Alter MJ, Kruszon-Moran D, Nainan OV, et al. The prevalence of hepatitis C virus infection in the United States, 1988 through 1994. N Engl J Med 1999;341: 556–62.

36. Jhaveri R, Grant W, Kauf TL, et al. The burden of hepatitis C virus infection in children; estimated direct medical costs over a ten year period. J Pediatr 2006;148:353–8.

37. Nainan OV, Alter MJ, Kruszon-Moran D, et al. Hepatitis C virus genotypes and viral concentrations in participants of a general population survey in the United States. Gastroenterology 2006;131:478–84.

38. Luban NL, Colvin CA, Mohan P, et al. The epidemiology of transfusion-associated hepatitis C in a children's hospital. Transfusion 2007;47:615-20.
39. Granot E, Sokal EM. Hepatitis C virus in children: deferring treatment in expectation of direct-acting antiviral agents. Isr Med Assoc J 2015;17:707-11.
40. Pergam SA, Wang CC, Gardella CM, et al. Pregnancy complications associated with hepatitis C: data from a 2003-2005 Washington state birth cohort. Am J Obstet Gynecol 2008;199:38.e1-9.
41. Mok J, Pembrey L, Tovo PA, et al, European Paediatric Hepatitis C Virus Network. When does mother to child transmission of hepatitis C virus occur? Arch Dis Child Fetal Neonatal Ed 2005;90:F156-60.
42. Lin HH, Kao JH, Hsu HY, et al. Absence of infection in breast-fed infants born to hepatitis C virus-infected mothers. J Pediatr 1995;126:589-91.
43. Kumar RM, Shahul S. Role of breastfeeding in transmission of hepatitis C virus to infants of HCV-infected mothers. J Hepatol 1998;29:191-7.
44. Ruiz-Extremera A, Salmeron J, Torres C, et al. Follow-up of transmission of hepatitis C to babies of human immunodeficiency virus negative women: the role of breastfeeding in transmission. Pediatr Infect Dis J 2000;19:511-6.
45. Granovsky MO, Minkoff HL, Tess BH, et al. Hepatitis C virus infection in the mothers and infants cohort study. Pediatrics 1998;102:355-9.
46. Resti M, Azzari C, Mannelli F, et al. Mother-to-child transmission of hepatitis C virus: prospective study of risk factors and timing of infection in children born to women seronegative for HIV-1. BMJ 1998;317:437-41.
47. Resti M, Bortolotti F, Vajro P, et al. Guidelines for the screening and follow-up of infants born to anti-HCV positive mothers. Dig Liver Dis 2003;35:453-7.
48. Resti M, Jara P, Hierro L, et al. Clinical features and progression of perinatally acquired hepatitis C virus infection. J Med Virol 2003;70:373-7.
49. Yeung LT, To T, King SM, et al. Spontaneous clearance of childhood hepatitis C virus infection. J Viral Hepat 2007;14:797-805.
50. Bortolotti F, Verucchi G, Camma C, et al. Long-term course of chronic hepatitis C in children: from viral clearance to end-stage liver disease. Gastroenterology 2008;134:1900-7.
51. Chen ST, Ni YH, Chen PJ, et al. Low viraemia at enrollment in children with chronic hepatitis C favours spontaneous viral clearance. J Viral Hepat 2009; 16:796-801.
52. Casiraghi MA, De PM, Romano L, et al. Long-term outcome (35 years) of hepatitis C after acquisition of infection through mini transfusions of blood given at birth. Hepatology 2004;39:90-6.
53. Vogt M, Lang T, Frosner G, et al. Prevalence and clinical outcome of hepatitis C infection in children who underwent cardiac surgery before the implementation of blood-donor screening. N Engl J Med 1999;341:866-70.
54. Locasciulli A, Testa M, Pontisso P, et al. Prevalence and natural history of hepatitis C infection in patients cured of childhood leukemia. Blood 1997;90: 4628-33.
55. Farmand S, Wirth S, Loffler H, et al. Spontaneous clearance of hepatitis C virus in vertically infected children. Eur J Pediatr 2012;171:253-8.
56. Schwarz KB, Gonzalez-Peralta RP, Murray KF, et al, Peds-C Clinical Research Network. The combination of ribavirin and peginterferon is superior to peginterferon and placebo for children and adolescents with chronic hepatitis C. Gastroenterology 2011;140:450-8.e1.

57. Alter HJ, Seeff LB. Recovery, persistence, and sequelae in hepatitis C virus infection: a perspective on long-term outcome. Semin Liver Dis 2000;20: 17–35.

58. González-Peralta RP, Langham MR Jr, Andres JM, et al. Hepatocellular carcinoma in 2 young adolescents with chronic hepatitis C. J Pediatr Gastroenterol Nutr 2009;48:630–5.

59. Nishiguchi S, Kuroki T, Nakatani S, et al. Randomised trial of effects of interferon-alpha on incidence of hepatocellular carcinoma in chronic active hepatitis C with cirrhosis. Lancet 1995;346:1051–5.

60. Nishiguchi S, Shiomi S, Nakatani S, et al. Prevention of hepatocellular carcinoma in patients with chronic active hepatitis C and cirrhosis. Lancet 2001;357:196–7.

61. Ghany MG, Strader DB, Thomas DL, et al. Diagnosis, management, and treatment of hepatitis C: an update. Hepatology 2009;49:1335.

62. Centers for Disease Control and Prevention (CDC). Testing for HCV infection: an update of guidance for clinicians and laboratorians. MMWR Morb Mortal Wkly Rep 2013;62:362.

63. American Academy of Pediatrics. Medical evaluation of internationally adopted children for infectious diseases. In: Kimberlin DW, Brady MT, Jackson MA, et al, editors. Red book: 2015 report of the committee on infectious diseases. 30th edition. Elk Grove Village (IL): American Academy of Pediatrics; 2015. p. 194.

64. Hepatitis C virus infection. American Academy of Pediatrics. Committee on Infectious Diseases. Pediatrics 1998;101:481–5.

65. Gretch DR. Diagnostic tests for hepatitis C. Hepatology 1997;26:43S.

66. Maheshwari A, Thuluvath PJ. Management of acute hepatitis C. Clin Liver Dis 2010;14:169.

67. Stockman LJ, Guilfoye SM, Benoit AL, et al. Rapid hepatitis C testing among persons at increased risk for infection–Wisconsin, 2012-2013. MMWR Morb Mortal Wkly Rep 2014;63:309.

68. Chevaliez S, Bouvier-Alias M, Brillet R, et al. Overestimation and underestimation of hepatitis C virus RNA levels in a widely used real-time polymerase chain reaction-based method. Hepatology 2007;46:22.

69. Murray KF, Richardson LP, Morishima C, et al. Prevalence of hepatitis C virus infection and risk factors in an incarcerated juvenile population: a pilot study. Pediatrics 2003;111:153.

70. Nelson DR, Davis GL, Jacobson I, et al. Hepatitis C virus: a critical appraisal of approaches to therapy. Clin Gastroenterol Hepatol 2009;7:397–414.

71. Jacobson KR, Murray K, Zellos A, et al. An analysis of published trials of interferon in children with chronic hepatitis C. J Pediatr Gastroenterol Nutr 2002;34: 52–8.

72. Schwarz KB, Mohan P, Narkewicz MR, et al. Safety, efficacy and pharmacokinetics of peginterferon alpha2a (40 kd) in children with chronic hepatitis C. J Pediatr Gastroenterol Nutr 2006;43:499–505.

73. Wirth S, Pieper-Boustani H, Lang T, et al. Peginterferon alfa-2b plus ribavirin treatment in children and adolescents with chronic hepatitis C. Hepatology 2005;41:1013–8.

74. Mack CL, Gonzalez-Peralta RP, Gupta N, et al. NASPGHAN practice guidelines: diagnosis and management of hepatitis C infection in infants, children, and adolescents. J Pediatr Gastroenterol Nutr 2012;54:838–55.

75. Druyts E, Thorlund K, Wu P, et al. Efficacy and safety of pegylated interferon alfa-2a or alfa-2b plus ribavirin for the treatment of chronic hepatitis C in children

and adolescents: a systematic review and meta-analysis. Clin Infect Dis 2013; 56:961–7.

76. Wörle H, Maass E, Köhler B, et al. Interferon alpha-2a therapy in haemangiomas of infancy: spastic diplegia as a severe complication. Eur J Pediatr 1999;158:344.

77. Jonas MM, Balistreri W, Gonzalez-Peralta RP, et al. Pegylated interferon for chronic hepatitis C in children affects growth and body composition: results from the pediatric study of hepatitis C (PEDS-C) trial. Hepatology 2012;56: 523–31.

78. Haber B, Alonso E, Pedreira A, et al. Long-term follow-up of children treated with peginterferon and ribavirin for hepatitis C virus infection. J Pediatr Gastroenterol Nutr 2017;64(1):89–94.

79. Narkewicz MR, Rosenthal P, Schwarz KB, et al. Ophthalmologic complications in children with chronic hepatitis C treated with pegylated interferon. J Pediatr Gastroenterol Nutr 2010;51:183–6.

80. Te HS, Randall G, Jensen DM. Mechanism of action of ribavirin in the treatment of chronic hepatitis C. Gastroenterol Hepatol 2007;3:218–26.

81. Castellvi P, Navinés R, Gutierrez F, et al. Pegylated interferon and ribavirin-induced depression in chronic hepatitis C: role of personality. J Clin Psychiatry 2009;70:817–28.

82. Karnsakul W, Alford MK, Schwarz KB. Managing pediatric hepatitis C: current and emerging treatment options. Ther Clin Risk Manag 2009;5:651–60.

83. Jacobson IM, McHutchison JG, Dusheiko G, et al. Telaprevir for previously untreated chronic hepatitis C virus infection. N Engl J Med 2011;364:2405–16.

84. Poordad F, McCone J Jr, Bacon BR, et al. Boceprevir for untreated chronic HCV genotype 1 infection. N Engl J Med 2011;364:1195–206.

85. Brown NA. Progress towards improving antiviral therapy for hepatitis C with hepatitis C virus polymerase inhibitors. Part I: nucleoside analogues. Expert Opin Investig Drugs 2009;18:709–25.

86. Masci P, Bukowski RM, Patten PA, et al. New and modified IFN alfas: preclinical and clinical data. Curr Oncol Rep 2003;5:108–13.

87. Everson G, Cooper C, Hezode C, et al. DAUPHINE: a randomized phase II study of danoprevir/ritonavir plus peginterferon alpha-2a/ribavirin in HCV genotypes 1 or 4. Liver Int 2014;35:108–19.

88. Fried MW, Buti M, Dore GJ, et al. Once-daily simeprevir (TMC435) with pegylated interferon and ribavirin in treatment-naive genotype 1 hepatitis C: the randomized PILLAR study. Hepatology 2013;58:1918–29.

89. Lawitz E, Sulkowski MS, Ghalib R, et al. Simeprevir plus sofosbuvir, with or without ribavirin, to treat chronic infection with hepatitis C virus genotype 1 in non-responders to pegylated interferon and ribavirin and treatment-naïve patients: the COSMOS randomised study. Lancet 2014;384:1756–65.

90. Gentile I, Buonomo AR, Zappulo E, et al. Interferon-free therapies for chronic hepatitis C: toward a hepatitis C virus-free world? Expert Rev Anti Infect Ther 2014;12:763–73.

91. Murray KF, Finn LS, Taylor SL, et al. Liver histology and alanine aminotransferase levels in children and adults with chronic hepatitis C infection. J Pediatr Gastroenterol Nutr 2005;41:634–8.

92. Afdhal N, Zeuzem S, Kwo P, et al. Ledipasvir and sofosbuvir for untreated HCV genotype 1 infection. N Engl J Med 2014;370:1889–98.

93. Berenguer M, Prieto M, Palau A, et al. Severe recurrent hepatitis C after liver re-transplantation for hepatitis C virus-related graft cirrhosis. Liver Transpl 2003;9: 228–35.

94. Delgado-Borrego A, Healey D, Negre B, et al. Influence of body mass index on outcome of pediatric chronic hepatitis C virus infection. J Pediatr Gastroenterol Nutr 2010;51:191–7.

95. Eltayeb AA, Abdou MA, Abdel-aal AM. Vitamin D status and viral response to therapy in hepatitis C infected children. World J Gastroenterol 2015;21:1284–91.

96. Villar LM, Del Campo JA, Ranchal I, et al. Association between vitamin D and hepatitis C virus infection: a meta-analysis. World J Gastroenterol 2013;19: 5917–24.

97. Goodman ZD, Makhlouf HR, Liu L, et al. Pathology of chronic hepatitis C in children: liver biopsy findings in the Peds-C Trial. Hepatology 2008;47:836–43.

98. Lee CK, Perez-Atayde AR, Mitchell PD, et al. Serum biomarkers and transient elastography as predictors of advanced liver fibrosis in a United States cohort: the Boston children's hospital experience. J Pediatr 2013;163:1058–64.

99. Domagalski K, Pawlowska M, Tretyn A, et al. Impact of IL-28B polymorphisms on pegylated interferon plus ribavirin treatment response in children and adolescents infected with HCV genotypes 1 and 4. Eur J Clin Microbiol Infect Dis 2013; 32:745–54.

100. Rodrigue JR, Balistreri W, Haber B, et al. Impact of hepatitis C virus infection on children and their caregivers: quality of life, cognitive, and emotional outcomes. J Pediatr Gastroenterol Nutr 2009;48:341–7.

101. Sarrazin C, Dvory-Sobol H, Svarovskaia ES, et al. Prevalence of resistance-associated substitutions in HCV NS5A, NS5B, or NS3 and outcomes of treatment with ledipasvir and sofosbuvir. Gastroenterology 2016;151:501–12.

Nonalcoholic Fatty Liver Disease in Children

Hepatic and Extrahepatic Complications

Praveen Kumar Conjeevaram Selvakumar, MD[a],
Mohammad Nasser Kabbany, MD[a], Valerio Nobili, MD[b],
Naim Alkhouri, MD[c],*

KEYWORDS

- Nonalcoholic fatty liver disease • Extrahepatic complications
- Hepatic complications • Metabolic syndrome • Obesity complications in children

KEY POINTS

- Nonalcoholic fatty liver disease (NAFLD) includes a broad spectrum of liver diseases ranging from simple steatosis to nonalcoholic steatohepatitis with further progression to fibrosis or cirrhosis.
- Liver biopsy still remains the gold standard for the diagnosis of NAFLD.
- Noninvasive diagnostic methods, such as serum markers or imaging, are still not well established or validated for children with NAFLD.
- NAFLD is associated with multiple extrahepatic complications, such as cardiovascular disease, type 2 diabetes, sleep disorders, and osteoporosis.
- Clinicians should be aware of these extrahepatic complications to ensure prompt screening and treatment.

INTRODUCTION

With the increasing trend in obesity, nonalcoholic fatty liver disease (NAFLD) has now become the most common cause of chronic liver disease in children and adolescents, with a prevalence of 3% to 10% in the general pediatric population increasing to up to 70% in obese children.[1,2] NAFLD is a clinicopathologic entity that encompasses a broad spectrum of liver injury ranging from accumulation of fat in the liver (simple

Conflict of Interest: None to disclose.
[a] Department of Pediatric Gastroenterology and Hepatology, Cleveland Clinic, Cleveland, OH, USA; [b] Liver Unit, IRCCS Bambino Gesù Children's Hospital, IRCCS, Rome, Italy; [c] Department of Pediatric Gastroenterology and Hepatology, Digestive Disease Institute, Cleveland Clinic Cleveland, Cleveland Clinic Main Campus, Mail Code A111, 9500 Euclid Avenue, Cleveland, OH 44195, USA
* Corresponding author.
E-mail address: alkhouri@txliver.com

steatosis) to the potentially progressive form of nonalcoholic steatohepatitis (NASH) characterized by hepatocyte ballooning and inflammation, and is often associated with fibrosis. NAFLD can cause decompensated cirrhosis requiring liver transplantation and hepatocellular carcinoma even in children.[3–5]

Although NAFLD increases the risk of liver-related mortality and morbidity, the most common causes of death among patients with NAFLD are cardiovascular disease (CVD) and extrahepatic malignancy.[6] This has led to an increasing awareness of extrahepatic complications associated with NAFLD. NAFLD is often considered a hepatic manifestation of metabolic syndrome (MetS); however, emerging data indicate that NAFLD can be a risk factor for the development of MetS, type 2 diabetes mellitus (DM), and CVD.[7–9] Similarly, NAFLD is shown to be associated with other extrahepatic complications, such as chronic kidney disease, hypothyroidism, polycystic ovarian syndrome, obstructive sleep apnea (OSA), osteoporosis, and colorectal cancer in adults.[10,11] In children, recent evidence suggests that pediatric NAFLD is associated with individual extrahepatic complications, such as CVD, type 2 DM, retinopathy, vitamin D deficiency, and low bone mineral density.

HEPATIC COMPLICATIONS
Clinical Manifestations

Children with NAFLD are usually diagnosed because of incidental elevation in liver enzymes or evidence of steatosis on ultrasound done either as a part of routine screening test in obese children or for evaluation of other diseases. Children remain asymptomatic and present clinically once the liver disease has progressed or with concurrent extrahepatic manifestations of MetS. The mean age of diagnosis of NAFLD in children is reported to be between 11 and 13 years.[12] Clinical manifestations of NAFLD include nonspecific right upper quadrant abdominal pain from stretching of liver capsule (approximately 42%–59% of the patients), fatigue, and irritability. Physical examination may reveal acanthosis nigricans from insulin resistance (IR); hepatomegaly in up to 50% of the patients, which might be difficult to assess because of abdominal obesity; and, rarely, splenomegaly.[13,14]

Diagnostic Methods

Liver enzymes

In spite of the high prevalence of NAFLD in children, screening and diagnostic approaches in pediatric NAFLD are not well defined. The American Academy of Pediatrics recommends biannual screening of children 10 years of age or older who are overweight with other risk factors for NAFLD or obese even without risk factors with alanine aminotransferase (ALT) and aspartate aminotransferase (AST) levels and further referral to pediatric hepatologist if ALT or AST levels are 2 times the upper limit of normal levels.[15] However, the European Society for Pediatric Gastroenterology Hepatology and Nutrition recommends screening in obese children 3 years of age or older with both liver enzymes and ultrasound.[14] Analysis of data from the National Health and Nutrition Examination Survey between 1999 and 2006 in the SAFETY study showed that the 95th percentiles for ALT in healthy weight, metabolically normal, and liver disease–free children were 26 U/L in boys and 22 U/L in girls in comparison with the median upper limit of normal of 53 U/L (range 30–90 U/L) used at different children's hospitals in the United States.[16] Hence, lower cutoff of ALT to screen for NAFLD should be used to improve its sensitivity.

Imaging

Ultrasound is a widely used screening tool for hepatic steatosis with a sensitivity of approximately 80% and specificity of approximately 50% to 60%.[17,18] However, ultrasound has decreased sensitivity in patients with mild steatosis.[19] Moreover, ultrasound cannot accurately distinguish between simple steatosis and NASH or fibrosis. Newer imaging techniques, such as controlled attenuation parameter and MRI with proton density fat fraction, are shown to be more accurate in assessing hepatic steatosis.[20,21] Imaging techniques that measure liver stiffness using elastography to assess hepatic fibrosis have been developed recently.[22] Although these recent imaging techniques are more accurate than conventional ultrasound, their use is currently limited because of cost and the lack of validated cutoff values in children.

Liver biopsy

Liver biopsy remains the gold standard in the evaluation of steatosis, NASH, and NAFLD-related liver fibrosis. Simple steatosis is defined as macrovesicular steatosis in ≥5% of the hepatocytes after excluding other causes of hepatic steatosis, such as viral hepatitis, Wilson disease, or autoimmune hepatitis.[23] NASH is characterized by hepatocyte injury (ballooning) and neutrophilic infiltration of the liver (lobular and portal inflammation). In a retrospective analysis of children with biopsy-proven NAFLD, 2 distinctive patterns of histology were identified. Steatosis, ballooning degeneration, lobular inflammation, and perisinusoidal fibrosis were categorized as type 1 (adult type) NASH, whereas steatosis, portal inflammation, and portal fibrosis were categorized as type 2 (pediatric type) NASH. Type 2 NASH was found to be the most common histologic pattern seen in younger children with NAFLD.[24]

Progression of Liver Disease

Limited data exist on pediatric NAFLD progression from simple steatosis to NASH, to fibrosis and cirrhosis. The presence of advanced liver fibrosis is shown to be a predictor of overall and liver-related mortality irrespective of other histologic features.[25] The prevalence of advanced liver fibrosis in children with NAFLD is variable. In a study by Alkhouri and colleagues,[26] only 15% of 67 children with biopsy-proven NAFLD were found to have significant fibrosis (stage 2–3). In a retrospective review of liver histology from 742 children who had autopsy for sudden expected death, NASH was observed in approximately 23% of the children with fatty liver of which only 9% of them had bridging fibrosis or cirrhosis.[27] In a multicenter retrospective cohort study including 108 children with biopsy-proven NAFLD, stage 3 fibrosis was observed in approximately 20% of the children at the time of presentation.[28] In another multicenter study involving 92 children with biopsy-proven NAFLD, approximately 24% of them had stage 3 fibrosis.[29] Therefore, approximately 10% to 25% of children diagnosed with NAFLD can progress to advanced fibrosis.

Long-term follow-up studies to assess liver and overall outcomes in children with NAFLD are lacking. A retrospective longitudinal follow-up of 66 children with NAFLD over 20 years demonstrated a standardized mortality ratio of 13.6 of whom 3% of them needed liver transplantation (LT). The observed LT-free survival was significantly lower than expected survival of the US population of same age and gender.[3] In a data analysis from United Network for Organ Sharing database of 330 children and young adults who underwent LT for NASH cirrhosis between 1987 and 2012, 14 patients had LT when younger than 18 years, 20 had LT between 18 and 25 years of age, and 13 needed re-transplantation due to NASH recurrence.[4] Therefore, it is very clear that pediatric NAFLD can progress to end-stage liver disease requiring LT in childhood and young adults.

Multiple adult studies have shown that NAFLD is a risk factor for the development of hepatocellular carcinoma (HCC) even in the absence of cirrhosis.[30] One of the follow-up studies involving adults with cirrhosis showed that the yearly cumulative incidence of HCC in patients with NASH cirrhosis was 2.6%.[31] HCC has been reported in a pe-diatric patient in the setting of obesity and steatosis without evidence of fibrosis or cirrhosis.[5] Pediatric NAFLD might lead to increased risk of HCC in adulthood, but this association has not been studied. Development of HCC in the absence of cirrhosis or fibrosis might indicate the potential role of other factors, such as metabolic syn-drome, obesity, IR, or oxidative stress in the pathogenesis of HCC in patients with NAFLD.[32]

EXTRAHEPATIC COMPLICATIONS

Mechanisms involved in the development of extrahepatic complications in children with NAFLD are not completely understood. It is hypothesized to be caused by an interplay of many factors such as proinflammatory mediators, oxidative stress, IR, and lipotoxicity. Different studies evaluating different extrahepatic complications (**Fig. 1**) of pediatric NAFLD are outlined in **Table 1**.

Cardiovascular Disease

In recent years, there has been a tremendous interest in understanding the association between NAFLD and CVD and potential role of NAFLD in the pathophysiology of

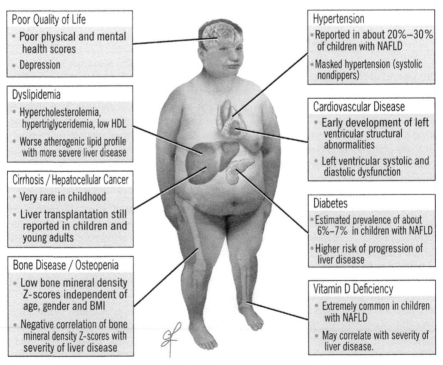

Fig. 1. Extrahepatic complications in children with NAFLD. (Reprinted with permission, Cleveland Clinic Center for Medical Art & Photography © 2016. All Rights Reserved).

Table 1
Studies of extrahepatic complications in children with NAFLD

References	Study Population	Diagnosis of NAFLD	Variable of Interest	Results
Cardiovascular diseases				
Schwimmer et al,[37] 2008	Obese children with (n = 150) and without NAFLD (n = 150)	Liver biopsy	Dyslipidemia Impaired fasting glucose Hypertension	Children with NAFLD had significantly higher TC, LDL-C, TG, fasting glucose and blood pressures than those without NAFLD.
Nobili et al,[39] 2010	Children with NAFLD (n = 18)	Liver biopsy	Atherogenic lipid profile	NAFLD activity and fibrosis scores had a significant positive correlation with TG/HDL-C, TC/HDL-C, and LDL-C/HDL-C ratios even after the adjustment for BMI, insulin resistance, impaired glucose intolerance and MetS.
Corey et al,[40] 2015	Children with NAFLD in TONIC trial (n = 173). Children with and without histologic improvement are compared	Liver biopsy	Dyslipidemia	Children with histologic improvement had significant decreases in TC, LDL-C and non-HDL-C compared with children with no histologic improvement.
Pacifico et al,[41] 2008	Obese children with (n = 29) and without NAFLD (n = 33) and lean subjects (n = 30)	Liver ultrasound	CIMT	CIMT was significantly higher in obese children with NAFLD compared to age-matched and sex-matched obese children without NAFLD and healthy controls. There was also a significant association between higher CIMT and severity of hepatic steatosis.

(continued on next page)

Table 1
(*continued*)

References	Study Population	Diagnosis of NAFLD	Variable of Interest	Results
Demircioğlu et al,[42] 2008	Study groups: Controls (n = 30) Obese children without hepatic steatosis (n = 26) Obese children with grade 1 hepatic steatosis (n = 32) Obese children with grade 2 or 3 hepatic steatosis (n = 22)	Liver ultrasound	CIMT	CIMT was significantly higher in obese children with NAFLD and correlated with grades of steatosis.
Manco et al,[43] 2010	Study groups: Obese children with NAFLD (n = 31) Obese children matched for gender, age and BMI without NAFLD (n = 49)	Liver biopsy	CIMT	There was no significant association between CIMT and NAFLD or grades of steatosis.
Schwimmer et al,[44] 2014	Children with NAFLD (n = 484) from NASH CRN Children assessed both at enrollment and 48 wk afterward	Liver biopsy	Hypertension	Prevalence of hypertension was approximately 36% at baseline and 21% at 48-wk follow-up. Children with hypertension had more severe grades of steatosis than children without hypertension. Girls with NAFLD had higher risk of having persistent hypertension at 48-wk follow-up.

Study	Population	Method	Outcome measure	Findings
Giordanno et al,[45] 2014	Children with NAFLD (n = 101)	Liver biopsy	Systolic and diastolic dipping by ambulatory blood pressure monitoring	Systolic nondippers had significantly impaired oral glucose tolerance and higher insulin resistance compared with systolic dippers.
Sert et al,[46] 2012	Obese adolescents with and without NAFLD (n = 80) Lean subjects (n = 37)	Liver ultrasound and ALT	Left ventricular mass	Significantly higher left ventricular mass with impaired diastolic function in obese children with NAFLD compared with obese children with no NAFLD and lean subjects.
Pacifico et al,[47] 2014	Obese children with (n = 54) and without (n = 54) NAFLD. Lean healthy subjects (n = 18)	MRI	Left ventricular function	Obese children with NASH had more severe left ventricular systolic and diastolic dysfunction compared with obese children with simple steatosis and obese children with no NAFLD.
Fintini et al,[48] 2014	Children with NAFLD (n = 50)	Liver biopsy	Cardiac function and geometry	Left ventricular hypertrophy, concentric remodeling and left atrial dilatation were seen in 50 children with biopsy-proven NAFLD. Significantly lower cardiac alterations in children with simple steatosis compared with those with NASH.
Type 2 DM and abnormal glucose metabolism				
Manco et al,[53] 2008	Children with NAFLD (n = 120)	Liver biopsy	MetS	Prevalence of type 2 DM was approximately 2% in children with NAFLD. Significant association was found between histologic severity and component of MetS.
Schwimmer et al,[54] 2003	Children with NAFLD (n = 43)	Liver biopsy	Insulin resistance Type 2 DM	Insulin resistance was present in 95% of subjects and prevalence of type 2 DM was found to be 14%.
Carter-Kent et al,[55] 2009	Children with NAFLD (n = 130)	Liver biopsy	Type 2 DM	Prevalence of type 2 DM was approximately 7% in children with NAFLD.

(continued on next page)

Table 1
(continued)

References	Study Population	Diagnosis of NAFLD	Variable of Interest	Results
Xanthakos et al,[56] 2015	Adolescents undergoing bariatric surgery (n = 148)	Liver biopsy	Type 2 DM	Prevalence of type 2 DM was found to be approximately 14% and diabetes was found to be the only significant predictor of presence of liver fibrosis.
Newton et al,[57] 2016	Children with NAFLD (n = 675)	Liver biopsy	Prediabetes Type 2 DM	Prevalence of prediabetes and diabetes were 23.4% and 6.5%, respectively. Girls with NAFLD had higher risk of developing prediabetes and type 2 DM than boys with NAFLD. Children with prediabetes and diabetes had significantly higher odds for developing NASH.
Vitamin D deficiency				
Nobili et al,[61] 2014	Children with NAFLD (n = 73)	Liver biopsy	Vitamin D deficiency	Children with NASH had significantly lower vitamin D levels than those without NASH. Low vitamin D levels also correlated with the severity of liver fibrosis.
Hourigan et al,[62] 2015	Children with NAFLD (n = 102)	Liver biopsy	Vitamin D deficiency	Prevalence of vitamin D deficiency and insufficiency was high in patients with NAFLD. There was no relationship between vitamin D levels and histologic severity of NAFLD.
Osteopenia and osteoporosis				
Pirgon et al,[64] 2011	Obese children with or without NAFLD (n = 82) Lean controls (n = 30)	Liver ultrasound	BMD	Children with hepatic steatosis on ultrasound had lower spine BMD Z-scores compared with children with no hepatic steatosis.
Pardee et al,[65] 2012	Obese children with (n = 38) and without (n = 38) NAFLD Age, gender, weight, and height matched	Liver biopsy	BMD	BMD Z-scores are significantly lower in obese children with NAFLD compared with those without NAFLD. Children with NASH had lower BMD Z-scores than those without NASH.

Study	Population	Method	Outcome	Findings
Pacifico et al,[66] 2013	Obese children with (n = 44) and without (n = 44) NAFLD Age, gender, pubertal stage and BMI matched	MRI Liver biopsy in a subset of NAFLD patients	BMD	Obese children with NAFLD had lower BMD Z-scores than those without NAFLD. Children with NASH had lower BMD than those without NASH.
OSA				
Sundaram et al,[68] 2014	Obese children with NAFLD (n = 25)	Liver biopsy	OSA	Prevalence of OSA was approximately 60%. OSA is associated with severe hepatic fibrosis.
Nobili et al,[69] 2014	Obese children with NAFLD (n = 65)	Liver biopsy	OSA	Approximately 60% of the children with NAFLD had OSA. OSA was associated with presence of NASH and fibrosis.
QOL				
Kistler et al,[72] 2010	Obese children with NAFLD (n = 240) Healthy controls (n = 5480)	Liver biopsy	QOL	39% of children with biopsy-proven NAFLD had impaired QOL scores. Children with NAFLD had worse total, physical, and psychosocial scores compared with healthy children.
Kerkar et al,[73] 2013	Children with NAFLD (n = 48) Obese controls without NAFLD (n = 40)	At least 3 of the following: BMI >97th percentile ALT >50 IU/L, positive liver ultrasound Liver biopsy	QOL	Children with NAFLD had higher levels of depression compared with obese controls without NAFLD.

Abbreviations: ALT, alanine aminotransferase; BMD, bone mineral density; BMI, body mass index; CIMT, carotid intima media thickness; CRN, Clinical Research Network; DM, diabetes mellitus; HDL-C, high-density lipoprotein cholesterol; LDL-C, low-density lipoprotein cholesterol; MetS, metabolic syndrome; NAFLD, nonalcoholic fatty liver disease; NASH, nonalcoholic steatohepatitis; OSA, obstructive sleep apnea; QOL, quality of life; TC, total cholesterol; TG, triglycerides.

cardiovascular changes. Evidence from multiple studies in adults suggest that NAFLD is an independent risk factor for CVD and has been found to be associated with endothelial dysfunction, increased carotid intima thickness, and higher prevalence of coronary artery plaques.[33–36] However, studies evaluating CVD in pediatric NAFLD are limited. In a case-control study, obese children with biopsy-proven NAFLD had significantly higher total cholesterol (TC), low-density lipoprotein cholesterol (LDL-C), triglycerides (TG), fasting glucose, and blood pressure than children with obesity alone, indicating a higher cardiovascular risk profile in children with NAFLD.[37]

Atherosclerosis can begin as early as in childhood, with the deposition of fatty streaks in the coronary and carotid arteries.[38] Assessment of subclinical atherosclerosis and CVD risk in children can be accomplished with lipid profile and examination of vascular structures, such as carotid intima media thickness (CIMT) or endothelial dysfunction. In a study that recruited consecutive children with biopsy-proven NAFLD, Nobili and colleagues[39] found that NAFLD activity and fibrosis scores had a significant positive correlation with TG/HDL-C, TC/HDL-C, and LDL-C/HDL-C ratios even after the adjustment for body mass index (BMI), IR, impaired glucose intolerance, and MetS. This positive correlation between atherogenic profile and histologic severity has also been demonstrated in data analysis from the Treatment of NAFLD in Children (TONIC) trial. Children with histologic improvement in the TONIC trial had significant decreases in TC, LDL-C, and non–HDL-C compared with children with no histologic improvement.[40]

Many studies have assessed CIMT in children with NAFLD with contradictory results. A case-control study demonstrated that CIMT was significantly higher in obese children with NAFLD diagnosed with ultrasound compared with age-matched and sex-matched obese children without NAFLD and healthy controls. There was also a significant association between higher CIMT and severity of hepatic steatosis.[41] Similar results were also found in another prospective case-control study.[42] Conversely, a more recent case-control study involving age, BMI, and sex-matched obese children with and without biopsy-proven NAFLD reported no significant association between CIMT and NAFLD.[43] These differences in results could be from different study designs, research methodologies, and small sample sizes.

Children with NAFLD are also reported to have hypertension as a part of the metabolic syndrome. In a longitudinal study including 382 children with biopsy-proven NAFLD, prevalence of hypertension was approximately 36% at baseline and 21% at 48-week follow-up. Children with hypertension had more severe grades of steatosis than children without hypertension. Girls with NAFLD had higher risk of having persistent hypertension at 48-week follow-up.[44] Ambulatory blood pressure monitoring performed in 101 children with biopsy-proven NAFLD in a study by Giordano and colleagues[45] showed significant impaired glucose tolerance and IR in systolic nondippers compared with systolic dippers.

Multiple pediatric studies have consistently demonstrated a significant association between NAFLD and structural and functional abnormalities of the heart. Sert and colleagues[46] reported significantly higher left ventricular mass with impaired diastolic function in obese children with NAFLD compared with obese children with no NAFLD and lean subjects. Few studies also have reported positive correlation between cardiac dysfunction and histologic severity. Doppler echocardiography in 108 obese children in a study by Pacifico and colleagues[47] showed more severe left ventricular systolic and diastolic dysfunction in obese children with NASH compared with obese children with simple steatosis and obese children with no NAFLD. Similarly Fintini and colleagues[48] reported left ventricular hypertrophy, concentric remodeling, and left atrial dilatation in 50 children with biopsy-proven

NAFLD with significantly lower cardiac alterations in children with simple steatosis compared with those with NASH.

Type 2 Diabetes Mellitus and Abnormal Glucose Metabolism

IR plays an important role in the pathogenesis of NAFLD and therefore abnormal glucose metabolism is very frequent among patients with NAFLD. Multiple adult studies reported significantly higher odds of developing type 2 DM in patients with NAFLD.[10] Type 2 DM is also proven to be an independent risk factor for the progression of NAFLD to NASH and advanced fibrosis.[49] Hepatic steatosis in children has been shown to increase the risk of IR and glucose dysregulation.[50,51]

Although metabolic syndrome and IR are more prevalent in children with NAFLD,[37,52] prevalence of type 2 DM or prediabetes in children with NAFLD is not well established. The prevalence of type 2 DM in a group of 122 children with biopsy-proven NAFLD was found to be approximately 2% in a study by Manco and colleagues.[53] A retrospective review of 43 children with biopsy-proven NAFLD found the prevalence of type 2 DM to be approximately 14%.[54] In another retrospective multicenter study including children with biopsy-proven NAFLD, prevalence of type 2 DM was approximately 7%.[55] These studies were limited by small sample size, lack of correlation with histologic severity, and cross-sectional nature of the study. The relationship between prevalence and histologic severity was addressed by a prospective multicenter cohort study including adolescents undergoing bariatric surgery. In this study, overall prevalence of diabetes was found to be approximately 14%, but more importantly, diabetes was found to be the only significant predictor of presence of liver fibrosis (odds ratio = 3.56).[56] This relationship between type 2 DM and histologic severity was confirmed by a more recent multicenter cross-sectional study including 675 children with biopsy-proven NAFLD enrolled in the NASH Clinical Research Network (CRN). In this study, prevalence of prediabetes and diabetes were 23.4% and 6.5%, respectively. Interestingly, girls with NAFLD had higher risk of developing prediabetes and type 2 DM than boys with NAFLD. A key finding is that children with prediabetes and diabetes had significantly higher odds for developing NASH.[57] Thus, recently emerging pediatric studies indicate that type 2 DM is a risk factor for the progression of liver disease in NAFLD with possible increase in liver-related mortality and morbidity. Longitudinal studies are needed to understand the cause-effect relationship between NAFLD and type 2 DM.

Vitamin D Deficiency

Vitamin D deficiency has been associated with obesity in adults[58] and children.[59] Adult patients with NAFLD are found to have a high prevalence of vitamin D deficiency with low levels of vitamin D, correlating with histologic severity of NAFLD.[60] Similarly, pediatric studies also have reported high prevalence in children with NAFLD but correlation with histologic severity is contradictory. In a cross-sectional Italian study including obese and overweight children with biopsy-proven NAFLD, children with NASH had significantly lower vitamin D levels than those without NASH. Moreover, low vitamin D levels also correlated with the severity of liver fibrosis.[61] More recent data analysis from NASH CRN involving children with biopsy-proven NAFLD showed high prevalence of vitamin D deficiency and insufficiency; however, there was no relationship between vitamin D levels and histologic severity of NAFLD.[62] These are cross-sectional studies with limited sample size and lack of healthy controls, so the pathophysiology of vitamin D deficiency in pediatric NAFLD could not be inferred.

Osteopenia and Osteoporosis

Osteoporosis is more frequent in patients with chronic liver disease.[63] There is accumulating evidence to support the impact of NAFLD on bone health in both adults and children.[10] The relationship between bone mineral density (BMD) and pediatric NAFLD was first evaluated in a Turkish study involving obese children with or without hepatic steatosis (diagnosed with liver ultrasound). Children with hepatic steatosis on ultrasound had lower spine BMD Z-scores compared with children with no hepatic steatosis.[64] Pardee and colleagues[65] evaluated BMD in obese children with (biopsy-proven) and without NAFLD and found that BMD Z-scores are significantly lower in obese children with NAFLD compared with those without NAFLD independent of age, gender, ethnicity, weight, and height. Moreover, among children with NAFLD, children with NASH had lower BMD Z-scores than those without NASH. Similar results were demonstrated in a case-control study in which obese children with NAFLD (diagnosed with MRI) had lower BMD Z-scores than age, gender, BMI, and pubertal stage–matched obese children without NAFLD. In a subgroup analysis of children who had biopsy-proven NAFLD, those with NASH had lower BMD than children without NASH.[66] Despite these findings, the role of NAFLD in osteoporosis and risk of fractures in children with NAFLD is not clearly understood due to the lack of longitudinal studies.

Obstructive Sleep Apnea

OSA has been recognized as a risk factor for NAFLD, NASH, and fibrosis independent of age, sex, and BMI in adults.[67] In 2 pediatric studies, polysomnographic evaluation of children with biopsy-proven NAFLD showed a prevalence of approximately 60%. In addition, OSA was significantly associated with NASH and severity of liver fibrosis.[68,69] It is postulated that progression of NAFLD in the setting of OSA could be either from hypoxemia, which can create an oxidative stress, or alternating hypoxemia and normoxia, which might produce a ischemic-reperfusion type of injury to the liver.[70] OSA can significantly affect children's school performance and activity levels, so it is important to screen for OSA in children with NAFLD.

Quality of Life

With the increasing comorbidities associated with NAFLD, patients with NAFLD can have poor quality of life (QOL). Comparison of QOL data between adults with NAFLD and US population with and without chronic illness showed worse physical and mental health scores in patients with NAFLD. Moreover, lower physical health score were associated with severity of the liver disease among patients with NAFLD.[71] Few pediatric studies have also addressed the psychosocial issues in children with NAFLD. In a study by Kistler and colleagues,[72] approximately 39% of children with biopsy-proven NAFLD had impaired QOL scores and children with NAFLD had worse total, physical, and psychosocial scores compared with healthy children; however, no association was found between QOL scores and histologic severity among children with NAFLD. In another case-control study, children with NAFLD had higher levels of depression compared with obese controls without NAFLD.[73] Poor QOL in pediatric NAFLD can increase the burden of illness in both children and parents. Hence, it is important to screen for psychosocial problems and address them accordingly.

SUMMARY

Although NAFLD is a leading cause of chronic liver disease in children and adolescents in developed countries, several aspects of pediatric NAFLD remain unclear.

Most of the pediatric studies on NAFLD are cross-sectional with limited sample size. This limits our understanding of the natural history of the disease in NAFLD. Despite the significant burden of the disease and its potential of progression to cirrhosis even in children and young adults, well-established screening methods are still lacking. Noninvasive biomarkers and imaging techniques in evaluation of NAFLD are being extensively studied, but validation of these tools is lacking. Furthermore, treatment options for liver-related disease in pediatric NAFLD are limited. Currently, lifestyle modification, including healthy dietary habits, weight loss, and physical activity, remains the only effective treatment method.

Multiple adult and pediatric studies have broadened the spectrum of NAFLD to include numerous extrahepatic complications. Long-term prospective longitudinal studies are needed to understand the complex interplay of factors involved in the development of these extrahepatic complications. Nevertheless, it is important for clinicians to recognize these complications associated with pediatric NAFLD. Proper guidelines for screening of these complications in children with NAFLD should be established, as this might have an effect on the long-term morbidity and mortality of the disease.

REFERENCES

1. Patton HM, Sirlin C, Behling C, et al. Pediatric nonalcoholic fatty liver disease: a critical appraisal of current data and implications for future research. J Pediatr Gastroenterol Nutr 2006;43(4):413–27.
2. Roberts EA. Pediatric nonalcoholic fatty liver disease (NAFLD): a "growing" problem? J Hepatol 2007;46(6):1133–42.
3. Feldstein AE, Charatcharoenwitthaya P, Treeprasertsuk S, et al. The natural history of non-alcoholic fatty liver disease in children: a follow-up study for up to 20 years. Gut 2009;58(11):1538–44.
4. Alkhouri N, Hanouneh IA, Zein NN, et al. Liver transplantation for nonalcoholic steatohepatitis in young patients. Transpl Int 2016;29(4):418–24.
5. Nobili V, Alisi A, Grimaldi C, et al. Non-alcoholic fatty liver disease and hepatocellular carcinoma in a 7-year-old obese boy: coincidence or comorbidity? Pediatr Obes 2014;9(5):e99–102.
6. Ong JP, Pitts A, Younossi ZM. Increased overall mortality and liver-related mortality in non-alcoholic fatty liver disease. J Hepatol 2008;49(4):608–12.
7. Anstee QM, Targher G, Day CP. Progression of NAFLD to diabetes mellitus, cardiovascular disease or cirrhosis. Nat Rev Gastroenterol Hepatol 2013;10(6): 330–44.
8. Byrne CD, Targher G. NAFLD: a multisystem disease. J Hepatol 2015;62(1 Suppl):S47–64.
9. Miele L, Targher G. Understanding the association between developing a fatty liver and subsequent cardio-metabolic complications. Expert Rev Gastroenterol Hepatol 2015;9(10):1243–5.
10. Armstrong MJ, Adams LA, Canbay A, et al. Extrahepatic complications of nonalcoholic fatty liver disease. Hepatology 2014;59(3):1174–97.
11. VanWagner LB, Rinella ME. Extrahepatic manifestations of nonalcoholic fatty liver disease. Curr Hepatol Rep 2016;15(2):75–85.
12. Berardis S, Sokal E. Pediatric non-alcoholic fatty liver disease: an increasing public health issue. Eur J Pediatr 2014;173(2):131–9.
13. AlKhater SA. Paediatric non-alcoholic fatty liver disease: an overview. Obes Rev 2015;16(5):393–405.

14. Vajro P, Lenta S, Socha P, et al. Diagnosis of nonalcoholic fatty liver disease in children and adolescents. J Pediatr Gastroenterol Nutr 2012;54(5):700–13.
15. Barlow SE. Expert committee recommendations regarding the prevention, assessment, and treatment of child and adolescent overweight and obesity: summary report. Pediatrics 2007;120(Suppl 4):S164–92.
16. Schwimmer JB, Dunn W, Norman GJ, et al. SAFETY study: alanine aminotransferase cutoff values are set too high for reliable detection of pediatric chronic liver disease. Gastroenterology 2010;138(4):1357–64.e2.
17. Shannon A, Alkhouri N, Carter-Kent C, et al. Ultrasonographic quantitative estimation of hepatic steatosis in children with NAFLD. J Pediatr Gastroenterol Nutr 2011;53(2):190–5.
18. Awai HI, Newton KP, Sirlin CB, et al. Evidence and recommendations for imaging liver fat in children, based on systematic review. Clin Gastroenterol Hepatol 2014; 12(5):765–73.
19. Saadeh S, Younossi ZM, Remer EM, et al. The utility of radiological imaging in nonalcoholic fatty liver disease. Gastroenterology 2002;123(3):745–50.
20. Sasso M, Miette V, Sandrin L, et al. The controlled attenuation parameter (CAP): a novel tool for the non-invasive evaluation of steatosis using Fibroscan®. Clin Res Hepatol Gastroenterol 2012;36(1):13–20.
21. Schwimmer JB, Middleton MS, Behling C, et al. Magnetic resonance imaging and liver histology as biomarkers of hepatic steatosis in children with nonalcoholic fatty liver disease. Hepatology 2015;61(6):1887–95.
22. Nobili V, Vizzutti F, Arena U, et al. Accuracy and reproducibility of transient elastography for the diagnosis of fibrosis in pediatric nonalcoholic steatohepatitis. Hepatology 2008;48(2):442–8.
23. Yeh MM, Brunt EM, Day CP, et al. Pathological features of fatty liver disease. Gastroenterology 2014;147(4):754–64.
24. Schwimmer JB, Behling C, Newbury R, et al. Histopathology of pediatric nonalcoholic fatty liver disease. Hepatology 2005;42(3):641–9.
25. Ekstedt M, Hagström H, Nasr P, et al. Fibrosis stage is the strongest predictor for disease-specific mortality in NAFLD after up to 33 years of follow-up. Hepatology 2015;61(5):1547–54.
26. Alkhouri N, Sedki E, Alisi A, et al. Combined paediatric NAFLD fibrosis index and transient elastography to predict clinically significant fibrosis in children with fatty liver disease. Liver Int 2013;33(1):79–85.
27. Schwimmer JB, Deutsch R, Kahen T, et al. Prevalence of fatty liver in children and adolescents. Pediatrics 2006;118(4):1388–93.
28. Carter-Kent C, Brunt EM, Yerian LM, et al. Relations of steatosis type, grade, and zonality to histological features in pediatric nonalcoholic fatty liver disease. J Pediatr Gastroenterol Nutr 2011;52(2):190–7.
29. Mansoor S, Yerian L, Kohli R, et al. The evaluation of hepatic fibrosis scores in children with nonalcoholic fatty liver disease. Dig Dis Sci 2015;60(5):1440–7.
30. Paradis V, Zalinski S, Chelbi E, et al. Hepatocellular carcinomas in patients with metabolic syndrome often develop without significant liver fibrosis: a pathological analysis. Hepatology 2009;49(3):851–9.
31. Ascha MS, Hanouneh IA, Lopez R, et al. The incidence and risk factors of hepatocellular carcinoma in patients with nonalcoholic steatohepatitis. Hepatology 2010;51(6):1972–8.
32. Guzman G, Brunt EM, Petrovic LM, et al. Does nonalcoholic fatty liver disease predispose patients to hepatocellular carcinoma in the absence of cirrhosis? Arch Pathol Lab Med 2008;132(11):1761–6.

33. Targher G, Bertolini L, Padovani R, et al. Prevalence of nonalcoholic fatty liver disease and its association with cardiovascular disease among type 2 diabetic patients. Diabetes Care 2007;30(5):1212–8.
34. Villanova N, Moscatiello S, Ramilli S, et al. Endothelial dysfunction and cardiovascular risk profile in nonalcoholic fatty liver disease. Hepatology 2005;42(2): 473–80.
35. Koskinen J, Magnussen CG, Kähönen M, et al. Association of liver enzymes with metabolic syndrome and carotid atherosclerosis in young adults. The Cardiovascular Risk in Young Finns Study. Ann Med 2012;44(2):187–95.
36. VanWagner LB, Ning H, Lewis CE, et al. Associations between nonalcoholic fatty liver disease and subclinical atherosclerosis in middle-aged adults: the Coronary Artery Risk Development in Young Adults Study. Atherosclerosis 2014;235(2): 599–605.
37. Schwimmer JB, Pardee PE, Lavine JE, et al. Cardiovascular risk factors and the metabolic syndrome in pediatric nonalcoholic fatty liver disease. Circulation 2008;118(3):277–83.
38. Stary HC. Lipid and macrophage accumulations in arteries of children and the development of atherosclerosis. Am J Clin Nutr 2000;72(5 Suppl):1297S–306S.
39. Nobili V, Alkhouri N, Bartuli A, et al. Severity of liver injury and atherogenic lipid profile in children with nonalcoholic fatty liver disease. Pediatr Res 2010;67(6): 665–70.
40. Corey KE, Vuppalanchi R, Vos M, et al. Improvement in liver histology is associated with reduction in dyslipidemia in children with nonalcoholic fatty liver disease. J Pediatr Gastroenterol Nutr 2015;60(3):360–7.
41. Pacifico L, Cantisani V, Ricci P, et al. Nonalcoholic fatty liver disease and carotid atherosclerosis in children. Pediatr Res 2008;63(4):423–7.
42. Demircioğlu F, Koçyiğit A, Arslan N, et al. Intima-media thickness of carotid artery and susceptibility to atherosclerosis in obese children with nonalcoholic fatty liver disease. J Pediatr Gastroenterol Nutr 2008;47(1):68–75.
43. Manco M, Bedogni G, Monti L, et al. Intima-media thickness and liver histology in obese children and adolescents with non-alcoholic fatty liver disease. Atherosclerosis 2010;209(2):463–8.
44. Schwimmer JB, Zepeda A, Newton KP, et al. Longitudinal assessment of high blood pressure in children with nonalcoholic fatty liver disease. PLoS One 2014;9(11):e112569.
45. Giordano U, Della Corte C, Cafiero G, et al. Association between nocturnal blood pressure dipping and insulin resistance in children affected by NAFLD. Eur J Pediatr 2014;173(11):1511–8.
46. Sert A, Pirgon O, Aypar E, et al. Relationship between left ventricular mass and carotid intima media thickness in obese adolescents with non-alcoholic fatty liver disease. J Pediatr Endocrinol Metab 2012;25(9–10):927–34.
47. Pacifico L, Di Martino M, De Merulis A, et al. Left ventricular dysfunction in obese children and adolescents with nonalcoholic fatty liver disease. Hepatology 2014; 59(2):461–70.
48. Fintini D, Chinali M, Cafiero G, et al. Early left ventricular abnormality/dysfunction in obese children affected by NAFLD. Nutr Metab Cardiovasc Dis 2014;24(1): 72–4.
49. Loomba R, Abraham M, Unalp A, et al. Association between diabetes, family history of diabetes, and risk of nonalcoholic steatohepatitis and fibrosis. Hepatology 2012;56(3):943–51.

50. Cali AMG, De Oliveira AM, Kim H, et al. Glucose dysregulation and hepatic steatosis in obese adolescents: is there a link? Hepatology 2009;49(6):1896–903.

51. D'Adamo E, Cali AMG, Weiss R, et al. Central role of fatty liver in the pathogenesis of insulin resistance in obese adolescents. Diabetes Care 2010;33(8):1817–22.

52. Patton HM, Yates K, Unalp-Arida A, et al. Association between metabolic syndrome and liver histology among children with nonalcoholic fatty liver disease. Am J Gastroenterol 2010;105(9):2093–102.

53. Manco M, Marcellini M, Devito R, et al. Metabolic syndrome and liver histology in paediatric non-alcoholic steatohepatitis. Int J Obes (Lond) 2008;32(2):381–7.

54. Schwimmer JB, Deutsch R, Rauch JB, et al. Obesity, insulin resistance, and other clinicopathological correlates of pediatric nonalcoholic fatty liver disease. J Pediatr 2003;143(4):500–5.

55. Carter-Kent C, Yerian LM, Brunt EM, et al. Nonalcoholic steatohepatitis in children: a multicenter clinicopathological study. Hepatology 2009;50(4):1113–20.

56. Xanthakos SA, Jenkins TM, Kleiner DE, et al. High prevalence of nonalcoholic fatty liver disease in adolescents undergoing bariatric surgery. Gastroenterology 2015;149(3):623–34.e8.

57. Newton KP, Hou J, Crimmins NA, et al. Prevalence of prediabetes and type 2 diabetes in children with nonalcoholic fatty liver disease. JAMA Pediatr 2016; 170(10):e161971.

58. Bellia A, Garcovich C, D'Adamo M, et al. Serum 25-hydroxyvitamin D levels are inversely associated with systemic inflammation in severe obese subjects. Intern Emerg Med 2013;8(1):33–40.

59. Harel Z, Flanagan P, Forcier M, et al. Low vitamin D status among obese adolescents: prevalence and response to treatment. J Adolesc Health 2011;48(5): 448–52.

60. Targher G, Bertolini L, Scala L, et al. Associations between serum 25-hydroxyvitamin D3 concentrations and liver histology in patients with non-alcoholic fatty liver disease. Nutr Metab Cardiovasc Dis 2007;17(7):517–24.

61. Nobili V, Giorgio V, Liccardo D, et al. Vitamin D levels and liver histological alterations in children with nonalcoholic fatty liver disease. Eur J Endocrinol 2014; 170(4):547–53.

62. Hourigan SK, Abrams S, Yates K, et al. Relation between vitamin D status and nonalcoholic fatty liver disease in children. J Pediatr Gastroenterol Nutr 2015; 60(3):396–404.

63. Collier J. Bone disorders in chronic liver disease. Hepatology 2007;46(4):1271–8.

64. Pirgon O, Bilgin H, Tolu I, et al. Correlation of insulin sensitivity with bone mineral status in obese adolescents with nonalcoholic fatty liver disease. Clin Endocrinol (Oxf) 2011;75(2):189–95.

65. Pardee PE, Dunn W, Schwimmer JB. Non-alcoholic fatty liver disease is associated with low bone mineral density in obese children. Aliment Pharmacol Ther 2012;35(2):248–54.

66. Pacifico L, Bezzi M, Lombardo CV, et al. Adipokines and C-reactive protein in relation to bone mineralization in pediatric nonalcoholic fatty liver disease. World J Gastroenterol 2013;19(25):4007–14.

67. Musso G, Cassader M, Olivetti C, et al. Association of obstructive sleep apnoea with the presence and severity of non-alcoholic fatty liver disease. A systematic review and meta-analysis. Obes Rev 2013;14(5):417–31.

68. Sundaram SS, Sokol RJ, Capocelli KE, et al. Obstructive sleep apnea and hypoxemia are associated with advanced liver histology in pediatric nonalcoholic fatty liver disease. J Pediatr 2014;164(4):699–706.e1.

69. Nobili V, Cutrera R, Liccardo D, et al. Obstructive sleep apnea syndrome affects liver histology and inflammatory cell activation in pediatric nonalcoholic fatty liver disease, regardless of obesity/insulin resistance. Am J Respir Crit Care Med 2014;189(1):66–76.

70. Henrion J, Colin L, Schapira M, et al. Hypoxic hepatitis caused by severe hypoxemia from obstructive sleep apnea. J Clin Gastroenterol 1997;24(4):245–9.

71. David K, Kowdley KV, Unalp A, et al. Quality of life in adults with nonalcoholic fatty liver disease: baseline data from the nonalcoholic steatohepatitis clinical research network. Hepatology 2009;49(6):1904–12.

72. Kistler KD, Molleston J, Unalp A, et al. Symptoms and quality of life in obese children and adolescents with non-alcoholic fatty liver disease. Aliment Pharmacol Ther 2010;31(3):396–406.

73. Kerkar N, D'Urso C, Van Nostrand K, et al. Psychosocial outcomes for children with nonalcoholic fatty liver disease over time and compared with obese controls. J Pediatr Gastroenterol Nutr 2013;56(1):77–82.

Pediatric Liver Transplantation

Nidhi Rawal, MD[a], Nada Yazigi, MD[b],*

KEYWORDS

- Liver • Failure • Pediatric • Transplant

KEY POINTS

- Liver transplantation is the standard of treatment for many end-stage pediatric liver disorders.
- Long-term outcomes are excellent for both patient and graft survival.
- Active research is ongoing to optimize immunosuppression protocols to decrease medications side effects and foster immune tolerance.
- Long-term compliance hurdles and transition to adult care are emerging as the new frontiers of pediatric liver transplantation.
- The growing population of pediatric liver transplant recipients begs for new health system streams that meet the complexity of the needed care.

EVOLVING TRENDS IN LIVER TRANSPLANTATION

Excellent outcomes over the last 3 decades have made liver transplantation the treatment of choice for many advanced liver disorders. This success also opened liver transplantation to new indications such as liver tumors, metabolic disorders, postoncologic liver disease, and cystic fibrosis liver disease. The emergence of such new indications for liver transplantation is bringing on a new stream of patients along with their disease-specific challenges.

The timing of referral to transplantation remains crucial to assure timely access to organs and an optimized postoperative survival. Disparities in organ demand and supply persist, resulting in a growing number of pediatric patients on the transplant wait list. A change in national allocation priority helped decrease mortality for those on

Disclosure Statement: The authors have nothing to disclose.
[a] Division of Gastroenterology, Hepatology and Nutrition, Department of Pediatrics, University of Maryland Medical Center, 22 South Green Street, Baltimore, MD 21201, USA; [b] Pediatric Transplant Hepatology, Department of Transplantation, MedStar Georgetown University Hospital, MedStar Georgetown Transplant Institute, PHC#2, 3800 Reservoir Road, Northwest, Washington, DC 20007, USA
* Corresponding author.
E-mail address: nada.a.yazigi@gunet.georgetown.edu

Pediatr Clin N Am 64 (2017) 677–684
http://dx.doi.org/10.1016/j.pcl.2017.02.003
0031-3955/17/© 2017 Elsevier Inc. All rights reserved.

the pediatric wait list; still, many pediatric patients require exception points to receive a liver transplant offer in a timely fashion. The number of liver transplant recipients is peaking, requiring novel systems of health care delivery that meet the needs of this special patient population.

LIVER TRANSPLANTATION INDICATIONS AND EPIDEMIOLOGY
Liver Transplantation Indications

The classical indication for liver transplantation is liver failure causing a life-threatening situation resulting in a mortality risk greater than 90% at 1 year. With improving diagnostic tools and treatment support for end-stage liver disorders, the historical indications for liver transplantation are changing. End-stage liver disease from biliary atresia remains the most common cause of liver disease leading to transplantation. With a growing obesity epidemic, nonalcoholic fatty liver disease is becoming one of the leading causes of liver transplantation in adults and young adolescents. Improving liver transplantation outcomes is allowing consideration of transplantation for patients with metabolic disorders in whom liver transplantation proves to be a reliable treatment modality improving their overall outcomes. Indeed, liver transplantation is now indicated in those with metabolic disorders, in whom a healthy liver can bring enough enzymatic activity to stabilize a metabolic disease like seen in some urea cycle defects and organic acidurias. Finally, advances in oncologic care are allowing hepatoblastomas and hepatocellular carcinomas to be considered for primary transplantation in case they present as unresectable liver tumors.

Pediatric transplants account for about 7% to 8% of total number of liver transplants performed in the country and remain relatively steady at about 500 cases a year. Most transplants are done at less than 2 years of age; another pediatric transplantation peak age is seen in adolescence (**Fig. 1**).[1]

Contraindications to Liver Transplantation

With improved supportive measures and medical expertise, relative contraindications to liver transplantation related to comorbidities are decreasing. Some absolute contraindications, however, remain and consist mostly in systemic disorders that cannot be cured or can be worsened by transplantation, such as ongoing infections, cancers, severe metabolic disorders, or in advanced cardiopulmonary diseases such as seen in severe pulmonary disease or heart failure.

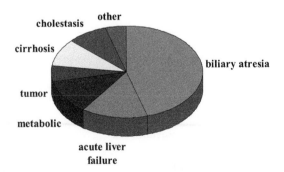

Fig. 1. Common indications for pediatric liver transplantation in the United States.

REFERRAL AND TRANSPLANTATION EVALUATION
Referral

A timely referral to transplant evaluation is a crucial step to assure good success in both early and long-term phases. Such a referral does not necessarily always lead to transplantation, rather it empowers the transplant team to rule out any treatable causes that can avoid transplantation and to put in place a detailed and supportive care plan in case transplant is needed.

It is imperative to refer a patient to the transplant center as soon as acute liver failure or an irreversible liver disease is diagnosed. The healthier a patient is at presentation to the transplant center, the better are the chances to optimize their status and get them if needed, to transplantation in a timely fashion.

Transplantation Evaluation and Wait List

The transplant evaluation is carried out by a multidisciplinary team that includes the primary care physician, primary pediatric gastrointestinal doctor, and the pediatric liver transplant team. The goal is to complete liver disease diagnosis; treat all possible causes of liver failure; rule out any absolute indications to transplantation; palliate to any treatable comorbidities; optimize vaccination, nutrition, and education; and define and foster family and patient education and psychosocial and economic support. A complex care plan is created at the end of the evaluation that puts in motion all that is needed to optimize short- and long-term transplantation outcomes. In some instances, such an evaluation identifies a treatable condition and helps avoid transplantation (**Box 1**).[2]

Box 1
Goals of liver transplant evaluation

- Define indications for transplant.
- Define best timing for listing.
- Identify specialized treatments that can avoid or delay the need for transplantation.
- Plan for care and support needed to minimize risk at transplantation.
- Anticipate long-term outcomes and support needed to optimize them.

Once a patient is on the transplant list, close follow-up is carried out in the transplant center along strict pretransplant protocols. This follow-up allows fine tuning of the care and optimizing of health in anticipation of transplantation. The emphasis in this period is on anticipating complications and on prevention and early treatment. Although it is often not possible to reverse deterioration, every effort is placed to get these children as healthy as possible to transplantation. In addition, this approach allows active wait list management that facilitates a timely transplantation (**Box 2**).

Box 2
Health topics managed while on the wait list

- Malnutrition
  - Protein-energy
  - Fat soluble vitamins
  - Water soluble vitamins
- Portal hypertension
  - Gastrointestinal bleeding
  - Ascites/spontaneous bacterial peritonitis
  - Hypersplenism

- Infectious prevention and treatment
- Vascular access/loss
- Hepatopulmonary syndrome
- Hepatorenal syndrome
- Developmental delay and rehabilitation support
- Hearing loss
- Family/socioeconomic support
- Teaching

TRANSPLANTATION

Patient survival after liver transplantation is currently 95% and 85% at 1 and 5 years after transplantation, respectively. Survival is clearly negatively affected by the severity of a patient's presentation to transplantation and by the presence of comorbidities, with survival rates decreasing to 65% to 70% at 1 year in the case of an acute liver failure presentation.[1] Liver transplantation, therefore, clearly is beyond an experimental phase and has rightfully gained momentum worldwide as a valid life-saving procedure.

In the United States, on average, half of the recipients receive an entire organ, whereas the other half receives an anatomic variant, often from a cadaveric "split" liver or from a living donor. Split-liver grafting involves the preparation of 2 allografts from a single donor, and usually the left lateral segment allograft is transplanted to small children. Outcomes are comparable between different types of grafts, and are mostly affected by timeliness of transplantation and the expertise of the transplant team. This is especially important in infants' transplantations, in which special technical expertise and medical support and experience are crucial.

Early Outcomes: The First 3 Months

The early posttransplantation period is dominated by the surgical recovery. The average pediatric intensive care unit stay is 3 to 5 days. The average length of stay in the hospital after transplantation is 15 to 20 days. Readmissions within the first 3 months are needed in about a third of patients, usually for sepsis or rejection. Acute rejection happens in 30% of patients during this period and usually responds nicely to adjusting immune modulators. Infectious incidence is 10% to 20% and is rarely life threatening in the current era of prophylactic measures. Vascular complications like hepatic artery thrombosis, hepatic vein thrombosis, and portal vein thrombosis average an incidence of 5% to 10%. Biliary leakage or stenosis occur 10% to 20% in most pediatric series. Vascular and biliary complications are more common in recipients weighing less than 10 kg. Although these complications are most common in the first year, they can present at any time after transplantation (**Box 3**).

The approach to the patient in the early phase after transplantation should always be comprehensive. Special considerations are given to the graft, immunosuppression, and prophylactic medications. It is also crucial to continuously assess the patient's and family's coping. Teaching of care should continue and build on that done in the pretransplant clinic.

Box 3
Parameters to watch in the pediatric intensive care unit: is the graft working?

- Hemodynamic stability
- Awake and normal neurologic examination
- Increasing factors V, VII levels
- Normalization of international normalized ratio
- Clearance of lactic acidosis
- Resolution of hypoglycemia
- Normalization of aspartate aminotransferase/alanine aminotransferase/bilirubin
- Confirmation of hepatic vessels patency by Doppler ultrasound scan

---

Long-Term Follow-up

The long-term transplant follow-up is characterized by a progressive shift of care from the transplant center to the primary gastrointestinal and primary care teams.[3] Strict protocols continue to guide all the transplant-related topics. Medications are slowly peeled off; the patient comes off steroids by 3 months and off most prophylactic medications by 6 months. Return to school or day care is allowed at 3 month after transplant. As long as no complications arise, the recipient should move to only yearly follow-up in the transplant center thereafter. Although immunosuppression currently still needs to continue lifelong, it is common practice to decrease it past the first year to the minimal needed to control rejection. This is only feasible if compliance is pristine and laboratory tests are done for monitoring at least every 2 months.

Long-term complications are less commonly seen than in the past but still affect 30% to 50% of children. Based on site-specific outcome measures and seminal work looking at the North American database registry, the Studies of Pediatric Liver Transplantation,[4–7] all programs have implemented new protocols aimed at kidney and bone protection, immunosuppression minimization, proactive vaccination, nutritional support, and psycho-social support (**Box 4**).

Box 4
Long-term complications

- Graft
  - Late acute rejection
  - Chronic rejection
  - Vascular complication
  - Biliary complication
  - Recurrent disease
- Infections
  - Viral
  - Opportunistic
  - Sexually transmitted diseases
- Malignancy
  - Posttransplant lymphoproliferative disease
  - Skin
  - Other (eg, colon, pancreas)

- Gastrointestinal
  - Diarrhea
  - Eosinophilic gastroenteritis
  - Pancreatic insufficiency
  - Motility disorders
  - Feeding disorder

- Cardiovascular
  - Hypertension
  - Kidney dysfunction
  - Hyperlipidemia
  - Insulin resistance
  - Obesity

- Bone health

- Chronic disease state
  - Growth
  - Psychological
  - Social
  - Economic
  - Quality of life

The Achilles heel of liver transplantation remains compliance, especially in the adolescent patients, and is closely linked to quality-of-life measures.[8–10] Low executive functions and quality-of-life markers were found in liver transplant recipients, similar to those seen in other chronic disease conditions. These factors make transitioning to adult care challenging.[11–13] Finally, long-term insurance hurdles remain forbidding in the United States and account also for major compliance breaks in the care of recipients reaching young adulthood.

IMPROVING LIVER TRANSPLANT OUTCOMES

Liver transplantation is coming of age. It is a life-saving treatment offered to a growing number of patients with end-stage liver disease. Its success is highlighted by a growing number of survivors that are currently presenting new challenges to our

---

Box 5
Next steps in improving liver transplantation care

- Improved donor selection

- Improved recipient selection

- Critical event analysis for ongoing improvements

- Sharing data with other transplant centers

- Technical improvements

- Improved immunosuppression: "tailored immunosuppression"

- Achieve tolerance

- Improved organ availability to allow better/earlier access to transplant improving transplant benefit

- Improved infectious prophylaxis and treatment

- Pre-emptive assessment of and palliation to psychosocial and economic issues

- Improved access to care—social policies and advocacy

community. These include but are not limited to long-term complications, recurrent disease, compliance, and quality-of-life issues. It is imperative that we continue to improve on perioperative and long-term care. This improvement is done through innovation and research. Inclusion and involvement of the primary team, family, and society in the care of those patients is crucial for the success of what is clearly a treatment that "takes a village" (**Box 5**).

Indeed, what started as a heroic medical act has now become a successful complex care that merits everyone's consideration and its place in the treatment of rare pediatric liver disorders.

REFERENCES

1. Kim WR, Lake JR, Smith JM, et al. OPTN/SRTR 2015 annual data report: liver. Am J Transplant 2017;17(Suppl 1):174–251.
2. Squires RH, Ng V, Romero R, et al, American Association for the Study of Liver Diseases, American Society of Transplantation, North American Society for Pediatric Gastroenterology, Hepatology, and Nutrition. Evaluation of the pediatric patient for liver transplantation: 2014 practice guideline by the American Association for the Study of Liver Diseases, American Society of Transplantation and the North American Society for Pediatric Gastroenterology, Hepatology, and Nutrition. J Pediatr Gastroenterol Nutr 2014;59(1):112–31.
3. Yazigi NA. Long term outcomes after pediatric liver transplantation [review]. Pediatr Gastroenterol Hepatol Nutr 2013;16(4):207–18.
4. Campbell KM, Yazigi N, Ryckman FC, et al. High prevalence of renal dysfunction in long-term survivors after pediatric liver transplantation. J Pediatr 2006;148(4): 475–80.
5. Ng VL, Alonso EM, Bucuvalas JC, et al. Studies of Pediatric Liver Transplantation (SPLIT) Research Group. Health status of children alive 10 years after pediatric liver transplantation performed in the US and Canada: report of the studies of pediatric liver transplantation experience. J Pediatr 2012;160(5):820–6.e3.
6. Ng VL, Fecteau A, Shepherd R, et al, Studies of Pediatric Liver Transplantation Research Group. Outcomes of 5-year survivors of pediatric liver transplantation: report on 461 children from a north american multicenter registry. Pediatrics 2008;122(6):e1128–35.
7. Kelly D, Verkade HJ, Rajanayagam J, et al. Late graft hepatitis and fibrosis in pediatric liver allograft recipients: Current concepts and future developments [review]. Liver Transpl 2016;22(11):1593–602 [Erratum appears in Liver Transpl 2017;23(2):270].
8. Sorensen LG, Neighbors K, Martz K, et al, Studies of Pediatric Liver Transplantation (SPLIT) Research Group and the Functional Outcomes Group (FOG). Longitudinal study of cognitive and academic outcomes after pediatric liver transplantation. J Pediatr 2014;165(1):65–72.e2.
9. Konidis SV, Hrycko A, Nightingale S, et al. Health-related quality of life in long-term survivors of paediatric liver transplantation. Paediatr Child Health 2015; 20(4):189–94.
10. Parmar A, Vandriel SM, Ng VL. Health related quality of life after pediatric liver transplantation: a systematic review [review]. Liver Transpl 2016. [Epub ahead of print].
11. Foster BJ, Dahhou M, Zhang X, et al. High risk of liver allograft failure during late adolescence and young adulthood. Transplantation 2016;100(3):577–84.

12. Wright J, Elwell L, McDonagh JE, et al. Parents in transition: experiences of parents of young people with a liver transplant transferring to adult services. Pediatr Transplant 2017;21(1).

13. Fredericks EM, Magee JC, Eder SJ, et al. Quality improvement targeting adherence during the transition from a pediatric to adult liver transplant clinic. J Clin Psychol Med Settings 2015;22(2–3):150–9.

Pancreatic Disorders

Aliye Uc, MD[a],*, Douglas S. Fishman, MD[b]

KEYWORDS

- Acute pancreatitis • Acute recurrent pancreatitis • Chronic pancreatitis
- Pancreatic insufficiency • Diabetes

KEY POINTS

- Once considered rare, pancreatic diseases, specifically acute, acute recurrent, and chronic pancreatitis, are increasingly recognized in children.
- Etiologies and risk factors of adult and pediatric pancreatitis are very different; therefore it is expected that their management, natural history, and response to therapy would also be different; however, studies on pediatric pancreatitis are limited.
- Genetic risk factors seem to play a role in the progression from acute recurrent to chronic pancreatitis; disease burden is high in chronic pancreatitis.
- Cystic fibrosis is the most common cause of exocrine pancreatic insufficiency in children; chronic pancreatitis and Shwachman Diamond syndrome are second most common.
- There is an urgent need for an exocrine pancreatic function that would be simple to perform, accurate, reliable, reproducible, and noninvasive.

Pediatric pancreatic diseases are increasingly recognized in childhood, possibly because of increased awareness among physicians.[1] Acute pancreatitis (AP) is estimated to occur at an incidence approaching that of adults. Although AP resolves without complications in most children, a subset continues to have recurrent attacks of pancreatitis (acute recurrent pancreatitis or ARP), and some progress to chronic pancreatitis (CP). In contrast to the adult population, most children with ARP or CP have genetic mutations; environmental risk factors are rare. Disease burden is significant in CP. Cystic fibrosis (CF) is the most common cause of exocrine pancreatic insufficiency (EPI) in childhood, followed by Shwachman-Diamond syndrome (SDS) and CP. Long-term effects of pancreatic diseases in children include possible nutritional deficiencies, pancreatogenic diabetes, and potentially pancreatic cancer later in life.

Disclosure Statement: None.
Funded by: NIH. Grant number(s): DK096327; DK097820; DK108334.
[a] Division of Pediatric Gastroenterology, Stead Family Department of Pediatrics, University of Iowa Carver College of Medicine, BT 1120-C, 200 Hawkins Drive, Iowa City, IA 52242, USA;
[b] Section of Pediatric Gastroenterology, Hepatology, and Nutrition, Texas Children's Hospital, Baylor College of Medicine, 6701 Fannin Street, Clinical Care Tower, 1010, Houston, TX 77030, USA
* Corresponding author.
E-mail address: aliye-uc@uiowa.edu

ACUTE PANCREATITIS
Risk Factors/Etiologies

Recent studies estimate the incidence of AP at between 3.6 and 13.2 cases per 100,000 children per year,[1] which is similar to incidences reported in adults.[2] **Box 1** lists etiologies of AP in children.

There are unique differences between risk factors of adult and pediatric AP.[3–17] In adults, alcohol use and gallstones account for the majority of cases, while etiologies in children are broad and variable. Biliary/obstructive factors, systemic illness, and medications are commonly identified in childhood AP; 15% to 30% cases are idiopathic. AP triggered by genetic mutations, metabolic factors, trauma, or alcohol is uncommon in children. In infants and toddlers, systemic illness is the leading cause.[3]

Pathophysiology

Pancreatitis may occur in the setting of an inciting factor (eg, medication, obstruction, genetic mutation) that triggers a cascade of events. There are several competing mechanisms of pancreatic inflammation including

The traditional trypsin-dependent theory (activation of the enzymes leading to destruction of pancreas)[18]
Inflammatory pathways (supported by animal models lacking trypsinogen and still developing inflammation)[19]
Endoplasmic reticulum stress (independent of trypsin activation)[20]

Models that mimic human disease are needed to better dissect the mechanisms of pancreatic inflammation.

Clinical Manifestations

The most common symptoms of AP are abdominal pain and vomiting. Young children may present with vague symptoms and/or irritability; thus diagnosis in this age group requires a high degree of suspicion.[3] Signs and symptoms of cholangitis may be present in gallstone pancreatitis, but mild jaundice and liver enzyme elevations may occur in nonbiliary pancreatitis due to significant inflammatory changes in the distal bile duct as it traverses through the head of the pancreas.

Diagnosis

AP is a clinical diagnosis based on a combination of history, physical examination, laboratory testing, and imaging findings as listed in **Table 1**.[21]

Laboratory findings

Amylase and lipase are the most commonly used biochemical markers of pancreatic inflammation. Amylase and lipase elevations are not specific for AP, but lipase appears to be a more sensitive marker for pancreatitis. In the absence of a known etiology or family history, liver indices (aminotransferases, conjugated and unconjugated bilirubin and GGT), along with fasting glucose, triglycerides, and calcium are recommended laboratory studies for the first episode of AP.

Imaging findings

Imaging may be done to confirm AP and/or its complications, assessing pancreatic parenchyma and the surrounding organs and vasculature. Imaging may include transabdominal ultrasound (TUS), contrast-enhanced computed tomography (CECT), MRI of the abdomen including magnetic resonance cholangiopancreatography (MRCP), and endoscopic ultrasound (EUS).

Box 1
Etiologies of pediatric acute pancreatitis

Biliary/obstructive factors (10%–30%)

Gallstones/biliary sludge

Choledocholithiasis

Choledochal cyst

Ampullary obstruction

Pancreas divisum

Anomalous biliopancreatic junction (union)

Annular pancreas

Systemic diseases/inflammation/infection (10%–50%)

Shock/hypoperfusion state

Inflammatory bowel disease

Hemolytic–uremic syndrome

Henoch-Schonlein purpura

Inflammatory bowel disease

Kawasaki disease

Malnutrition/anorexia nervosa

Primary sclerosing cholangitis

Sickle cell disease

Autoimmune pancreatitis

Sepsis/bacteremia

Bacterial infections
  Campylobacter jejuni
  Mycoplasma
  Staphylococcus aureus

Viral infections
  Adenovirus
  Coxsackie
  Cytomegalovirus
  Epstein-Barr virus
  Echovirus
  Human immunodeficiency syndrome
  Mumps
  Herpes simplex virus

Medications (5%–25%)

Valproic acid

6-mercaptopurine/azathioprine

L-asparaginase

Mesalamine

Trimethoprim/sulfamethoxazole

Furosemide

Tacrolimus

Steroids

Trauma (10%–20%)

Blunt abdominal trauma/child abuse

Duodenal hematoma

Post-ERCP pancreatitis

Metabolic diseases (5%–10%)

Diabetes mellitus/diabetic ketoacidosis

Hypertriglyceridemia

Glycogen storage disease

Organic acidemia (eg, methylmalonic acidemia)

Hypercalcemia

Idiopathic (15%–30%)

Genetic mutations (rare)
  PRSS1
  CFTR
  SPINK1
  CTRC
  CPA1
  CEL
  CEL-HYB

Malignancy (rare)
  Lymphoma
  Neuroblastoma

Abbreviations: CEL, carboxylesterlipase; CEL-HYB, CEL-Hybrid; CFTR, cystic fibrosis transmembrane generator; CPA1, carboxypeptidase 1; CTRC, chymotrypsin-C; PRSS1, cationic trypsinogen; SPINK1, serine protease inhibitor Kazal type I.
  Data from Refs.[3–17,88]

In children, TUS is the first-line study based on its diagnostic yield and safety profile.[22] In AP, the pancreas may appear normal on TUS, or difficult to visualize because of intestinal air; echogenicity may be variable. The advantages of TUS are its lower cost compared with other modalities, no need for sedation, and no ionizing radiation. TUS is useful for identifying biliary tract disease, including gallstones, choledochal cyst, common bile duct stones, or biliary tract dilation. TUS can also identify acute fluid collections, peripancreatic inflammation, and masses. The use of Doppler may delineate splenic vein thrombosis or other vascular changes.

Cross-sectional imaging such as CECT and MRI have a limited role in AP.[23] CECT can provide high-resolution images and assess pancreatic parenchyma, peripancreatic tissues, and nearby vessels and organs, but it is not effective in assessing nondilated pancreatic ducts. CECT is routine in adult patients with pancreatitis, but because of risks of ionizing radiation, it is not routinely performed in pediatrics.[24,25] Of note, recent adult guidelines recommend deferring CECT and/or MRI for the first 48 to 72 hours unless the diagnosis is in question or in those who fail to demonstrate clinical improvement.[26]

MRI/MRCP is not typically ordered for AP. The 2 most common scenarios in which MRI, specifically MRCP, is useful in children are (1) young children with pancreatitis to identify significant pancreatic anomalies[27] and (2) patients with gallstone pancreatitis with inconsistent laboratory and ultrasound findings.[28] The most significant risk–benefit assessment for pediatric patients in using MRI is the possible need for

Table 1	
Definitions of pancreatitis in children (INSPPIRE criteria)	
	Clinical Definition
AP	Requires at least 2 out of 3 criteria: 1. Abdominal pain suggestive of, or compatible with AP 2. Serum amylase and/or lipase activity at least 3 times greater than the upper limit of normal 3. Imaging findings characteristic of, or compatible with AP
ARP	Requires at least 2 distinct episodes of AP, plus: • Complete resolution of pain ($\geq$1 mo pain-free interval between the diagnoses of AP). Or • Complete normalization of amylase and lipase in between episodes.
CP	Requires at least 1 of the following 3: 1. Abdominal pain consistent with pancreatic origin and imaging findings suggestive of chronic pancreatic damage[a] 2. Evidence of exocrine pancreatic insufficiency and suggestive pancreatic imaging findings[a] 3. Evidence of endocrine pancreatic insufficiency and suggestive pancreatic imaging findings[a]

Ductal changes: irregular contour of the main pancreatic duct or its radicles; intraductal filling defects; calculi, stricture or dilation; Parenchymal changes: generalized or focal enlargement, irregular contour (accentuated lobular architecture), cavities, calcifications, heterogeneous echotexture.

[a] "Suggestive" imaging findings of CP include.

From Morinville VD, Husain SZ, Bai H, et al. Definitions of pediatric pancreatitis and survey of present clinical practices. J Pediatr Gastroenterol Nutr 2012;55:261–5.

sedation/anesthesia for completion of the study. MRCP does not require contrast, but gadolinium and related magnetic resonance contrast agents should be used with caution in those with renal impairment or allergy to the agents.

Complications

In general, AP has a mild course in childhood and resolves without significant complications. When complications occur, they can be local or systemic. Local complications include acute peripancreatic fluid collection, pancreatic pseudocyst (**Fig. 1**), acute necrotic collection, and walled-off necrosis (**Table 2**). They should be suspected when there is persistence or recurrence of abdominal pain, secondary increases in pancreatic enzymes, organ dysfunction, or signs and symptoms of sepsis, such as fever and leukocytosis.[29] Other local complications are poor gastric motility, splenic and portal vein thrombosis, and colonic necrosis. Systemic complications include organ failure, most commonly respiratory, cardiovascular, and renal. The 2012 Atlanta classification grades AP severity as mild, moderately severe, or severe (**Box 2, Fig. 2**).[29]

The scoring systems to assess the severity of pancreatitis in adults (Ranson, Glasgow, modified Glasgow, Bedside Index of Severity in Acute Pancreatitis [BISAP], and Acute Physiology and Chronic Health Evaluation [APACHE], II) cannot be easily applicable to children. The DeBanto scoring system was the first system to assess severity in a pediatric cohort.[30] A more recent scoring system proposes using lipase, albumin, and white blood cell count (WBC) obtained within 24 hours of admission to predict severity.[31] Developing a severity score in pediatrics is challenging, as severe complications are uncommon, and death is very rare.

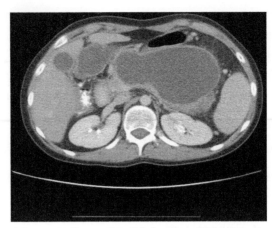

Fig. 1. CT scan showing pancreatic pseudocyst following a PEG-asparaginase induced AP in a child.

Management

The most important component in the management of AP is fluid therapy (**Fig. 3**). Fluid resuscitation is thought to maintain pancreatic microcirculation and prevent major complications, such as necrosis and organ failure. Lactated ringer has been shown to reduce systemic inflammation and thus prevent complications in adults with AP compared to saline.[32] Early and aggressive fluid resuscitation in children with normal saline and 5% dextrose is safe and well-tolerated, but has not been compared with other fluids.[33] The rates of intravenous fluid in pediatric AP have also not been assessed. One study showed that a combination of early enteral nutrition (<48 hours) and aggressive fluid management (>1.5–2× maintenance within the first 24 hours) decreased length of stay and complications.[33]

In both children and adults, the initial nutritional management of AP remains controversial. The American College of Gastroenterology recommends oral feedings for mild AP when patients' symptoms are significantly improved, and feeding with a low-fat solid diet appears as safe as a clear liquid diet.[26] Overall, it is agreed that children with mild-to-moderate disease require minimal to no additional nutritional support; enteral nutrition is preferred over parenteral nutrition, and nutritional support should begin within 48 to 72 hours.[34] For patients with severe AP, enteral nutrition is recommended to prevent infectious complications, decrease inflammatory response, reduce mortality, and improve outcome. Early enteral nutrition appears to be safe in children,[33] but more studies are needed.

Pain is managed with opioids, specifically intravenous morphine initially. Despite earlier concerns about Sphincter of Oddi dysregulation with morphine, there is no clinical evidence to support this theory.[35] Once tolerating oral feedings, patients may transition to oral acetaminophen or nonsteroidal anti-inflammatory drugs (NSAIDs) alone or combined with an opioid.

Endoscopic procedures for AP are limited to EUS and ERCP. ERCP is recommended in gallstone pancreatitis with choledocholithiasis, cholangitis, or in those with concern for biliary obstruction.[36,37] In adults with gallstone pancreatitis, EUS and MRCP are preferred in those without jaundice or cholangitis; however, this has not been formally

Table 2
Morphologic classification of acute pancreatitis

Morphologic Type	Definition	Contrast Enhanced CT Findings
IEP	Acute inflammation of the pancreatic parenchyma and peripancreatic tissues without recognizable tissue necrosis	• Pancreatic parenchyma enhanced by intravenous contrast • No peripancreatic necrosis
Necrotizing Pancreatitis	Inflammation associated with pancreatic parenchymal necrosis and/or peripancreatic necrosis	• Pancreatic parenchyma not enhanced by intravenous contrast and/or • Presence of peripancreatic necrosis (ANC and WON)
Acute Peripancreatic Fluid Collection (APFC)	• Peripancreatic fluid associated with interstitial edematous pancreatitis with no associated peripancreatic necrosis. • Only applies to fluid seen within the first 4 wk and without features of a pseudocyst	• Occurs in the setting of IEP • Homogenous collection with fluid density, no nonliquid component • Confined by normal peripancreatic fascial planes • No definable wall encapsulating the collection • Adjacent to pancreas (without intrapancreatic extension)
Pancreatic pseudocyst (**Fig. 1**)	• An encapsulated collection of fluid with a well-defined inflammatory wall • Usually outside the pancreas with minimal or no necrosis.	• Occurs after IEP • Homogenous fluid density • No nonliquid component • Well defined wall (completely encapsulated) • Usually >4 wk after onset of AP
Acute Necrotic Collection	• Collection containing variable amounts of both fluid and necrotic material • Associated with necrotizing pancreatitis • Involves pancreatic parenchyma or peripancreatic tissues • Rare in children	• Occurs only with acute necrotizing pancreatitis • Heterogeneous and nonliquid density of varying degrees in different locations • No definable wall encapsulating the collection • Intrapancreatic and/or extrapancreatic
Walled-Off Necrosis (WON)	• Mature encapsulated collection of pancreatic and/or peripancreatic necrosis • Usually occurs >4 wk after onset of necrotizing pancreatitis • Rare in children	• Heterogeneous with liquid and nonliquid density, varying degrees of loculations • Well-defined wall, completely encapsulated • Intrapancreatic and/or extrapancreatic

Adapted from Banks PA, Bollen TL, Dervenis C, et al. Classification of acute pancreatitis—2012: revision of the Atlanta classification and definitions by international consensus. Gut 2013;62:102–11.

studied in children. EUS drainage via endoscopic cystgastrostomy has become the standard modality for drainage of pancreatic pseudocysts and pancreatic necrosis in adults and children.[38] Surgery for AP is infrequently performed, and typically for pseudocyst drainage, debridement of necrosis or cholecystectomy. Recent studies show that early cholecystectomy after mild biliary pancreatitis is safe in children and reduces readmissions.[39–41]

> **Box 2**
> **Grades of pancreatitis severity**
>
> *Mild AP*
>
> No organ failure
>
> No local or systemic complications
>
> *Moderately severe AP*
>
> Organ failure that resolves within 48 hours (transient)
>
> Local or systemic complications without persistent organ failure
>
> *Severe AP*
>
> Persistent organ failure more than 48 hours (either single or multiple organ failure)
>
> *Adapted from* Banks PA, Bollen TL, Dervenis C, et al. Classification of acute pancreatitis—2012: revision of the Atlanta classification and definitions by international consensus. Gut 2013;62:102–11.

ACUTE RECURRENT AND CHRONIC PANCREATITIS
Risk Factors/Etiologies

A subset of children with AP (15%–35%) develops recurrent episodes of AP and may progress to CP.[21] Definitions of ARP and CP are listed in **Table 1**. Because ARP and CP are rare, large cohorts and multicenter studies are needed to characterize these diseases.[42] Conditions that predispose children to ARP then CP are listed in **Box 3**; genetic risks are the most common. In the large multicenter INSPPIRE (INternational Study Group of Pediatric Pancreatitis: In search for a cuRE) cohort, approximately 50% of children with ARP and approximately 75% of children with CP had genetic mutations in the cationic trypsinogen (PRSS1), CF transmembrane generator (CFTR), serine protease inhibitor Kazal type I (SPINK1), chymotrypsin-C (CTRC); PRSS1, SPINK1 mutations were more common in CP.[43,44] Moreover, carboxypeptidase 1 (CPA1) mutations were associated with early onset CP.[45] The genetic variants in the carboxylesterlipase (CEL) and CEL-Hybrid[46,47] increase the risk for CP in adults.

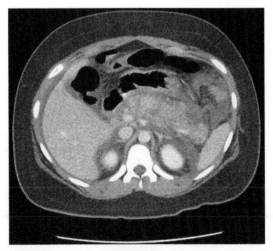

Fig. 2. CT scan in moderately severe pancreatitis in a teenager with gallstone pancreatitis. Pancreatic and peripancreatic inflammatory changes are seen.

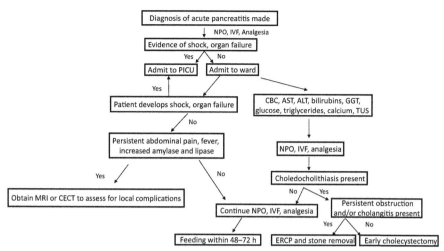

Fig. 3. Algorithm for management of AP and complications.

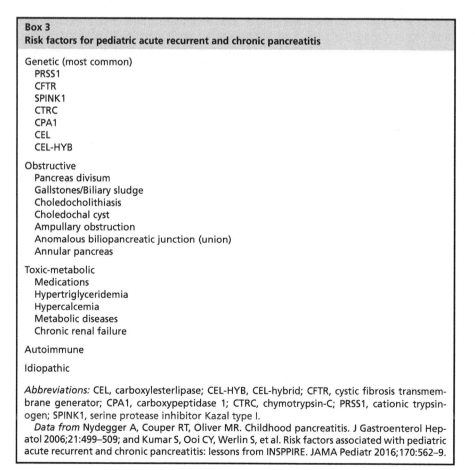

Box 3
Risk factors for pediatric acute recurrent and chronic pancreatitis

Genetic (most common)
    PRSS1
    CFTR
    SPINK1
    CTRC
    CPA1
    CEL
    CEL-HYB

Obstructive
    Pancreas divisum
    Gallstones/Biliary sludge
    Choledocholithiasis
    Choledochal cyst
    Ampullary obstruction
    Anomalous biliopancreatic junction (union)
    Annular pancreas

Toxic-metabolic
    Medications
    Hypertriglyceridemia
    Hypercalcemia
    Metabolic diseases
    Chronic renal failure

Autoimmune

Idiopathic

Abbreviations: CEL, carboxylesterlipase; CEL-HYB, CEL-hybrid; CFTR, cystic fibrosis transmembrane generator; CPA1, carboxypeptidase 1; CTRC, chymotrypsin-C; PRSS1, cationic trypsinogen; SPINK1, serine protease inhibitor Kazal type I.
Data from Nydegger A, Couper RT, Oliver MR. Childhood pancreatitis. J Gastroenterol Hepatol 2006;21:499–509; and Kumar S, Ooi CY, Werlin S, et al. Risk factors associated with pediatric acute recurrent and chronic pancreatitis: lessons from INSPPIRE. JAMA Pediatr 2016;170:562–9.

Environmental risk factors (ie, medications, alcohol, smoking, chronic renal failure, and hypercalcemia) are uncommon in pediatric ARP or CP (<10%).[43] It is not known whether obstructive factors and specifically pancreas divisum are sufficient to cause ARP or CP in children. Autoimmune pancreatitis (AIP) is rare in the pediatric population.

Clinical Manifestations

Children with ARP suffer from recurrent attacks of AP, but are in normal health in between episodes. Children with CP suffer from pain that ranges from mild to severe, episodic to constant.[43] Need for pain medications, disease burden (emergency department visits, hospitalizations, missed school days, medical, endoscopic, and surgical interventions) and health care cost were much higher in CP compared with ARP in the INSPPIRE cohort.[44,48]

Over time, children with CP can develop EPI and pancreatogenic diabetes mellitus (T3cDM). Diabetes occurs in approximately 5% of patients with hereditary pancreatitis by 10 years after the onset of symptoms, and 18% by 20 years.[49] Although the mechanism of this diabetes is unknown, partial or complete insulin deficiency is observed. In the INSPPIRE cohort, 1% of children already had diabetes at the time of enrollment.[43]

Diagnosis

The guidelines for causal evaluation of ARP and CP were recently published by the INSPPIRE group.[50] The diagnosis of ARP and CP requires a careful past medical and family history, inquiry of past pancreatitis attacks, abdominal pain, hospitalizations, emergency room visits, and possible complications of AP. Family history for AP, ARP and CP, pancreatic cancer, and diabetes have to be explored (**Box 4**). Testing for autoimmune pancreatitis may not be straightforward, as most children have type 2 disease and typically normal serum immunoglobulin (Ig)G4.

Box 4
Diagnostic approach to pediatric acute recurrent and chronic pancreatitis

History

- Past and current medical history (recurrent abdominal pain, emergency room visits, hospitalizations, medications)
- Family history of pancreatitis, pancreatic cancer, gallbladder disease

Biochemistry

- AST, ALT, GGT, total and direct bilirubin, serum triglycerides, calcium, tissue transglutaminase
- Consider: stool ova and parasites, serum aminoacids and urine organic acids, esophagogastroduodenoscopy, and colonoscopy in select cases

Genetic testing

- PRSS1, CFTR, SPINK1, CTRC, CPA1, CEL, CEL-HYB

Imaging

- TUS, MRI/MRCP

Other tests

- Sweat Cl, nasal potential difference (if available)

Abbreviations: CEL, carboxylesterlipase; CEL-HYB, CEL-Hybrid; CFTR, cystic fibrosis transmembrane generator; CPA1, carboxypeptidase 1; CTRC, chymotrypsin-C; PRSS1, cationic trypsinogen; SPINK1, serine protease inhibitor Kazal type I.

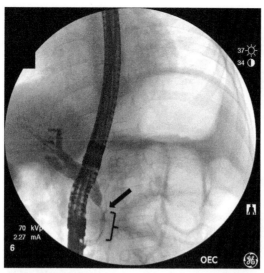

Fig. 4. ECRP study in a 5-year-old child showing anomalous biliopancreatic union. The bracket demonstrates the common channel greater than 1.5 cm, and the black arrow denotes the branch point of the pancreatic duct.

Imaging studies play an important role in the work-up to evaluate obstructive risk factors and explore the presence of AP/CP (**Figs. 4** and **5**). TUS is the first imaging test of choice, but it may not clearly delineate the pancreas anatomy. CT can detect advanced changes in CP, including calcifications, pancreas atrophy, and fat replacement, but it has poor sensitivity to identify ductal abnormalities and subtle parenchymal changes. MRI/MRCP can reliably detect pancreas atrophy, ductal dilatations, small filling defects, strictures, irregularities of the main pancreatic duct, and irregularity of side branches,[51] and it has become the diagnostic imaging method of choice in children.[52] Secretin may increase the detectability of the normally small pancreatic ducts on MRCP.[53] EUS can assist with the diagnosis in ARP and CP, specifically in microlithiasis and pancreatic anomalies (eg, pancreas divisum). However, specific criteria (Rosemont and Cambridge) available for EUS descriptions of CP in adults[54] have not been validated in children. Finally, ERCP should be reserved for therapeutic purposes.

Management

Medical

In the INSPPIRE cohort, approximately 80% of children with ARP or CP reported pain within the previous year that was of variable frequency and severity; one-third of children with CP were using narcotic analgesics.[43,44] Pediatric experience is limited for the treatment of pain in ARP/CP. Because of increased greater understanding about pain mechanisms in pancreatitis as well as the significant burden of addiction, there has been a significant emphasis on opioid-free therapies, such as GABA-analogues (eg, gabapentin and pregabalin).[55] Pediatric studies are needed to study the efficacy and safety of these medications in children. There are no data to support the benefit of antioxidant preparations or pancreatic enzyme supplementation in pediatric ARP/CP. There are also limited data on calorie/energy requirements, nutritional needs, and macronutrient and micronutrient deficiencies in children with ARP or CP.

Endoscopic

ERCP is reserved as therapeutic modality for ARP or CP. ERCP can also provide short-term symptom relief in pediatric patients.[56–58] Sphincterotomy, stent

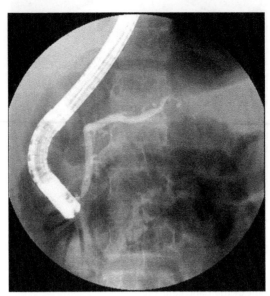

Fig. 5. ERCP study in a child showing dilated ventral pancreatic duct, along with secondary and tertiary side branch dilation.

placement, and stone removal are the most common therapies. Overall, ERCP is safe in children, but risk of anesthesia/sedation, post-ERCP pancreatitis, and ionizing radiation should be considered. Extracorporeal shock wave lithotripsy has been used in pediatric patients with large pancreatic duct stones,[57] but it is not available in most centers.

Surgical

Surgery for CP involves drainage procedures and partial or total resections. Surgical drainage procedures typically require the presence of a dilated pancreatic duct greater than 5 to 6 mm. In the majority of cases, a Puestow-type procedure (longitudinal pancreatojejunostomy that involves opening the pancreatic duct throughout the body and tail of the gland) is used. Drainage procedures are discouraged if the patient will undergo total pancreatectomy and islet autotransplantation (TPIAT) in the future, since they adversely affect the islet yield from the pancreas.[59,60]

TPIAT is increasingly performed in specialized centers for pediatric ARP/CP intractable to other therapies. Within a year of this operation, 50% to 80% of patients became narcotic independent on follow-up.[60–65] The pain improvement was largely sustained at 10-year follow-up, whereby 10% to 20% of patients continued to take narcotics.[61,64] Similarly, insulin independence was also sustained over the 10-year follow-up in the majority of children (∼40%).[61] Both children and adults demonstrated significant improvement in physical and mental health after TPIAT.[60,63,64,66] Prospective studies are needed to study the long-term effects of TPIAT in children.

EXOCRINE PANCREATIC INSUFFICIENCY

The pancreas is a resilient organ. Clinically significant EPI causing steatorrhea develops only after a large portion of pancreatic acini (>90%) is permanently damaged. The causes of EPI in childhood are listed in **Box 5**.

| **Box 5** |
| **Etiologies of exocrine pancreatic insufficiency in childhood** |
| CF (most common) |
| CP |
| SDS |
| Johanson-Blizzard syndrome |
| Pearson syndrome |
| Jeune syndrome |
| Pancreatic aplasia |
| Pancreatic hypoplasia |
| Isolated enzyme deficiencies |

Cystic Fibrosis

CF is by far the most common cause of EPI in childhood. Caused by mutations in the CF transmembrane regulator protein (CFTR), pancreas involvement begins in utero in children with CF and progresses into childhood. CFTR is typically expressed in pancreatic duct epithelia and controls anion secretion into the lumen. Loss of CFTR function impairs fluid and anion secretion, which then leads to acidic luminal contents, plugging of ducts, and eventual destruction of the pancreas. The type of CFTR mutations greatly influences the degree of exocrine pancreatic involvement; 85% are pancreatic insufficient and depend on pancreatic enzymes to maintain adequate growth and nutrition, while 15% are pancreatic sufficient. Pancreatic status is directly linked to genotype.[30] Patients with homozygous or compound heterozygous mutations that belong to class I-III or VI mutations that severely alter CFTR function suffer from EPI, versus patients with class IV or V mutations who are usually pancreatic sufficient.[67,68] Pancreas-sufficient patients are prone to recurrent attacks of pancreatitis and may eventually become pancreatic insufficient.[69] In a rare instance, pancreatitis may be the first manifestation of CF. Ooi and colleagues estimated the risk of EPI and pancreatitis for the most common CF-causing mutations by using pancreatic insufficiency prevalence (PIP) score. The score is higher for the severe mutations and lower for mild mutations.[70]

Shwachman-Diamond Syndrome

SDS is a rare autosomal-recessive disorder characterized by congenital anomalies, EPI, bone marrow defects, and short stature.[71] Ninety percent of children with SDS have mutations in the Shwachman-Bodian-Diamond Syndrome (SBDS) gene located on chromosome 7q11. In contrast to CF, pancreatic ductal function is normal in SDS.

The presentation of SDS may be variable. Neutropenia is the most common hematologic abnormality at presentation ($\sim$80%), but it may be intermittent or develop over time.[71] Two-thirds of patients present with failure to thrive; only 50% describe diarrhea. Pancreatic lipomatosis is not universal; low fecal elastase levels may be present in approximately 80% of patients at presentation. Skeletal abnormalities are the most common congenital abnormality, reported in approximately one-third of patients.[72] Various congenital anomalies involving the cardiac, gastrointestinal, renal, neurologic, urologic, and other systems have been reported. Over time, patients are prone to developing myelodysplasia and leukemia. Poor growth does not usually improve despite adequate pancreatic replacement therapy. EPI is often transient, and steator-rhea may spontaneously improve over time. Recurrent infections are common and a frequent cause of death.

Diagnosis of SDS is often made clinically by documenting the presence of EPI and hematologic abnormalities, excluding other causes of EPI and bone marrow failure. Consensus guidelines have been developed to facilitate early diagnosis and therapy.[73]

Chronic Pancreatitis

Exocrine pancreatic insufficiency develops in 50% to 80% of adults after a diagnosis of 5.6 to 13.1 years.[74,75] The exact prevalence of EPI in pediatric CP is unknown, but 34% of children with CP in the INSPPIRE cohort were exocrine pancreatic insufficient at the time of enrollment.[43] Typically, the diagnosis of CP is made prior to the diagnosis of EPI. Interestingly, in a Norwegian family, EPI was diagnosed after the diagnosis of maturity-onset diabetes of the young (MODY) and discovery of CEL mutations.[76]

Johanson-Blizzard Syndrome

This rare autosomal-recessive disorder is caused by mutations in ubiquitin ligase (UBR1) gene that lead to destruction of pancreatic acini in utero.[77] Pancreatic ductal function is unaffected. Patients usually present with EPI, multiple congenital anomalies, hypothyroidism, and developmental delay. Diabetes may develop over time. In contrast to SDS, children with Johanson-Blizzard syndrome do not have bone marrow and skeletal abnormalities. Milder phenotypes have been described; thus the absence of multiple congenital anomalies or mental retardation does not rule out this syndrome.[78,79]

Pearson Syndrome

This is a rare multisystem disorder caused by defects in the oxidative phosphorylation due to sporadic mutations in the mitochondrial DNA.[80] Patients typically present in infancy with severe, transfusion-dependent, hypoplastic macrocytic anemia; variable degree of neutropenia and thrombocytopenia; and normal or reduced bone marrow cellularity with vacuolated precursors. Other features are exocrine and endocrine pancreas dysfunction, hyperlipidemia, liver steatosis, proximal renal tubular insufficiency, metabolic acidosis, and failure to thrive. Pearson Syndrome is distinguished from SDS by the presence of sideroblastic anemia, bone marrow changes, pancreatic fibrosis rather than lipomatosis, and absence of bone lesions. Diagnosis is confirmed by Southern blot analysis that detects mtDNA rearrangements. There is no specific treatment available, and patients usually succumb to death in infancy or early childhood because of metabolic disorders and/or infections.

Other Causes

Jeune syndrome, pancreatic aplasia, pancreatic hypoplasia, and isolated pancreatic enzyme deficiencies (pancreatic lipase deficiency or PNLIP) are rare causes of EPI in childhood.

Clinical manifestations

EPI presents primarily as fat malabsorption defined by a fecal fat greater than 7% of oral fat intake in 3- to 5-day fat balance studies. Fat malabsorption, steatorrhea (bulky, foul-smelling stools), and malnutrition are the hallmarks of EPI. Patients suffer from poor weight gain or weight loss, diarrhea, steatorrhea, bloating, and flatulence. Fat malabsorption can lead to deficiencies of fat-soluble vitamins A, D, E, and K.

Diagnosis

Tests for EPI are classified as direct and indirect tests (**Box 6**). The direct pancreatic function tests (PFTs) involve the stimulation of the pancreas with pancreatic secretagogues followed by collection of duodenal fluid and analysis of its contents for pancreatic enzymes (acinar cell function), and/or fluid volume and electrolytes (ductal cell function). The direct pancreatic function tests are more sensitive and specific than indirect tests, but they are invasive and difficult to perform. Indirect tests are widely available and easier to perform but have low sensitivity and specificity. Although the indirect tests are useful to diagnose EPI, they cannot accurately measure the pancreatic acinar cell reserve and ductal cell function.

Direct tests include

- Secretin-stimulated MRI/MRCP—exocrine pancreas function is studied by changes in pancreatic duct caliber, anteroposterior diameter of the pancreas, signal intensity ratio between pancreas and spleen on T1-weighted, and arterial-venous enhancement ratios and duodenal filling before and after secretin. The study is highly subjective and operator dependent and lacks sensitivity and specificity.[81] This test has not yet been validated in children.
- Dreiling tube method— in this test, pancreatic fluid is collected as it is secreted into the duodenum and measured for volume, pancreatic enzymes and electrolytes before and after stimulation with cholecystokinin and/or secretin.[82] Although it is considered gold standard' to quantify the exocrine pancreatic function, the invasive and complex nature of the test (placement of nasoduodenal catheter, intravenous cannulation, sedation, and radiation exposure) limits its routine clinical use.
- Endocsopic pancreatic function test (ePFT)— the collection of the duodenal fluid via the endoscope[83] is becoming increasingly popular in the pediatric age group. In these tests, duodenal fluid is aspirated during an upper gastrointestinal endoscopy procedure before and after stimulation with a pancreatic secretagogue. ePFT leads to prolonged sedation or anesthesia, and samples are likely to be diluted with gastric fluid. There is a lack of standardization between protocols among the centers about which secretagogues to use and type and frequency of samples to collect. In 1 study, ePFT underestimated the pancreatic secretory capacity and led to erroneous classification of patients as pancreatic insufficient.[82]

Box 6
Tests for exocrine pancreatic insufficiency

Direct tests

- Secretin-stimulated MRI

- Dreiling tube method

- Endoscopic pancreatic function test

Indirect tests

- 72 h fecal fat test

- Fecal elastase

- ^{13}C-mixed triglyceride breath test

Box 7
Pancreatic enzyme therapy for exocrine pancreatic insufficiency

Infants
  2000 to 4000 units per 120 mL of infant formula or per breast feeding

Less than 4 years of age
  1000 lipase units/kg per meal and 500 lipase units/kg per snacks

Greater than 4 years of age.
  500 lipase units/kg per meal and 250 lipase units/kg per snacks

---

Indirect tests include

- 72-hour fecal fat test—steatorrhea can be measured by a 72-hour stool collection and calculation of coefficient of fat absorption (CFA: ([grams of fat ingested–grams of fat excreted)/(grams of fat ingested) $\times100$]. In children younger than 6 months of age, a fecal fat greater than 15% of fat intake is considered abnormal; this value is 7% for children over 6 months of age. It is not a specific test for EPI, as it can be abnormal in other diseases causing fat malabsorption. The test is not easy to perform; stool samples may be missed, and dietary documentation may be incomplete.
- Fecal elastase-1 (FE1)— This widely available enzyme-linked immunosorbent assay (ELISA)-based stool test is the preferred method to diagnose EPI.[84] A value of less than100 µg/g is considered diagnostic. The test is only useful to detect severe EPI. Results may be falsely low when the stool is diluted in cases of diarrhea.
- ^{13}C-mixed triglyceride breath test—this test relies on the hydrolysis of ingested triglycerides by pancreatic lipase and measurement of $^{13}CO_2$ released to breath. Numerous factors such as rate of gastric emptying, degree of solubilization by bile acids, mucosal absorption, endogenous CO_2 production, and pulmonary excretion may influence the results. The test is not available in the United States.

Management

Pancreatic enzyme replacement therapy

EPI is managed with exogenous pancreatic enzyme replacement therapy (PERT) (**Box 7, Fig. 6**). Dosing is based on the number of lipase units administered per meal. For children who cannot swallow capsules, delayed-release capsules containing enteric coated microspheres or microtablets may be opened and the contents sprinkled on soft food with low pH (applesauce, gelatins, pureed apricot, banana, or sweet potatoes). Foods with a pH greater than 7.3 (milk, custard, or ice cream) should be avoided as a vehicle for the sprinkled enzymes, because the protective enteric coating can dissolve in these foods, leaving the enzymes vulnerable to inactivation by gastric acid. Pancrealipase tablets or capsules should not be crushed or chewed. Concurrent administration with H_2 antagonists or proton pump inhibitors may enhance enzyme efficacy.

Vitamin Supplementation

Children with EPI are prone to fat malabsorption that may lead to deficiencies of the fat-soluble vitamins A, D, E, and K. Children with CF should receive supplementation of these vitamins, and vitamin levels should be monitored annually.[85–87] There are no guidelines for EPI caused by other diseases.

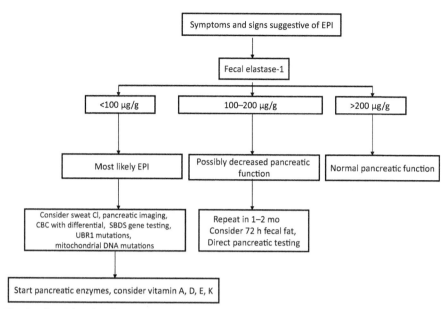

Fig. 6. Algorithm for diagnosis and management of exocrine pancreatic insufficiency.

REFERENCES

1. Nydegger A, Heine RG, Ranuh R, et al. Changing incidence of acute pancreatitis: 10-year experience at the Royal Children's Hospital, Melbourne. J Gastroenterol Hepatol 2007;22:1313–6.

2. Corfield AP, Cooper MJ, Williamson RC. Acute pancreatitis: a lethal disease of increasing incidence. Gut 1985;26:724–9.

3. Kandula L, Lowe ME. Etiology and outcome of acute pancreatitis in infants and toddlers. J Pediatr 2008;152:106–10, 110.

4. Bai HX, Lowe ME, Husain SZ. What have we learned about acute pancreatitis in children? J Pediatr Gastroenterol Nutr 2011;52:262–70.

5. Park A, Latif SU, Shah AU, et al. Changing referral trends of acute pancreatitis in children: a 12-year single-center analysis. J Pediatr Gastroenterol Nutr 2009;49:316–22.

6. Park AJ, Latif SU, Ahmad MU, et al. A comparison of presentation and management trends in acute pancreatitis between infants/toddlers and older children. J Pediatr Gastroenterol Nutr 2010;51:167–70.

7. Lopez MJ. The changing incidence of acute pancreatitis in children: a single-institution perspective. J Pediatr 2002;140:622–4.

8. Werlin SL, Kugathasan S, Frautschy BC. Pancreatitis in children. J Pediatr Gastroenterol Nutr 2003;37:591–5.

9. Sanchez-Ramirez CA, Larrosa-Haro A, Flores-Martinez S, et al. Acute and recurrent pancreatitis in children: etiological factors. Acta Paediatr 2007;96:534–7.

10. Fujishiro J, Masumoto K, Urita Y, et al. Pancreatic complications in pediatric choledochal cysts. J Pediatr Surg 2013;48:1897–902.

11. Nitsche C, Maertin S, Scheiber J, et al. Drug-induced pancreatitis. Curr Gastroenterol Rep 2012;14:131–8.

12. Trivedi CD, Pitchumoni CS. Drug-induced pancreatitis: an update. J Clin Gastroenterol 2005;39:709–16.
13. Spanier BW, Tuynman HA, van der Hulst RW, et al. Acute pancreatitis and concomitant use of pancreatitis-associated drugs. Am J Gastroenterol 2011;106:2183–8.
14. Berney T, Belli D, Bugmann P, et al. Influence of severe underlying pathology and hypovolemic shock on the development of acute pancreatitis in children. J Pediatr Surg 1996;31:1256–61.
15. Bai HX, Ma MH, Orabi AI, et al. Novel characterization of drug-associated pancreatitis in children. J Pediatr Gastroenterol Nutr 2011;53:423–8.
16. Lowe ME, Greer JB. Pancreatitis in children and adolescents. Curr Gastroenterol Rep 2008;10:128–35.
17. Lowe ME. Pancreatitis in childhood. Curr Gastroenterol Rep 2004;6:240–6.
18. Chiari H. Ueber Selbstverdauung des menschlichen Pankreas. Zeitschrift für Heilkunde 1896;17:69–96.
19. Sah RP, Dudeja V, Dawra RK, et al. Cerulein-induced chronic pancreatitis does not require intra-acinar activation of trypsinogen in mice. Gastroenterology 2013;144:1076–85.e2.
20. Szmola R, Sahin-Toth M. Pancreatitis-associated chymotrypsinogen C (CTRC) mutant elicits endoplasmic reticulum stress in pancreatic acinar cells. Gut 2010; 59:365–72.
21. Morinville VD, Husain SZ, Bai H, et al. Definitions of pediatric pancreatitis and survey of present clinical practices. J Pediatr Gastroenterol Nutr 2012;55:261–5.
22. Lin TK, Troendle DM, Wallihan DB, et al. Specialized imaging and procedures in pediatric pancreatology: a NASPGHAN clinical report. J Pediatr Gastroenterol Nutr 2017;64:472–84.
23. Shinagare AB, Ip IK, Raja AS, et al. Use of CT and MRI in emergency department patients with acute pancreatitis. Abdom Imaging 2015;40:272–7.
24. Nydegger A, Couper RT, Oliver MR. Childhood pancreatitis. J Gastroenterol Hepatol 2006;21:499–509.
25. Kinney TP, Freeman ML. Recent advances and novel methods in pancreatic imaging. Minerva Gastroenterol Dietol 2008;54:85–95.
26. Tenner S, Baillie J, DeWitt J, et al. American College of Gastroenterology guideline: management of acute pancreatitis. Am J Gastroenterol 2013;108:1400–15, 1416.
27. Wang DB, Yu J, Fulcher AS, et al. Pancreatitis in patients with pancreas divisum: imaging features at MRI and MRCP. World J Gastroenterol 2013;19:4907–16.
28. Hallal AH, Amortegui JD, Jeroukhimov IM, et al. Magnetic resonance cholangiopancreatography accurately detects common bile duct stones in resolving gallstone pancreatitis. J Am Coll Surg 2005;200:869–75.
29. Banks PA, Bollen TL, Dervenis C, et al. Classification of acute pancreatitis–2012: revision of the Atlanta classification and definitions by international consensus. Gut 2013;62:102–11.
30. Kristidis P, Bozon D, Corey M, et al. Genetic determination of exocrine pancreatic function in cystic fibrosis. Am J Hum Genet 1992;50:1178–84.
31. Szabo FK, Hornung L, Oparaji JA, et al. A prognostic tool to predict severe acute pancreatitis in pediatrics. Pancreatology 2016;16:358–64.
32. Wu BU, Hwang JQ, Gardner TH, et al. Lactated Ringer's solution reduces systemic inflammation compared with saline in patients with acute pancreatitis. Clin Gastroenterol Hepatol 2011;9:710–7.e1.

33. Szabo FK, Fei L, Cruz LA, et al. Early enteral nutrition and aggressive fluid resuscitation are associated with improved clinical outcomes in acute pancreatitis. J Pediatr 2015;167:397–402.e1.

34. Mirtallo JM, Forbes A, McClave SA, et al. International consensus guidelines for nutrition therapy in pancreatitis. JPEN J Parenter Enteral Nutr 2012;36:284–91.

35. Thompson DR. Narcotic analgesic effects on the sphincter of Oddi: a review of the data and therapeutic implications in treating pancreatitis. Am J Gastroenterol 2001;96:1266–72.

36. Troendle DM, Barth BA. ERCP can be safely and effectively performed by a pediatric gastroenterologist for choledocholithiasis in a pediatric facility. J Pediatr Gastroenterol Nutr 2013;57:655–8.

37. Fishman DS, Chumpitazi BP, Raijman I, et al. Endoscopic retrograde cholangiography for pediatric choledocholithiasis: assessing the need for endoscopic intervention. World J Gastrointest Endosc 2016;8:425–32.

38. Jazrawi SF, Barth BA, Sreenarasimhaiah J. Efficacy of endoscopic ultrasound-guided drainage of pancreatic pseudocysts in a pediatric population. Dig Dis Sci 2011;56:902–8.

39. Lin TK, Palermo JJ, Nathan JD, et al. Timing of cholecystectomy in children with biliary pancreatitis. J Pediatr Gastroenterol Nutr 2016;62:118–21.

40. Gurusamy KS, Nagendran M, Davidson BR. Early versus delayed laparoscopic cholecystectomy for acute gallstone pancreatitis. Cochrane Database Syst Rev 2013;(9):CD010326.

41. van Baal MC, Besselink MG, Bakker OJ, et al. Timing of cholecystectomy after mild biliary pancreatitis: a systematic review. Ann Surg 2012;255:860–6.

42. Morinville VD, Lowe ME, Ahuja M, et al. Design and implementation of INSPPIRE (International Study Group of Pediatric Pancreatitis: In Search for a Cure). J Pediatr Gastroenterol Nutr 2014;59(3):360–4.

43. Schwarzenberg SJ, Bellin M, Husain SZ, et al. Pediatric chronic pancreatitis is associated with genetic risk factors and substantial disease burden. J Pediatr 2015;166:890–6.e1.

44. Kumar S, Ooi CY, Werlin S, et al. Risk factors associated with pediatric acute recurrent and chronic pancreatitis: lessons from INSPPIRE. JAMA Pediatr 2016; 170:562–9.

45. Witt H, Beer S, Rosendahl J, et al. Variants in CPA1 are strongly associated with early onset chronic pancreatitis. Nat Genet 2013;45:1216–20.

46. Fjeld K, Weiss FU, Lasher D, et al. A recombined allele of the lipase gene CEL and its pseudogene CELP confers susceptibility to chronic pancreatitis. Nat Genet 2015;47(5):518–22.

47. Ragvin A, Fjeld K, Weiss FU, et al. The number of tandem repeats in the carboxyl-ester lipase (CEL) gene as a risk factor in alcoholic and idiopathic chronic pancreatitis. Pancreatology 2013;13:29–32.

48. Ting J, Wilson L, Schwarzenberg SJ, et al. Direct costs of acute recurrent and chronic pancreatitis in children in the INSPPIRE registry. J Pediatr Gastroenterol Nutr 2016;62:443–9.

49. Howes N, Lerch MM, Greenhalf W, et al. Clinical and genetic characteristics of hereditary pancreatitis in Europe. Clin Gastroenterol Hepatol 2004;2:252–61.

50. Gariepy CE, Heyman MB, Lowe ME, et al. The causal evaluation of acute recurrent and chronic pancreatitis in children: consensus from the INSPPIRE Group. J Pediatr Gastroenterol Nutr 2017;64(1):95–103.

51. Hansen TM, Nilsson M, Gram M, et al. Morphological and functional evaluation of chronic pancreatitis with magnetic resonance imaging. World J Gastroenterol 2013;19:7241–6.

52. Kolodziejczyk E, Jurkiewicz E, Pertkiewicz J, et al. MRCP Versus ERCP in the evaluation of chronic pancreatitis in children: which is the better choice? Pancreas 2016;45:1115–9.

53. Manfredi R, Lucidi V, Gui B, et al. Idiopathic chronic pancreatitis in children: MR cholangiopancreatography after secretin administration. Radiology 2002;224: 675–82.

54. Catalano MF, Sahai A, Levy M, et al. EUS-based criteria for the diagnosis of chronic pancreatitis: the Rosemont classification. Gastrointest Endosc 2009;69: 1251–61.

55. Olesen SS, Bouwense SA, Wilder-Smith OH, et al. Pregabalin reduces pain in patients with chronic pancreatitis in a randomized, controlled trial. Gastroenterology 2011;141:536–43.

56. Troendle DM, Barth BA. Pediatric considerations in endoscopic retrograde cholangiopancreatography. Gastrointest Endosc Clin N Am 2016;26:119–36.

57. Agarwal J, Nageshwar Reddy D, Talukdar R, et al. ERCP in the management of pancreatic diseases in children. Gastrointest Endosc 2014;79:271–8.

58. Oracz G, Pertkiewicz J, Kierkus J, et al. Efficiency of pancreatic duct stenting therapy in children with chronic pancreatitis. Gastrointest Endosc 2014;80:1022–9.

59. Kobayashi T, Manivel JC, Bellin MD, et al. Correlation of pancreatic histopathologic findings and islet yield in children with chronic pancreatitis undergoing total pancreatectomy and islet autotransplantation. Pancreas 2010;39:57–63.

60. Bellin MD, Freeman ML, Schwarzenberg SJ, et al. Quality of life improves for pediatric patients after total pancreatectomy and islet autotransplant for chronic pancreatitis. Clin Gastroenterol Hepatol 2011;9:793–9.

61. Chinnakotla S, Bellin MD, Schwarzenberg SJ, et al. Total pancreatectomy and islet autotransplantation in children for chronic pancreatitis: indication, surgical techniques, postoperative management, and long-term outcomes. Ann Surg 2014;260:56–64.

62. Bellin MD, Carlson AM, Kobayashi T, et al. Outcome after pancreatectomy and islet autotransplantation in a pediatric population. J Pediatr Gastroenterol Nutr 2008;47:37–44.

63. Wilson GC, Sutton JM, Salehi M, et al. Surgical outcomes after total pancreatectomy and islet cell autotransplantation in pediatric patients. Surgery 2013;154: 777–83 [discussion: 783–4].

64. Chinnakotla S, Radosevich DM, Dunn TB, et al. Long-term outcomes of total pancreatectomy and islet auto transplantation for hereditary/genetic pancreatitis. J Am Coll Surg 2014;218:530–43.

65. Sutherland DE, Radosevich DM, Bellin MD, et al. Total pancreatectomy and islet autotransplantation for chronic pancreatitis. J Am Coll Surg 2012;214:409–24 [discussion: 424–6].

66. Walsh RM, Saavedra JR, Lentz G, et al. Improved quality of life following total pancreatectomy and auto-islet transplantation for chronic pancreatitis. J Gastrointest Surg 2012;16:1469–77.

67. Welsh MJ, Smith AE. Molecular mechanisms of CFTR chloride channel dysfunction in cystic fibrosis. Cell 1993;73:1251–4.

68. Wilschanski M, Durie PR. Patterns of GI disease in adulthood associated with mutations in the CFTR gene. Gut 2007;56:1153–63.

69. De BK, Weren M, Proesmans M, et al. Pancreatitis among patients with cystic fibrosis: correlation with pancreatic status and genotype. Pediatrics 2005;115: e463–9.

70. Ooi CY, Dorfman R, Cipolli M, et al. Type of CFTR mutation determines risk of pancreatitis in patients with cystic fibrosis. Gastroenterology 2011;140: 153–61.

71. Myers KC, Bolyard AA, Otto B, et al. Variable clinical presentation of Shwachman-Diamond syndrome: update from the North American Shwachman-Diamond syndrome registry. J Pediatr 2014;164:866–70.

72. Dall'oca C, Bondi M, Merlini M, et al. Shwachman-Diamond syndrome. Musculoskelet Surg 2012;96:81–8.

73. Dror Y, Donadieu J, Koglmeier J, et al. Draft consensus guidelines for diagnosis and treatment of Shwachman-Diamond syndrome. Ann N Y Acad Sci 2011;1242: 40–55.

74. Ammann RW, Akovbiantz A, Largiader F, et al. Course and outcome of chronic pancreatitis. Longitudinal study of a mixed medical-surgical series of 245 patients. Gastroenterology 1984;86:820–8.

75. Layer P, Yamamoto H, Kalthoff L, et al. The different courses of early- and late-onset idiopathic and alcoholic chronic pancreatitis. Gastroenterology 1994;107: 1481–7.

76. Raeder H, Johansson S, Holm PI, et al. Mutations in the CEL VNTR cause a syndrome of diabetes and pancreatic exocrine dysfunction. Nat Genet 2006;38: 54–62.

77. Zenker M, Mayerle J, Lerch MM, et al. Deficiency of UBR1, a ubiquitin ligase of the N-end rule pathway, causes pancreatic dysfunction, malformations and mental retardation (Johanson-Blizzard syndrome). Nat Genet 2005;37:1345–50.

78. Atik T, Karakoyun M, Sukalo M, et al. Two novel UBR1 gene mutations in a patient with Johanson Blizzard syndrome: a mild phenotype without mental retardation. Gene 2015;570:153–5.

79. Ellery KM, Erdman SH. Johanson-Blizzard syndrome: expanding the phenotype of exocrine pancreatic insufficiency. JOP 2014;15:388–90.

80. Tumino M, Meli C, Farruggia P, et al. Clinical manifestations and management of four children with Pearson syndrome. Am J Med Genet A 2011;155A:3063–6.

81. Ketwaroo G, Brown A, Young B, et al. Defining the accuracy of secretin pancreatic function testing in patients with suspected early chronic pancreatitis. Am J Gastroenterol 2013;108:1360–6.

82. Schibli S, Corey M, Gaskin KJ, et al. Towards the ideal quantitative pancreatic function test: analysis of test variables that influence validity. Clin Gastroenterol Hepatol 2006;4:90–7.

83. Conwell DL, Zuccaro G Jr, Vargo JJ, et al. An endoscopic pancreatic function test with cholecystokinin-octapeptide for the diagnosis of chronic pancreatitis. Clin Gastroenterol Hepatol 2003;1:189–94.

84. Walkowiak J, Nousia-Arvanitakis S, Agguridaki C, et al. Longitudinal follow-up of exocrine pancreatic function in pancreatic sufficient cystic fibrosis patients using the fecal elastase-1 test. J Pediatr Gastroenterol Nutr 2003;36:474–8.

85. Tangpricha V, Kelly A, Stephenson A, et al. An update on the screening, diagnosis, management, and treatment of vitamin D deficiency in individuals with cystic fibrosis: evidence-based recommendations from the Cystic Fibrosis Foundation. J Clin Endocrinol Metab 2012;97:1082–93.

86. Cantin AM, White TB, Cross CE, et al. Antioxidants in cystic fibrosis. Conclusions from the CF antioxidant workshop, Bethesda, Maryland, November 11-12, 2003. Free Radic Biol Med 2007;42:15–31.

87. Borowitz D, Baker RD, Stallings V. Consensus report on nutrition for pediatric patients with cystic fibrosis. J Pediatr Gastroenterol Nutr 2002;35:246–59.

88. Pohl JF, Uc A. Paediatric pancreatitis. Curr Opin Gastroenterol 2015;31:380–6.

The Transition of the Gastrointestinal Patient from Pediatric to Adult Care

 CrossMark

Punyanganie S.A. de Silva, MBBS, MPH, MRCP(UK)[a],
Laurie N. Fishman, MD[b],*

KEYWORDS

- Transition • Transfer • Gastrointestinal • Adolescents

KEY POINTS

- Transition is the long process of developing independent self-management skills whereas transfer is the actual move from pediatric to adult-centered provider.
- Structured anticipated transition works best with timelines of tasks to master and discussion of the stylistic differences between pediatric and adult practices.
- Disease-specific issues need to be addressed, such as earlier timelines for diet-based therapies, parental support for critical illnesses, and differences in therapeutic strategies.

INTRODUCTION
Transition vs Transfer

Transition has increasingly been recognized as an important concept. As adolescents with chronic gastrointestinal (GI) illnesses mature to adulthood, it is crucial that their clinical care remains uninterrupted. The goal of transition is to ensure that adolescents and young adults receive optimal health care management as they transition from pediatric to adult-centered health care. Transition is a patient-centered process that seeks to maximize lifelong functioning and potential through the provision of high-quality, developmentally appropriate health care services that continue uninterrupted as an individual moves from adolescence to adulthood.[1]

Unlike transfer, which refers to the actual move from a pediatric to an adult health care provider, transition is a lengthy process of preparing adolescents for a life as an adult and receiving care from adult health care providers. As with other specialties, the ongoing support of the pediatric provider and the active participation of the parent remain integral factors that help ensure that the transitioning patient develops

[a] Division of Gastroenterology, Hepatology and Endoscopy, Brigham and Women's Hospital, Harvard Medical School, 75 Francis Street, Boston, MA 02115, USA; [b] Division of Pediatric Gastroenterology, Boston Children's Hospital, Harvard Medical School, 300 Longwood Avenue, Boston, MA 02115, USA
* Corresponding author.
E-mail address: laurie.fishman@childrens.harvard.edu

Pediatr Clin N Am 64 (2017) 707–720
http://dx.doi.org/10.1016/j.pcl.2017.02.001
0031-3955/17/© 2017 Elsevier Inc. All rights reserved.
pediatric.theclinics.com

the skills and confidence needed to deal with a chronic illness in adulthood. In addition, the adult health care provider and affiliated health care team need to take into account various physical, medical, developmental, social, and emotional needs of these patients and their families, in a manner that is different than for established adult patients.

Although transition used to predominantly be a pediatric concern, now more and more adult gastroenterologists acknowledge the importance of a seamless transition[2,3] and are aware that the transition process may be a lengthy one.[4,5] The age of transition in GI disease continues to vary according to geography and culture, ranging from as young as 16 in the United Kingdom and Australia to mid-20s in the United States.

Timing of Transition Preparation

It is recommended that discussion about transition start when an adolescent is 12 years to 13 years old and a transition plan developed when the child is 14 years to 15 years old, with the actual transfer taking place at 18 years of age or older.[6,7] One study of young patients with inflammatory bowel disease (IBD) and their caregivers,[8] however, found many survey respondents endorsed 16 years to 17 years as the best ages to initiate discussions about transition and 18 years or older as the best ages to transfer care. Patients need to know whether the transfer is based on age; milestones, such as marriage or graduation; or other parameters. The authors believe that reminders at every visit for the 3 to 5 visits preceding transfer help break through denial and gently establish reality.

Preparation for Differing Practice Style

An aspect of transfer that is often overlooked is the difference in style between those who provide care to children and those who care for adults. If not well prepared, a transitioning patient may be taken aback by the shift in culture across environments. The adult-style practice emphasizes autonomy and respect, centered on the individual, whereas pediatric-style practice favors nurturance, with possible paternalism, and centers on the family. There is also a different medical focus between pediatric and adult gastroenterologists, with pediatric care focused on growth and development and adult care directed toward cancer surveillance, sexual function, fertility, and pregnancy.[9,10] Misinterpretation of the differences between adult care and pediatric care can sometimes lead to unhappiness by patients, families, and providers. Adult providers may think that patients are unprepared and clingy, whereas pediatric patients may view adult providers as cold or less involved.[11] Discussion of the underlying principles can help support understanding across the transition gap (**Table 1**).

Table 1
Comparative perspective about adult-centered practices

Practice Change	Pediatric Provider View	Adult Provider View
Shorter visits	Rushed	Respecting patients time
Sees patient alone	Ignoring family	Respecting privacy
More patient choice regarding treatment	Not spending enough time to have patient make "correct choice"	Allowing autonomy Empowering patient
Infrequent visits	Not checking in enough	Trusting patient to follow through

Development of Self-Management

Many transition programs highlight knowledge, self-efficacy, decision making and problem solving, self-advocacy, and information gathering as key skills that need to be developed during the transition process for a patient to be transfer ready.[1] These categories of skills are also important for adolescent patients with chronic GI conditions to thrive in the adult world. Acquisition of these skills is not limited to a single encounter but rather should be a stepwise program, with age-appropriate checklists of tasks for patients as well as for the medical team.[9,10,12,13] These tasks should be introduced early during pediatric care, typically age 11 or 12, and paced according to individual response. The goal of this stepwise approach is to have patients practice and master the steps leading to full responsibility and independent self-management behaviors that are associated with ideal adult practice by the time they are ready to transfer to adult health care.

Assessing Transition Readiness

Transfer readiness occurs when patients have the comfort, confidence, and competency to understand their medical condition, follow self-management strategies, and communicate independently with the provider. It can be assessed by the patient, the pediatric providers, or, occasionally, the parents. Clinicians may assume that their overall sense of whether a patient is ready counts as an assessment. For example, at one institution, more than 90% of clinicians reported routinely doing informal assessment and transition counseling with adolescent patients.[14] But assessment of true readiness remains difficult to measure. Although no universal instrument or transition scale has emerged, there are multiple tools that have been developed.[15,16] Some, like the Transition Readiness Assessment Questionnaire (TRAQ),[17] the social-ecological model of adolescent and young adult readiness for transition (SMART),[18] and the University of North Carolina TRxANSITION scale,[16] can be used for all conditions. Other tools are disease specific.

Transfer

The actual transfer process can take place in a variety of ways. In some settings, the pediatric and adult gastroenterologists see the patient at the same visit; in others, pediatric and adult gastroenterologists meet annually to discuss patients in transition. Joint transition clinics with pediatric and adult service clinicians can be established for information delivery and generating trust in the new physician. In other cases, a

---

Transfer checklist

- Timing should be discussed multiple times, with clear understanding of whether the graduation to adult care is based on age or milestone, such as graduation.
- Ensure medical record reaches adult provider and ideally provide summary as well.
- Clarify whom to call for problems or prescriptions during interval between providers.
- Anticipate the different practice style and expect patient is less comfortable at the first few visits with new provider.
- Review advantages of adult-style care now that the patient is mature (avoid criticism).
- Allow emotions of sadness, nostalgia, and pride in patient's growth to be discussed.
- Explain how patient can communicate nonmedical updates, such as with cards or e-mails, to avoid feeling cut off abruptly from pediatric provider.

transition coordinator accompanies a patient from one setting to the other. One study demonstrated even a 2-day workshop to reinforce transitioning skills mastered over time improved self-efficacy, satisfaction, and transition competence.[19] Although the relative merits of each system can be debated, the reality is often dictated by politics of health care alliances, insurance coverage, facility locations, and provider schedules. Some aspects of transfer, however, are important regardless of the settings. The transfer needs to be structured and expected. If patients graduate from a practice at widely differing ages, there can be confusion and a concern about favoritism.

The Adult Health Care Provider Role

Adult-based health services expect that their adult patients are able to care for themselves and are capable of negotiating the hospital clinical system, yet not all pediatric patients are ready. There is a need to bridge the gap between pediatric and adult services.[20] If the transitioning patient does not possess adequate communication skills, then initial visits in the adult clinic with a parent is acceptable. It should be made clear to the patient and parents prior to transfer, however, that this is not encouraged as a long-term practice.[21] Although the bulk of preparation for transition to adult care lies with the pediatric provider, it is good practice for the adult provider to reiterate skills required to ensure good health maintenance and responsibility as an adult. This includes encouraging maturation of communication and decision-making skills, allowing patients to take responsibility for medical self-management, and education and counseling of the adolescent/young adult to avoid risk-taking behaviors.

The ability to maintain a good relationship with the new provider is important. Many transitioning patients and families fear that the adult provider and office will provide decreased support and availability for advice.[22] It is, therefore, encouraged that the new adult provider be accessible and sympathetic to the patient's requirements. Adolescents and young adults may have difficulty communicating with health providers so providers often have to be flexible and patient in their communication styles initially when working with these patients.[23] Easy accessibility is important and many younger patients prefer e-mail or portal access as a mode of communication rather than speaking on the phone.

IBD, celiac disease, eosinophilic esophagitis (EoE), and liver transplant are diagnostic groups that have started to explore transition from pediatric to adult care. These four groups are detailed. The same disease may present differently in pediatric and adult populations, leading to misunderstanding among providers.

INFLAMMATORY BOWEL DISEASE

The incidence of IBD in children is increasing[24] with very-early-onset disease more frequently recognized. Children with IBD characteristically have more aggressive and extensive disease, with a greater prevalence of disease complications already having occurred by the time children reach adulthood and adult care. Many cohort and population-based studies have highlighted that at diagnosis between 19% to 38% of all Crohn disease patients have complicated disease. After 10 years, 56% to 65% of patients have developed either stricturing or penetrating complications, and after 20 years, these numbers range from 61% to 88%.[25] Therefore, the adult gastroenterologist needs to recognize that pediatric-onset patients comprise a sicker patient cohort with a longer, more complex history of IBD and related medication use. The more aggressive nature of pediatric disease also increases the risk of relapse or surgery.[26]

Medical History

Adult patients are expected to know their own medical history. Yet, young IBD patients are often characterized as lacking basic knowledge about their own medical conditions and treatments. Expected knowledge for a patient includes basic medical history and the nature of the condition, the names and doses of medications, allergies, names of the medical team, and how to contact the team. A study from Toronto demonstrated that only 22% of adolescent patients could recall the location of their disease and only 55% could recall when they were diagnosed.[27] More than 55% of respondents from a national survey of adult gastroenterologists found that IBD patients transitioning from pediatric care had inadequate knowledge of their own disease.[4] Unfortunately, adult patients also have imperfect knowledge of their condition. Using the validated Crohn's and Colitis Knowledge Score[28] on a cohort of adult patients, only 21% to 23% knew that IBD ran in families, 26% to 46% knew that IBD can affect other parts of the body besides intestines, and 18% to 29% knew they were at increased risk for colon cancer. Only 68% to 74% were aware that they still would still have the disease if symptom-free for 3 years.[29] A recent review also did not find adult patients more knowledgeable than a decade ago.[29]

It is important to have medical records available to the receiving provider even if a patient can recall all relevant medical details to facilitate a successful transfer. Ideally, the pediatric provider knows which adult provider will see the patient and when this visit will occur. The pediatric provider can then provide a form or letter summarizing medical history, remind patients to sign releases for medical information, and call the new adult provider to convey any sensitive information. When patients are moving far away, have an emergent problem, or have not yet obtained health insurance, it can be difficult to know which adult provider is available. Patients may then be responsible for providing information about their own medical course until records can be obtained. An organized transition program should, therefore, incorporate an age-appropriate educational component to address deficits in adolescent patients' knowledge. If a patient's course is straightforward, it may be reasonable to have the patient learn and recite his or her own history. If it is complex, a written record to carry is more important, such as MyHealth Passport for IBD.[27]

Self-Management

In addition to medical knowledge, patients need to master self-management, which includes making healthy and informed choices regarding diet, lifestyle, adherence, and monitoring symptoms. Patients are more likely to be successful when they have increased self-efficacy — the belief in their own ability to complete specific tasks and reach goals. To encourage mastery and self-efficacy, substantial areas of self-management can be broken down into smaller tasks. For example, managing medications can first be discussed in terms of remembering name, then dose, and then timing of medication, or first just calling in refills, then picking up the medicines at the pharmacy, and scheduling follow-up appointments. Allowing repeated opportunities for success can help patients build confidence in their own ability to handle health-related tasks. At present, it seems that patients are taking over these health-promoting tasks very late from parents.[30] In 1 study looking at the development of independent behaviors, fewer than 20% of adolescents 16 years old to 18 year old order medication refills, 35% of the 19 year olds to 21 year olds schedule clinic visits, and 30% of 19 year olds to 21 year olds contact the provider between visits if there is a problem.[31]

Both pediatric and adult providers are encouraged to use problem-solving skills, engage in collaborative relationships, and help patients maintain their social support networks, all as ways of increasing overall self-management.[32]

Medication adherence is another sign of successful self-efficacy. Adolescents have multiple developmental reasons for poor adherence, however, such as denial, sense of invincibility, risk-taking, desire to emulate peers, and poor planning. Additionally, adherence seems to vary with disease severity. Individual studies have demonstrated that 75% of adults on biologics were adherent[33]; 74% of adolescents on thiopurines were adherent[34] but only one-quarter of adults with ulcerative colitis were adherent with 5-aminosalicylic acid medication.[35] Furthermore, there is evidence from other fields that transfer to adult health care caused significantly poorer outcome,[36,37] indicating that the change in provider and in setting may be an independent risk factor for some patients. This underscores the importance of a smooth transition.

Solo communication with providers is a skill that not all patients have mastered by the time of transfer. Hopefully, the pediatric provider has started a stepwise preparation for speaking alone with the patient, so that both patient and parent are comfortable with this when transfer to adult care occurs. Answering questions is a skill that is mastered before asking questions of the provider or coming in with prepared questions. Parents who typically allow the young adult patient to see the provider alone may be particularly anxious at the time of transition and may wish to meet the new provider at least once. Although many adolescents with chronic disease report that their parents' support and involvement are important components of a successful transition, it can be difficult to discuss sexuality, alcohol, or drugs in front of parents. Adolescents may hold back unreported symptoms to avoid recrimination for not reporting sooner or leave off concerning symptoms to avoid scaring parents. Seeing the provider alone may also help create a clearer picture of an adolescent's transition readiness because parents are often guilty of overestimating their child's capabilities. A recent study demonstrated that, in comparison with patient's self-assessment, parents thought that their child was more self-efficacious in knowledge of IBD and diagnostic tests, self-management of medication use, and transfer readiness.[14]

It has also become increasingly more important in IBD transition that patients be able to research their condition outside of the medical visit.[4] The physician; support groups; and now online resources, such as Crohnology,[38] are important sources of information. One study shows that 62% of older adolescents use the Internet to obtain information.[31] When transitioning patients with IBD, it has been shown that health literacy is an important prerequisite for a successful transition, and younger youth, nonwhites, and those of nondisadvantaged socioeconomic status may find this more challenging.[39]

Young adults with IBD have been shown to often be delayed in the attainment of life milestones, such as holidays without adults, jobs during secondary school and beyond, and falling in love for the first time.[40] It is important for the adult provider to be cognizant of these potential delays and address the psychosocial impact brought on by the burden of disease. Despite this, these resources are often poorly used, with prior studies demonstrating that in IBD care there is a very low usage (5%) of psychological services in both pediatric and adult cohorts. Furthermore, the adult provider must be willing to broach certain topics that may not have been covered in pediatric care (such as sexual relationships, screening and prevention of sexually transmitted diseases, and family planning).[41] Many patients also have a history of stress and anxiety. A recent 2016 study demonstrated a high prevalence of mood disturbance ranging up to 35% in transitioning patients.[41] The adult care provider may be expected to provide the psychological support necessary for the patient.

Assessing Readiness

General transition tools are discussed previously. Others, like the MyHealth Passport[14,27] and the checklist by Hait,[9] are specific to IBD. More recently, the iPad Emma[42] — an electronic, interactive iPad quiz game that could be used in a clinical setting, with the aims of measuring IBD-related knowledge and concomitant mood and quality of life — has been shown to evaluate gaps in IBD knowledge, assess emotional functioning, and increase patient engagement as a transition tool in the clinical setting. Despite all these developments however, a recent study demonstrated that age is the primary factor that drives transition readiness.[43]

Transition Models

At present there is no universally established model for transition in IBD.[16] Models that are used include joint adult and pediatric clinics, alternating visits, advance tours of the adult facilities, coordinator-initiated transition, preparation of patient using the assessment tools in pediatric clinics, and common transition clinics for patients with a variety of chronic diseases. Joint medical visits have been demonstrated to enable successful, well-coordinated transition to adult medical-care follow-up.[39,44] Infrastructure for this is variable, however, and greatly depends on patient circumstance. Virtual joint visits, however, may potentially be an option in the future, particularly for complex cases. Although many specialties also recommend a specifically designated transfer clinic in either the adult or pediatric clinic, this is less often seen in IBD, particularly in the United states.[45] At the present time, there have been no head-to-head trials of these different models to determine which is the most appropriate.

Rather than a universal model, each institution or practice needs to adapt a model that is most efficient given the geographic location, available resources, patient cohort, and existing services within both the local pediatric and adult care teams. Given the challenges faced by many IBD patients, proactive involvement of a social worker and psychologist/psychiatrist also can be extremely helpful in facilitating a seamless transition and better patient compliance.[46]

CELIAC DISEASE

Celiac disease is commonly diagnosed in childhood and requires lifelong medical monitoring, necessitating a seamless transition from pediatric to adult care. This chronic condition is characterized by duodenal villous atrophy and intraepithelial lymphocytosis. Inflammation occurs on exposure to gluten, a protein present in wheat, rye, barley, and possibly oats. Strict adherence to a gluten-free diet is, therefore, necessary to promote healing. Failure to avoid gluten can result in growth and developmental delays, osteopenia, iron deficiency anemia, and infertility. A more serious complication of long-term dietary noncompliance is enteropathy-associated T-cell lymphoma.

As with IBD, a recent consensus report recommends that patients with celiac disease should gradually assume exclusive responsibility for their care.[21] There are no clear benchmarks, however, for when a patient with celiac disease should be expected to manage various tasks. Unlike medication-based treatments, those conditions requiring dietary treatment need continuous self-monitoring. Once children attend elementary school or visit peers, the responsibility for choosing foods wisely begins to fall on their shoulders. When children move away from parents, for work or college, many young adults learn to shop for gluten-free foods and prepare gluten-free meals for the first time. Social pressures around eating can factor heavily into adolescent psychology. Thus, it is important to understand that that although parental support is still important, dietary adherence and the consequences of nonadherence should be discussed and reinforced during transition.[47]

Patients with celiac disease may lose touch with medical providers. There are no required visits for prescriptions, because the treatment is mainly dietary. Also, for a large proportion of patients, nonadherence does not cause symptoms and thus can lead adolescents, who have a sense of invincibility already, to have a false sense of health. Therefore, adolescents/young adults with celiac disease are at risk of being lost to follow-up prior to and during transfer. Despite many providers' best efforts, most patients diagnosed with celiac in childhood receive no medical or dietary supervision after transition to adulthood.[22]

Growth impairment is a known consequence of untreated or undertreated celiac disease as well as IBD. Some adolescents and young adults with celiac disease experience a delay in pubertal development and may continue to grow and sexually mature beyond the expected age of pubertal completion. This may result in delays in emotional maturity, sexual health, and menstrual regularity. At transfer the pediatric provider should provide data regarding the patient's history of physical development and should note whether the patient has achieved his or her final adult height. For some patients who have experienced significant pubertal delay, it may be advisable to coordinate transfer to an adult provider at the completion of puberty, particularly where other pediatric specialists, such as endocrinologists, continue to care for the patient to manage growth failure.

It is essential that patients understand that that there are chronic complications from celiac disease, including osteoporosis and lymphomas, and that regular attendance to a clinic for assessment and compliance with investigations are important.

EOSINOPHILIC ESOPHAGITIS

There has been a dramatic rise in the actual incidence and prevalence of EoE as well as recognition of this entity. Initially described in children, there has been increasing recognition by adult providers. It can be diagnosed in all ages but a vast majority are identified in the pediatric age range.[48] Because the condition was first described in the 1990s, the diagnosis is still relatively new and transition programs are limited. As with the other chronic GI diseases, patients with EoE should have a structured transition program and teaching of skills that incorporate self-management and adherence to therapy.

There are also disease-specific features, however, that complicate transfer in EoE. The condition itself may be distinct in the pediatric and adult populations. Children can often be treated with dietary therapy or steroids, whereas adults seem to have more fibrosis and often require dilations. Additionally, the structure of the provider group may differ. Typically, the pediatric providers are in a multidisciplinary team of gastroenterologists, allergists, and dieticians, whereas many adult GI providers do not have this option for care. Thus it is not a simple transition from 1 pediatric to 1 adult provider for EoE.

EoE patients typically require repeat upper endoscopic procedures more often than their celiac disease and IBD counterparts. A majority of endoscopic procedures in adult care are undertaken with conscious sedation rather than general anesthesia. Educating individuals regarding this change well ahead of the transition and allaying any fears that they may have regarding conscious sedation should be anticipated and addressed.

Studies evaluating transition readiness in EoE are few. One multicenter online study evaluated transfer readiness in adolescents/young adults with EoE ages 13 years to 25 years with the Self-Management and Transition to Adulthood with Rx = Treatment (STARx) Questionnaire (a 6-domain self-report tool with a score range of 0–90).[49] Of 75 patients diagnosed in childhood, 78% (n = 52) of the patients and 76% (n = 187) of 245 unrelated parents had no transfer knowledge. Mean transfer readiness score in adolescents/young adults (n = 50) was 30.4 ± 11.3, with higher scores in domains of provider communication and engagement during appointments. Mean parent-reported (n = 123) score was 35.6 ± 9.7, with higher scores in medication management and disease knowledge. The investigators concluded that there was a significant deficit in health care transfer knowledge and that transfer readiness scores were lower than other chronic health conditions.

Transition readiness is relevant because another study demonstrated that a majority of young adults diagnosed with EoE during childhood continue to require pharmacologic treatment and/or dietary modification for EoE.[50] A substantial proportion of this population experiences ongoing swallowing difficulties. Dietary quality of life, but not total quality of life, seems adversely affected. Therefore, it is important that the adult provider be able to provide the necessary dietary support and education often needed by these patients. Furthermore, the adult provider should be observant for signs of malnutrition and noncompliance with medications.

EoE patients are one of the newest groups to look at health care transition. Differences in pediatric and adult therapies need to be considered, and better ways to prepare patients for self-management and transfer are needed.

LIVER TRANSPLANT

Excellent survival rates in pediatric liver transplant have resulted in increasing numbers of young people transferring from pediatric to adult care. The need for daily medication to prevent graft rejection poses a significant hurdle for adolescents learning self-management. Unfortunately, a key component of ensuring good long-term outcomes is medication compliance. It has previously been suggested that transition to adult care is a vulnerable period for pediatric transplant recipients and is associated with reduced medication compliance and graft loss. In a single-center Australian study, it was shown that the 1-year and 5-year survival rates after transition were 100% and 92%, respectively, with no episodes of late rejection.[51] In total, 66.7% of patients were compliant with immunosuppression, and 61.1% of patients were compliant with clinic attendance, with a significant relationship between medication compliance and clinic attendance. In another study, however, 19% of transitioned patients reported being out of medication during transition.[52] Suggestions for improving compliance and thus outcomes range from increased flexibility on the part of adult providers to overlapping management of pediatric and adult providers to extending transition support for a year after transfer. Other investigators have suggested that liver transplant patients, with the severity of nonadherence complications, be transferred at an older age.[53]

It is not surprising that parents of transplant patients have higher rates of involvement than other parents. The severe nature of the condition and the serious ramifications of failure to comply require parents to pay attention to their children's treatment. Many parents also suffer from the emotional impact of transplantation, leading to a more protective attitude toward their child,[54] which can hinder the development of independence. It is, therefore, important that attention be given to parents, and they should be provided with support to enable them to move from a managerial to a

Table 2
Questions that help providers assess readiness

Question	Age to Start Asking
Do you know the name of your medications? Dose?	12–14
Have ever called in a refill?	15
Have you made a clinic appointment yourself?	15
How do you remember to take your medicines (besides parental reminder)?	15
Do you carry your insurance card in your wallet?	17
How will you reach me (or the office) if you have a problem?	17

supervisory role during transition, thereby facilitating the ability of the young adult to independently engage with the new health care team.

Studies in this field often focus on the patients believing that the most important aspect for their successful transfer is a good relationship with health care professionals and continuity of care.

Many of these young people experience difficulty ending relationships with pediatric clinicians and forming new relationships with adult clinicians. They often express frustrations over a perceived lack of continuity of care after transfer and a fear of the unknown nature of adult services.[55] Having an expected time course and discussing details of the transfer in advance can be reassuring to patients.

The actual impact of transfer on outcomes remains unclear. In a recent study to assess the effect of transfer on patient and graft survival, it was demonstrated that pediatric liver transplant recipients who undergo transfer to the adult service have good long-term outcomes.[56]

SUMMARY

The transition of the adolescent or young adult GI patient can be a protracted and challenging process. With appropriate planning, preparation, and communication between pediatric and adult care teams, however, successful transfer of a responsible and autonomous individual can be achieved. Variability in transition programming, practices, and policies reflect the emerging nature of clinical practice in this area. Understanding the current state of transition programming can inform future programming. Efforts to identify evidence-based practices in transition to adult care are needed (**Tables 2 and 3**).

Table 3
Celiac benchmarks

Task	Median Age of Mastery (y)
Able to recognize gluten-free symbol	8
Able to explain celiac to a friend	9.5
Able to explain celiac to a stranger	10
Able ask about gluten-free options in restaurant	12
Able to identify safe gluten-free domestic travel	14
Able to identify gluten exposure in job options	15

Data from Laurie N. Fishman, MD, unpublished data, 2016.

REFERENCES

1. American Academy of Pediatrics, American Academy of Family Physicians, American College of Physicians-American Society of Internal Medicine. A consensus statement on health care transitions for young adults with special health care needs. Pediatrics 2002;110(6 pt 2):1304–6.

2. Blum RW, Garell D, Hodgman CH, et al. Transition from child-centered to adult health-care systems for adolescents with chronic conditions. A position paper of the Society for Adolescent Medicine. J Adolesc Health 1993;14:570–6.

3. Baldassano R, Ferry G, Griffiths A, et al. Transition of the patient with inflammatory bowel disease from pediatric to adult care: recommendations of the North American Society for Pediatric Gastroenterology, Hepatology and Nutrition. J Pediatr Gastroenterol Nutr 2002;34:245–8.

4. Hait EJ, Barendse RM, Arnold JH, et al. Transition of adolescents with inflammatory bowel disease from pediatric to adult care: a survey of adult gastroenterologists. J Pediatr Gastroenterol Nutr 2009;48:61–5.

5. Sebastian S, Jenkins H, McCartney S, et al. The requirements and barriers to successful transition of adolescents with inflammatory bowel disease: differing perceptions from a survey of adult and paediatric gastroenterologists. J Crohns Colitis 2012;6:830–44.

6. Cooley WC, Sagerman PJ, American Academy of Pediatrics; American Academy of Family Physicians; American College of Physicians, Transitions Clinical Report Authoring Group. Supporting the health care transition from adolescence to adulthood in the medical home. Pediatrics 2011;128:182–200.

7. Husby S, Koletzko S, Korponay-Szabó IR, et al. European Society for Pediatric Gastroenterology, Hepatology, and Nutrition guidelines for the diagnosis of coeliac disease. J Pediatr Gastroenterol Nutr 2012;54:136–60.

8. Maddux MH, Ricks S, Bass J. Patient and caregiver perspectives on transition and transfer. Clin Pediatr (Phila) 2017;56(3):278–83.

9. Hait E, Arnold JH, Fishman LN. Educate, communicate, anticipate—practical recommendations for transitioning adolescents with IBD to adult health care. Inflamm Bowel Dis 2006;12:70–3.

10. Pinzon JL, Jacobson K, Reiss J. Say goodbye and say hello: the transition from pediatric to adult gastroenterology. Can J Gastroenterol 2004;18:735–42.

11. Abraham BP, Kahn SA. Transition of care in inflammatory bowel disease. Gastroenterol Hepatol (N Y) 2014;10(10):633–40.

12. Lugasi T, Achille M, Stevenson M. Patients' perspective on factors that facilitate transition from child-centered to adult-centered health care: a theory integrated metasummary of quantitative and qualitative studies. J Adolesc Health 2011; 48:429–40.

13. Leung Y, Heyman MB, Mahadevan U. Transitioning the adolescent inflammatory bowel disease patient: guidelines for the adult and pediatric gastroenterologist. Inflamm Bowel Dis 2011;17:2169–73.

14. Zijlstra M, De Bie C, Breij L, et al. Self-efficacy in adolescents with inflammatory bowel disease: a pilot study of the "IBD-yourself", a disease-specific questionnaire. J Crohns Colitis 2013;7(9):e375–85.

15. Van Walleghem N, Macdonald CA, Dean HJ. Evaluation of a systems navigator model for transition from pediatric to adult care for young adults with type 1 diabetes. Diabetes Care 2008;31:1529–30.

16. Ferris ME, Harward DH, Bickford K, et al. A clinical tool to measure the components of health-care transition from pediatric care to adult care: the UNC TRxAN-SITION scale. Ren Fail 2012;34:744–53.
17. Sawicki GS, Lukens-Bull K, Yin X, et al. Measuring the transition readiness of youth with special healthcare needs: validation of the TRAQ–Transition Readiness Assessment Questionnaire. J Pediatr Psychol 2011 Mar;36(2):160–71.
18. Schwartz LA, Tuchman LK, Hobbie WL, et al. A social-ecological model of readiness for transition to adult-oriented care for adolescents and young adults with chronic health conditions. Child Care Health Dev 2011;37(6):883–95.
19. Schmidt S, Herrmann-Garitz C, Bomba F, et al. A multicenter prospective quasi-experimental study on the impact of a transition-oriented generic patient education program on health service participation and quality of life in adolescents and young adults. Patient Educ Couns 2016;99(3):421–8.
20. Viner R. Transition from paediatric to adult care. Bridging the gaps or passing the buck? Arch Dis Child 1999;81:271–5.
21. Ludvigsson JF, Agreus L, Ciacci C, et al. Transition from childhood to adulthood in coeliac disease: the Prague consensus report. Gut 2016;65(8):1242–51.
22. O'Leary C, Wieneke P, Healy M, et al. Celiac disease and the transition from childhood to adulthood: a 28-year follow-up. Am J Gastroenterol 2004;99:2437–41.
23. Available at: http://www.healthychildren.org/English/health-issues/conditions/chronic/pages/Common-Coping-Styles-of-Teens-Who-Are-Chronically-Ill-or-Disabled.aspx. Accessed November 1, 2016.
24. Benchimol EI, Fortinsky KJ, Gozdyra P, et al. Epidemiology of pediatric inflammatory bowel disease: a systematic review of international trends. Inflamm Bowel Dis 2011;17:423–39.
25. Louis E. Epidemiology of the transition from early to late Crohn's disease. Dig Dis 2012;30(4):376–9.
26. Adamiak T, Walkiewicz-Jedrzejczak D, Fish D, et al. Incidence, clinical characteristics, and natural history of pediatric IBD in Wisconsin: a population-based epidemiological study. Inflamm Bowel Dis 2013;19(6):1218–23.
27. Benchimol EI, Walters TD, Kaufman M, et al. Assessment of knowledge in adolescents with inflammatory bowel disease using a novel transition tool. Inflamm Bowel Dis 2011;17(5):1131–7.
28. Eaden JA, Abrams K, Mayberry JF. The Crohn's and Colitis Knowledge Score: a test for measuring patient knowledge in inflammatory bowel disease. Am J Gastroenterol 1999;94(12):3560–6.
29. Wardle RA, Mayberry JF. Patient knowledge in inflammatory bowel disease: the Crohn's and Colitis Knowledge Score. Eur J Gastroenterol Hepatol 2014;26(1):1–5.
30. van Groningen J, Ziniel S, Arnold J, et al. When independent healthcare behaviors develop in adolescents with inflammatory bowel disease. Inflamm Bowel Dis 2012 Dec;18(12):2310–4.
31. Fishman LN, Barendse RM, Hait E, et al. Self-management of older adolescents with inflammatory bowel disease: a pilot study of behavior and knowledge as prelude to transition. Clin Pediatr (Phila) 2010;49(12):1129–33.
32. Plevinsky JM, Greenley RN, Fishman LN. Self-management in patients with inflammatory bowel disease: strategies, outcomes, and integration into clinical care. Clin Exp Gastroenterol 2016;9:259–67.
33. Lopez A, Billioud V, Peyrin-Biroulet C, et al. Adherence to anti-TNF therapy in inflammatory bowel diseases: a systematic review. Inflamm Bowel Dis 2013;19(7):1528–33.

34. LeLeiko NS, Lobato D, Hagin S, et al. 6-Thioguanine levels in pediatric IBD patients: adherence is more important than dose. Inflamm Bowel Dis 2013;19(12): 2652–8.

35. Mitra D, Hodgkins P, Yen L, et al. Association between oral 5-ASA adherence and health care utilization and costs among patients with active ulcerative colitis. BMC Gastroenterol 2012;12:132.

36. Watson AR, Harden P, Ferris M. Transition from pediatric to adult renal services: a consensus statement by the International Society of Nephrology (ISN) and the International Pediatric Nephrology Association. (IPNA). Pediatr Nephrol 2011;26: 1753–7.

37. Hilliard ME, Perlus JG, Clark LM, et al. Perspectives from before and after the pediatric to adult care transition: a mixed-methods study in type 1 diabetes. Diabetes Care 2014;37(2):346–54.

38. Available at: www.crohnology.com. Accessed November 1, 2016.

39. Webb N, Harden P, Lewis C, et al. Building consensus on transition of transplant patients from pediatric to adult healthcare. Arch Dis Child 2010;95:606–11.

40. Hummel TZ, Tak E, Maurice-Stam H, et al. Psychosocial developmental trajectory of adolescents with Inflammatory Bowel Disease. J Pediatr Gastroenterol Nutr 2013;57(2):219–24.

41. Bennett AL, Moore D, Bampton PA, et al. Outcomes and patients' perspectives of transition from paediatric to adult care in inflammatory bowel disease. World J Gastroenterol 2016;22(8):2611–20.

42. Tung J, Grunow JE, Jacobs N. Pilot development of an electronic pediatric inflammatory bowel disease quiz game. J Pediatr Gastroenterol Nutr 2015;61(3):292–6.

43. Rosen D, Annunziato R, Colombel JF, et al. Transition of inflammatory bowel disease care: assessment of transition readiness factors and disease outcomes in a young adult population. Inflamm Bowel Dis 2016;22(3):702–8.

44. Crowley R, Wolfe I, Lock K, et al. Improving the transition between paediatric and adult healthcare: a systematic review. Arch Dis Child 2011;96(6):548–53.

45. Goodhand J, Dawson R, Hefferon M, et al. Inflammatory bowel disease in young people: the case for transitional clinics. Inflamm Bowel Dis 2010;16:947–52.

46. Shanske S, Arnold J, Carvalho M, et al. Transition of patients with inflammatory bowel disease from pediatric to adult care. Gastroenterol Clin Biol 2008;32(5 Pt 1):451–9.

47. Ciclitira PJ, Moodie SJ. Transition of care between paediatric and adult gastroenterology. Coeliac disease. Best Pract Res Clin Gastroenterol 2003;17(2):181–95.

48. Dellon ES, Jones PD, Martin NB, et al. Health-care transition from pediatric to adult-focused gastroenterology in patients with eosinophilic esophagitis. Dis Esophagus 2013;26(1):7–13.

49. Eluri S, Book WM, Kodroff E, et al. Lack of knowledge and low readiness for healthcare transition in eosinophilic esophagitis and eosinophilic gastroenteritis. J Pediatr Gastroenterol Nutr 2016. [Epub ahead of print].

50. Menard-Katcher P, Marks KL, Liacouras CA, et al. The natural history of eosinophilic oesophagitis in the transition from childhood to adulthood. Aliment Pharmacol Ther 2013;37(1):114–21.

51. Mitchell T, Gooding H, Mews C, et al. Transition to adult care for pediatric liver transplant recipients: the Western Australian experience. Pediatr Transplant 2017;21(1):e12820.

52. Chandra S, Luetkemeyer S, Romero R, et al. Growing up: not an easy transition-perspectives of patients and parents regarding transfer from a pediatric liver transplant center to adult care. Int J Hepatol 2015;2015:765957.

53. Fredericks EM, Magee JC, Eder SJ, et al. Quality improvement targeting adherence during the transition from a pediatric to adult liver transplant clinic. J Clin Psychol Med Settings 2015;22(2–3):150–9.

54. Wright J, Elwell L, McDonagh JE, et al. Parents in transition: experiences of parents of young people with a liver transplant transferring to adult services. Pediatr Transplant 2017;21(1).

55. Wright J, Elwell L, McDonagh JE, et al. "Are these adult doctors gonna know me?" Experiences of transition for young people with a liver transplant. Pediatr Transplant 2016;20(7):912–20.

56. Sagar N, Leithead JA, Lloyd C, et al. pediatric liver transplant recipients who undergo transfer to the adult healthcare service have good long-term outcomes. Am J Transplant 2015;15(7):1864–73.

Index

Note: Page numbers of article titles are in **boldface** type.

A

Abdominal pain, **525–541**
    causes of, 526
    evaluation of, 526–529
    in functional gastrointestinal disorders, 529–537
    warning signs of, 528
Achalasia
    evaluation of, 593–603
    treatment of, 604–605
Acid suppression test, for GERD, 494
Adalimumab, for IBD, 585
Adefovir, for hepatitis B, 645–646
Adenocarcinomas, n caustic ingestions, 512
Adult care, pediatric care transition to, **707–720**
Aganglionosis, in Hirschprung disease, 606–607
Agile syndrome, cholestasis in, 627–629
Alanine aminotransferase, in NAFLD, 660
Algrove syndrome, 603
Alkali agents, ingestion of, 508–512
Allergy, eosinophilic disorders in, 475–485
Alpha-1 antitrypsin deficiency, 630–631
Alport syndrome, 603
5-Aminosalicylate, for IBD, 583
Amoxicillin, for *Helicobacter pylori* infections, 555
Amylase levels, in pancreatitis, 686
Angiography, for GI bleeding, 557
Anorectal manometry, 597
Antacids, for GERD, 498
Antibiotics
    for FDIGs, 535
    for IBD, 583–584
Antidepressants, for FDIGs, 535
Antireflux barrier, 487–488
Antireflux surgery, 498–499
Apnea
    in GERD, 493
    in NAFLD, 667, 670
Apparent life-threatening event, in GERD, 493
Aspartate aminotransferase, in NAFLD, 660
Asthma, GERD with, 489, 491
Atherosclerosis, in NAFLD, 668

Pediatr Clin N Am 64 (2017) 721–733
http://dx.doi.org/10.1016/S0031-3955(17)30057-3
0031-3955/17

Moving?

Make sure your subscription moves with you!

To notify us of your new address, find your **Clinics Account Number** (located on your mailing label above your name), and contact customer service at:

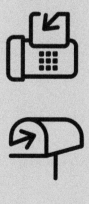

Email: journalscustomerservice-usa@elsevier.com

800-654-2452 (subscribers in the U.S. & Canada)
314-447-8871 (subscribers outside of the U.S. & Canada)

Fax number: 314-447-8029

Elsevier Health Sciences Division
Subscription Customer Service
3251 Riverport Lane
Maryland Heights, MO 63043

*To ensure uninterrupted delivery of your subscription, please notify us at least 4 weeks in advance of move.

Printed and bound by CPI Group (UK) Ltd, Croydon, CR0 4YY

03/10/2024

01040395-0008